FIXED BRIDGE PROSTHESES

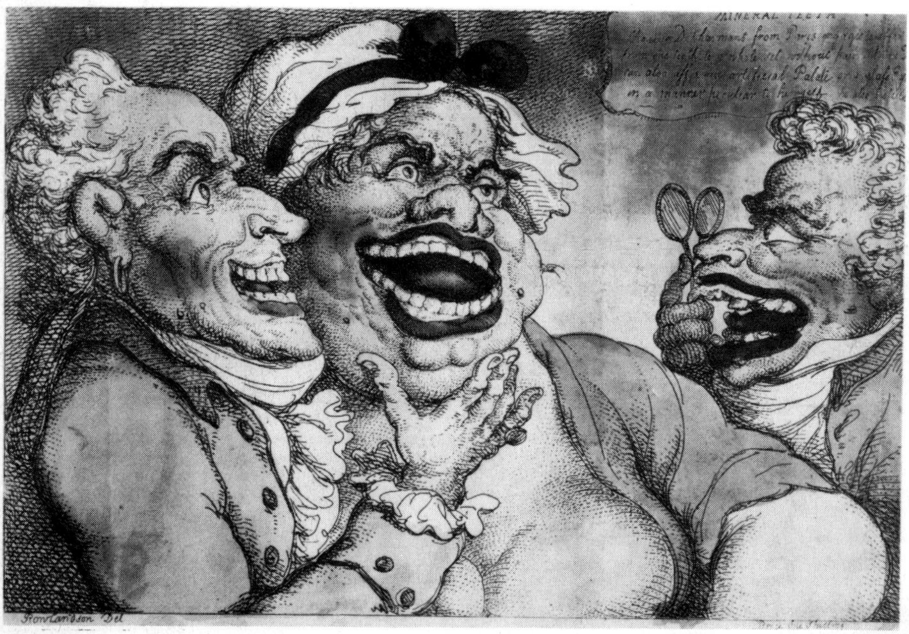

'One of the author's more successful fixed bridge prostheses.'
(A cartoon by Rowlandson. From T. Purland, *Dental Memoranda*; by courtesy of the Wellcome Trustees.)

16·25

D. H. ROBERTS FDS RCS (Eng)

Formerly of the Institute of Dental Surgery, Eastman Dental Hospital, London

With Sections by Professor Ian Davies, Mr B. J. Parkins and Mr W. M. Tay

FIXED BRIDGE PROSTHESES

Second Edition

John Wright & Sons Ltd, Bristol 1980

24 Shipbourne Road, Tonbridge, Kent,
England TN10 3DN.

Published by John Wright & Sons Ltd,
42–44 Triangle West, Bristol, England
BS8 1EX.

First edition, 1973
Second edition, 1980

British Library Cataloguing in Publication Data

Roberts, Derek Harry
Fixed bridge prostheses.—2nd ed.
1. Bridges (Dentistry)
I. Title
617.6'92 RK666

ISBN 0 7236 0545 9

PRINTED IN GREAT BRITAIN
BY JOHN WRIGHT & SONS LTD
AT THE STONEBRIDGE PRESS
BRISTOL

PREFACE TO SECOND EDITION

Despite substantial alterations to the second edition of *Fixed Bridge Prostheses,* the aim of the book remains exactly the same; to assist dental surgeons in assessing, designing, constructing and fitting fixed bridges with the minimum of difficulty for both themselves and their patients, and, above all, with the optimum long-term prognosis for both the prosthesis and the mouth in general.

With this latter point particularly in mind, we have expanded all matter relating to the correct assessment of the patient's dentition in general and the prosthesis in particular. Professor Ian Davies has kindly contributed a section on the periodontal preparation of the mouth prior to bridgework, which is obviously a prerequisite of any successful treatment plan. Details of periodontal techniques cannot be described in detail in a book of limited size such as this, but it should give readers a good idea of the approach which may be employed in virtually all cases.

To try to emphasize the importance of correct periodontal assessment, a case is illustrated (*Figs.* 15.1–15.9) of a patient, who, in her early twenties was advised by three independent dental surgeons to have a full clearance because of bone loss averaging 70–75 per cent. However, by careful instruction, motivation and treatment planning, she still has her teeth some twenty years later. Obviously, even more desirable would have been the prevention of the periodontal disease in the first instance.

To illustrate how some of the principles of bridgework are applied, Mr Parkins describes the assessment and treatment of one particular case and, indeed, throughout the book increasing emphasis is placed on all clinical procedures. The number of references to articles and research as well as manufacturers' products has also increased to make the book of as much practical assistance to the restorative dental surgeon as possible.

All recent advances have, so far as practical, been incorporated in this edition, including a section by Mr W. M. Tay on acid-etch bonding techniques, which will probably play an increasingly important role in the bridgework of the future.

As with the first edition, so much help has been given me so freely by my colleagues at the Institute and, indeed, everywhere not only in this country but also abroad, that in many ways I feel that this is a collective work. One of the most heartening features of dentistry in the last 5–10 years is its increasingly international nature with a very free exchange of ideas, research material and, indeed, lectures between various countries.

I should like to express my sincere thanks to Mr L. J. Leggett, Mr D. Setchell and Mr C. Sturridge who have given valuable advice on many of the clinical procedures and also on various sections of the text.

Dr J. W. McLean and Professor J. A. von Fraunhofer have greatly simplified the revision of the chapter on dental materials by making their very wide knowledge of this subject freely available to me.

Others who have given advice on the text or assisted by providing illustrations are Messrs D. A. Behrend, I. R. Cooper, B. W. Cope, F. J. Harty, D. Rule, M. J. Shaw, R. Simpson, R. Valentine and Dr D. Manson. Mr P. Russell and Mr T. R. Hill have kindly consented to let me use *Figs*. 6.18–6.25 and *Figs*. 6.26–6.36 respectively.

As with the first edition, this work would not have been possible without the help of our laboratory staff ably led by Mr J. A. Woodford and supported in particular by Mr E. S. Barden, who carried out the laboratory procedures for several of the cases illustrated.

Mr W. J. Morgan, Head of the Photographic Department, Messrs A. Johnson and P. Brown have given invaluable assistance with many of the new photographs contained in this book, and Mrs J. Halstead has produced several new illustrations and revised many of the existing ones for which I am very grateful. Mrs S. Morgan has kindly provided secretarial services and Mrs Cowperthwaite and Mrs I. Faulkner have assisted with numerous references.

I am very grateful to all the staff of John Wright & Sons Ltd for their assistance in the production of this book and in particular to Mr A. H. B. Symons for the care taken and detailed advice given in the preparation of the text.

If this book assists more operators to place more bridges with the minimum of effort and, above all, with the optimum prognosis, while decreasing the occurrence of bridge failures, which can be such a disaster both for operator and patient alike, then the effort involved in producing it will have been well worthwhile.

My wife's support and also her acceptance of the loss of 'free' time which the production of a book such as this inevitably entails, is a continual source of gratitude.

Should this book repay, even to some small extent, all the kindness, help and good comradeship extended to me by so many members of the dental profession over the last 25 years then I shall be well satisfied.

D.H.R.

PREFACE TO FIRST EDITION

Bridge work has always been one of the more controversial branches of dentistry, having fluctuated between being in and out of favour with the medical and dental professions several times during the past 100 years. However, with the continual improvement of techniques available and a better understanding of the basic problems of bridge design, all doubts about its desirability have gradually been swept aside. The controversy now centres around which of the ever increasing number of different types of partial prosthesis is best and also, where fixed bridges are placed, which specific design will yield the most favourable results. This applies particularly to fixed-fixed and fixed-movable bridges. Other debatable factors are the use of the cantilever and spring cantilever designs.

Experience of bridges constructed at the Institute of Dental Surgery over the past 20 years, including a detailed analysis of over 1000 cases, has led us to the conclusion that no one design is best in all instances. Each has its specific uses, the indications and reasons for which must be fully understood.

The purpose of this book is to try and illustrate the basic principles of bridge design and the reasons why a particular type is best in a given case. The specific replacements for the various teeth which may be lost are also discussed.

No attempt has been made to go into details of laboratory techniques, except where it is of direct concern to the dental surgeon, but rather to concentrate on the information required by the clinician to design and fit a satisfactory prothesis.

Sound clinical judgement based on many years of practical experience is the only sure path to good bridge work. However, it is hoped that this book, which has been based on the experience of a large number of operators over a span of twenty years, will provide sufficient basic knowledge for many dental surgeons to avoid having to learn numerous lessons, as we have, the hard way.

D.H.R.

ACKNOWLEDGEMENTS TO FIRST EDITION

So much help has been given me so freely by all my colleagues at the Institute of Dental Surgery, Eastman Dental Hospital, that I feel the authorship of this book is in many ways a collective one. Certainly it could not have been written without the knowledge and experience so painstakingly acquired by past and present members of the Department of Conservative Dentistry so ably led by Mr A. Kinghorn in the clinical field and Professor G. A. Morrant academically. I am particularly grateful to them both for having placed the facilities of the department at my disposal.

I should like to express my sincerest thanks to Mr B. L. Parkins for devoting such a large amount of his time to reading and advising on the text, and moreover for writing the section on occlusion. Mr R. Valentine has given invaluable assistance during the preparation of the chapter on precision retainers and supplied all the illustrations for this. Similarly Mr C. Sturridge was good enough to read and criticize the clinical sections of the book. His extensive practical experience of complex operative procedures has proved of great benefit.

Mr J. W. McLean kindly gave advice on the chapters on materials, pontics, and anterior bridges and also provided *Figs.* 82(a)–(e). Dr J. A. von Fraunhofer assisted on all matters relating to dental materials.

Mr P. L'Estrange read part of the draft and gave helpful advice on the section concerning removable prostheses. He also supplied *Figs.* 27, 28, 29, and 30 in Chapter 2. Professor A. O. Mack was good enough to let me have *Figs.* 20, 21, 22, and 24.

Others who gave assistance with the text or with the illustrations either by carrying out the work or supplying the photographs were: Mr D. N. Atkinson, Mr J. Catling, Mr F. J. Harty, Mr T. R. Hill, Mr J. Lavis, Mr L. J. Leggett, Professor L. I. Linkow, Mr P. C. Moloney, Mr E. Pullen-Warner, and last but by no means least the past and present members of our laboratory staff and in particular Mr E. A. Dennison, Mr J. Woodford, and Mr E. Barden.

Miss J. Middleton provided the majority of the illustrations and I am extremely grateful to her for the many hours devoted to their preparation and, above all, her tolerance, understanding, and attention to detail.

The photographs contained in this book were nearly all taken by the hospital's photographic team ably led by Mr J. Morgan and assisted by Mr J. A. Neligan, Mr J. H. Scally, and Miss J. Wright. My thanks are due to Mr A. Kinghorn for letting me make such free use of this department. I am also grateful to Miss S. Hayward for posing for clinical photographs in the section on occlusion and to Messrs Warren Jepson and Co. for their preparation of some of the black and white prints from colour slides.

Mr Derrick, editor of the *Dental Practitioner,* kindly gave his permission to use some of the material contained in Chapter 2, and Mr Donaldson, editor of the *British Dental Journal,* was good enough to allow me to reproduce much of the material in Chapter 4. I am grateful to Miss E. M. Spencer, Librarian of the British Dental Association, and Mrs P. Flor, Librarian of the Institute of Dental Surgery, for assisting with the references.

I should like to express my appreciation of the extremely efficient secretarial services provided by Mrs S. Morgan, who typed the whole text not just once but several times. Further secretarial assistance has been ably provided by Miss J. Fox and Miss H. Shepherd.

Much has been gained by me from my informal discussions with fellow members of Condent.

Finally, these acknowledgements would be far from complete without thanking Mr L. G. Owens, the former publishing director of John Wright & Sons Ltd, and the present director Mr H. A. Humphrey, his senior editor Mr A. N. Boyd, and the other members of the staff for the extremely efficient way in which they have handled the publication of this book.

My wife's continual assistance, tolerance and understanding during the long hot summer when the majority of this book was prepared is still a source of appreciation and gratitude to me.

CONTENTS

General Considerations	1	**1**	History of fixed bridge prostheses
	7	**2**	Replacement of missing teeth; Reasons and methods
	30	**3**	Indications and contraindications for bridges
	43	**4**	Materials
	68	**5**	Pontics
	81	**6**	Abutments and retainers
Bridge Types	129	**7**	Anterior bridges
	139	**8**	Posterior bridges
	146	**9**	The cantilever bridge
	151	**10**	The spring bridge
	162	**11**	Compound bridges
	166	**12**	The use of precision retainers in fixed bridge prostheses
	173	**13**	Adhesive bridges
Clinical Procedures	181	**14**	Periodontal preparation of the mouth
	191	**15**	General and case assessment; Tooth restoration and preparation
	210	**16**	Impression techniques, shade taking and temporary bridges
	229	**17**	Occlusal records
	238	**18**	Bridge placement and care
	249	**19**	Causes and treatment of bridge failures
	262	**20**	Specific replacements
	277		*Appendix: Metric and English equivalents*
	279		*Index*

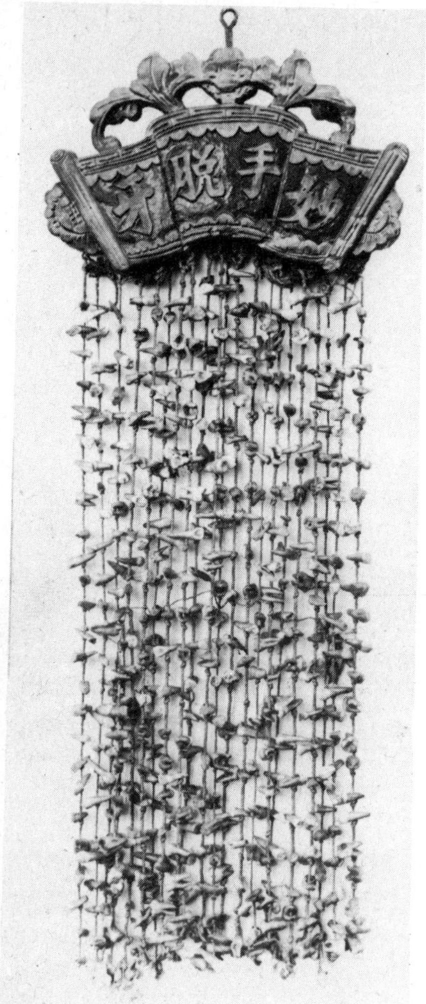

Fig. 1.1. *Early dental sign.*
(By courtesy of the Wellcome Museum.)

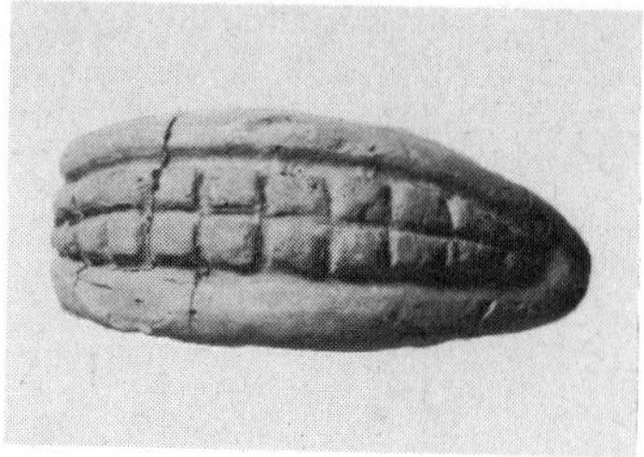

Fig. 1.3. *Votive offering of teeth made in pottery. Graeco-Roman. 3rd–1st century* B.C.
(By courtesy of the Wellcome Museum.)

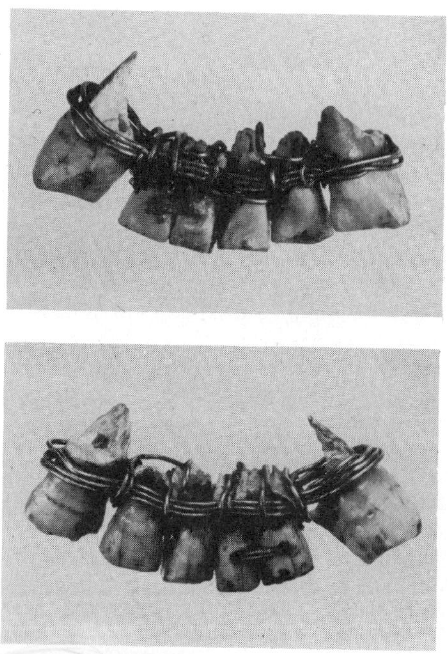

Fig. 1.4. *Fixed bridge replacing two incisors. Found in Sidon. Circa* 700 B.C.
(By courtesy of the Louvre, Paris.)

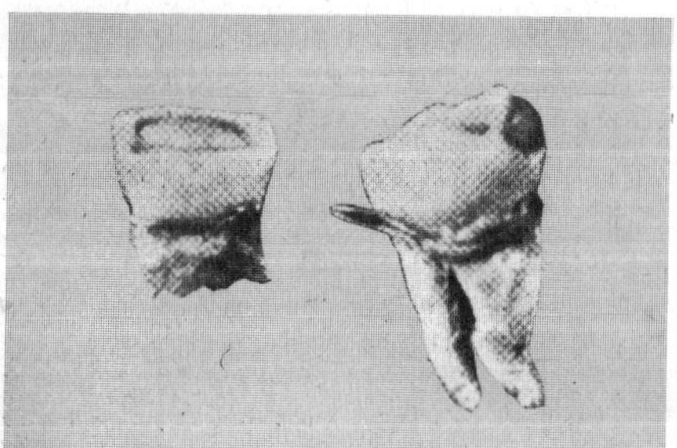

Fig. 1.2. *An early periodontal splint with* $\overline{|78}$ *wired together. Found at El Gizah. Probably around* 2500 B.C.

1

HISTORY OF FIXED BRIDGE PROSTHESES

It is somewhat humbling to realize that successful fixed dental prostheses were being placed long before the birth of Christ and that today, well over 2000 years later, we have still by no means perfected their design and construction.

The earliest medical and dental writings of ancient Egypt are the Ebers Papyri, some of which may date back as far as 3700 B.C. These contain references to a Hesi-Re being appointed Chief Toothist to the Pharaohs in 3000 B.C. However, according to M. D. K. Bremner in *The Story of Dentistry* there is no evidence to support the existence of any mechanical dentistry in ancient Egypt. This is somewhat surprising in view of the highly developed skills of the Egyptians in other fields. The only thing which has been shown is that they did wire teeth together.

The earliest dental appliances were made possible by the great craftsmanship of the Etruscan and other civilizations and by the discovery of the Nubian gold mines in 2900 B.C.

The fixed bridge was probably developed from the periodontal splint an example of which (*Fig.* 1.2) has been found in a tomb (No. 984) in the cemetery at El Gizah, near the Great Pyramids and the Sphinx. This, it is thought, goes back to 2500 B.C. It consists of the lower left second and third molars joined together by means of gold wire.

Fixed bridge work was certainly being constructed in the seventh century B.C. by the Phoenicians. They used soft or rolled gold and gold wire for their bridges. Soldering was also employed and impressions and models must almost certainly have been used. That they could take impressions and make models at that time is proved by the 'votive gifts' which have come down to us (*Fig.* 1.3). These were terracotta models of the donors' lips and teeth which were offered to the divinities for cures received or hoped for.

Ernest Renans (1823–1892) in his *Mission de Phoenicie* describes one of the discoveries of his medical assistant Dr Gaillardot as follows:

'. . . but that which was most interesting was one portion of the upper jaw of a woman showing the two canines and the four incisors united by wire [*Fig.* 1.4]. Two of these incisors seemed to have belonged to another person and to have been inserted here in order to replace those which are missing. This piece, however, which was discovered in one of the most ancient tombs, proves that the dental art was pretty well advanced in Sidon and also proves that the Scorbut de Terra (diseases of the gums) common at the present time in Sidon [1864] existed in those days.'

The Etruscans, who founded Rome in 754 B.C. and whose country was called Etruria (now Tuscany and parts of Umbria in Italy), were the most highly skilled craftsmen of that era. They produced quite complex bridges using gold bands soldered together and pontics made of human or animal teeth. These were held in place by gold rivets. Unfortunately, however, most of these bridges were destroyed by their conquerors together with other examples of their skills.

Weinberger, in his *An Introduction to the History of Dentistry*, when discussing the Mayer Relics, describes an Etruscan dental prosthesis dated around 600 B.C. in which a pair of missing centrals has been replaced by an ox tooth (*Fig.* 1.5). It is of fine workmanship, consisting of seven bands soldered together, five of which contain standing teeth. One band had held an artificial second premolar, now missing but with its pin still remaining, and one band contained a large tooth, that of an ox, which had been grooved in the centre to make it look like two teeth. This was retained by two pins.

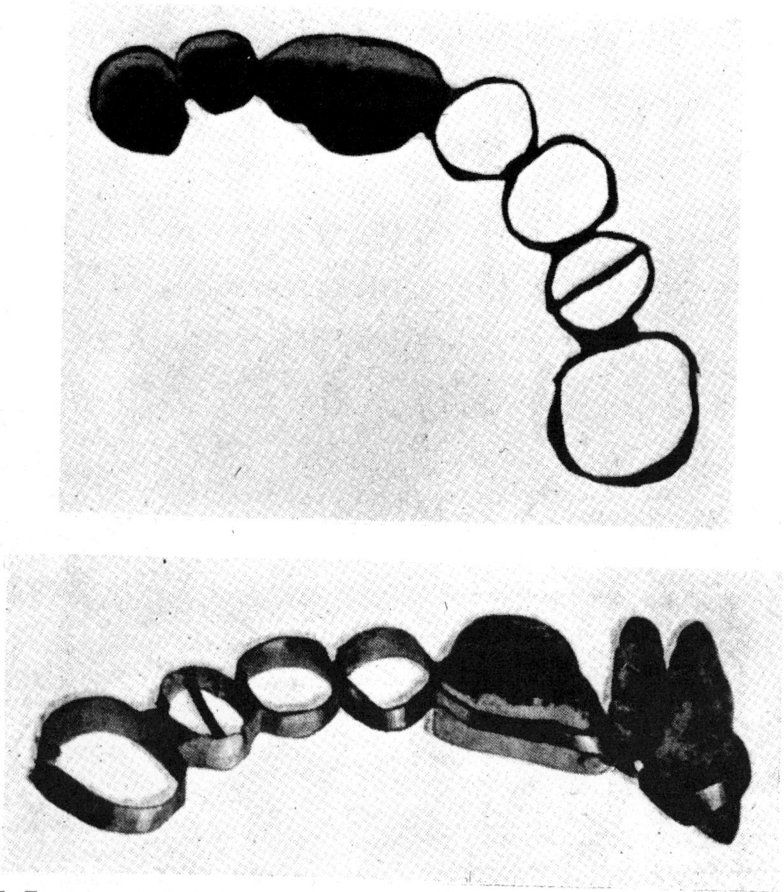

Fig. 1.5. *Etruscan prosthesis dated around* 600 B.C. *A pair of centrals has been replaced by an ox tooth grooved in the centre.*

Although several other Etruscan specimens similar to the above have also been discovered it is doubtful if the Greeks ever reached such a standard. However, Hippocrates in the third century B.C. makes mention of gold wires used for binding the teeth and in Attica, the heart of early Greek civilization, a bridge has been found which dates from the same period. It is somewhat similar to Etruscan workmanship, the teeth being held together by gold bands.

The Romans gained much of their knowledge of dentistry from the Etruscans and were probably the first people to use removable prostheses. It is interesting to note that the Laws of the Twelve Tables compiled in Rome in 450 B.C. state that although it was forbidden to offer burial gifts made of gold it was not unlawful to bury the dead 'with the gold with which the teeth may be perchance bound together'. This presumably refers to splinting but may apply to bridges.

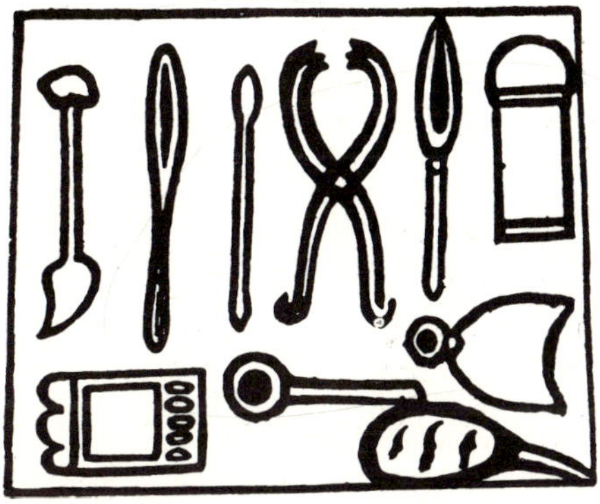

Fig. 1.6. *Dental and surgical instruments represented in a funeral marble in the Lateran Museum, Rome.*

An example of a bridge of Roman workmanship has been discovered dating back to 300 B.C. and there is evidence that gold shell crowns were in use in the first century B.C.

The Romans considered tooth loss a disaster and discoloration a grave misfortune. The following couplet from Martial makes this plain.

'How did it come about that Thais has black teeth and Laecaenia pearly white ones?' The answer: 'Thais has retained her own teeth, Laecaenia has purchased teeth.'

Elsewhere Martial mentions the use of bone, ivory and boxwood for false teeth. Similarly Horace (65 B.C.) in one of his satires depicts two courtesans, Sagona and Canidia, the former wearing a wig and the latter false teeth, probably an anterior gold bridge. It is likely that all the early dental prostheses were made for aesthetic purposes and were of little functional use.

Fig. 1.6 shows dental and surgical instruments depicted on a Roman funeral marble and *Fig.* 1.7 illustrates an early Christian tombstone, presumably of a dental surgeon.

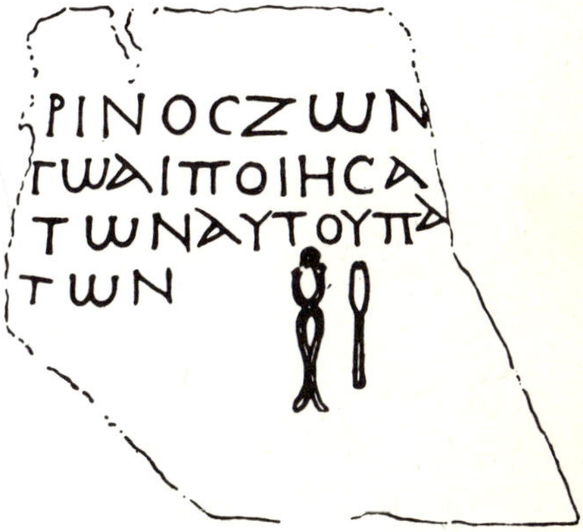

Fig. 1.7. *Dental instruments and inscription on the early Christian Roman tombstone of a dental surgeon.* (Reproduced with permission from Weinberger B. W. (1948) *An Introduction to the History of Dentistry, Vol.* 1, *St Louis, Mosby.*)

The ancient Hebrews copied from other races and it is possible that bridges were being made in Israel in the third century B.C. The Talmud, which was written during the second, fourth and sixth centuries A.D., consisted of the Rabbinical Law. In it, mention is made of prostheses fitted during the lifetime of Rabbi Zera (A.D. 279–320) constructed of gold, silver and wood. It also quotes Rashi the Rabbi as ruling that 'a gold tooth being valuable the woman may take it out of her mouth for display and meantime carry it in the street'. This indicates that, at least at that period, some of the prostheses were able to be removed by the patient.

The following extract from the Babylonian Talmud mentions one of the uses of bridges which has stayed unchanged to the present day.

'A certain maiden lady was rejected by a man she was betrothed to because she displayed an unsightly artificial tooth. She had an inserted tooth but Rabbi Ishmael (first century B.C.) had made for her one of gold to replace the inserted tooth, which so improved her appearance that the man accepted her in marriage.'

It is difficult to understand why, following an era spanning approximately 1000 years, during which time the Phoenicians, Etruscans, Greeks, and Romans had all fitted bridges, the principles of their construction were almost lost to civilization.

It is only the Arabians who were apparently using bridges in the Middle Ages. Albucasis, a Spanish Moor, in his *De Chirurgia* (tenth to eleventh century A.D.) mentions the splinting of the teeth by gold wire as the Phoenicians had done over 1000 years before. He also describes the replacement of missing teeth by animals' teeth or artificial ones made of bone and attached to the natural teeth by gold wire.

Guy de Chaliac, an eminent medical writer of the Middle Ages, made a few references to artificial teeth and Johann Jessenius Von Jessen (1566–1621) described carving ivory to fit the alveolus and wiring it in place. However, it is interesting to note that replacements were needed every few months.

Figure des Dents artificielles.

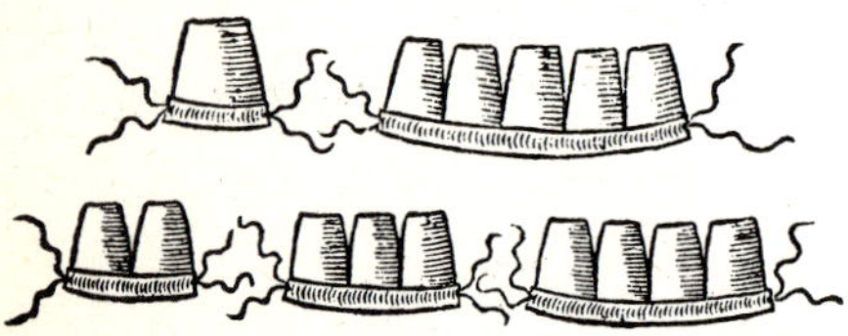

Fig. 1.8. *Dental prostheses held in place with gold or silver wire. Described by Ambroise Paré, 16th century* A.D. (By courtesy of the Wellcome Museum.)

The next known mention of a fixed prosthesis comes in the second half of the sixteenth century when Paré describes the placing of artificially made teeth. These were probably made of bone or ivory and fixed to the natural teeth by gold or silver wire (*Fig.* 1.8). There are also examples of bridges made of iron dating from the sixteenth to eighteenth centuries.

Pierre Fauchard (1678–1761) is considered by many to be the founder of modern scientific dentistry. In his book written in 1723 he describes both operative procedures and the making of prostheses. He used strips of gold, which he had enamelled and then riveted to bone, as artificial teeth. He also reamed out root canals so as to be able to place pivots made of gold or silver. These were used to retain crowns and bridges made of bone.

Transplantation and reimplantation were common in the eighteenth century and it was then that Philip Pfaff first described impression taking (1756). However, it was the beginning of the next century before the technique came into general use. A mixture of beeswax, shellac and white lead was used for this purpose until 1877 when Charles Stent invented composition.

One of the earliest examples of forensic dentistry concerns a Dr Joseph Warren. He had a bridge placed by Paul Revere in 1775 which was carved out of ivory and fastened to the teeth by silver wire. Revere subsequently identified his dead colleague by this prosthesis.

The use of human teeth as bridge pontics was continued comparatively late as is evidenced by the following advertisement in the *Independent Journal*, New York, 1783:

'Any person disposed to part with their front teeth may receive 2 guineas for each tooth by applying at No. 28, Maiden Lane.'

Even in 1844, P. B. Goddard in his textbook states that 'human teeth are best as artificial teeth with the exception of porcelain'. This material was first used in dentistry towards the end of the eighteenth century, although the extreme brittleness of the early porcelain delayed its acceptance. Colour matching has made slow but steady progress from then until the present day. The porcelain tube tooth was first employed in 1832.

The construction of bridges was described by J. B. Gariot of Paris in 1805 and he is possibly the first person to mention the use of the articulator for this purpose.

bridges made in this way had a longer life.

There have been many advances in the last 100 years which have greatly simplified the construction of bridges. Amongst the most important of these are our ability to provide profound analgesia to permit adequate tooth preparation and the use of radiography for diagnosis.

The advancement of dental engines (*Figs*. 1.9, 1.10) with an accompanying

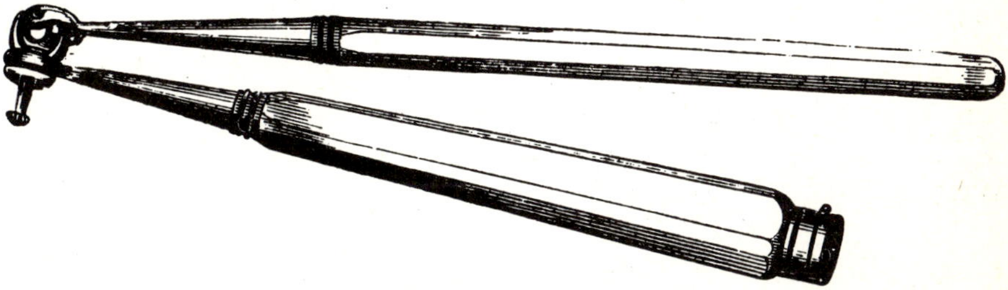

Fig. 1.9. *Dental drill mounted on a swivel handle. From S. Maw Son & Thompson, Surgical Instrument Catalogue, London,* 1882.
(By courtesy of the Wellcome Museum.)

The teachings of G. V. Black (1836–1915) raised dentistry to new standards and enabled the profession to appreciate many of the basic principles far more clearly than it had in the past. Even today most of his teaching is still valid.

By the end of the nineteenth century a large part of the theory of modern bridge work had been assimilated, although the equipment and materials necessary to construct the prostheses to the high standards possible today were not always available. Various arguments such as the use of fixed-fixed versus fixed-movable bridges were current even at that time. Thus Harris in 1889–90 was using mainly fixed-fixed designs, but it is interesting to note that he took great trouble to secure adequate retention, using full crowns, post crowns reinforced with gold skirts, and often even locked his gold inlays in place with cohesive gold.

However, in 1914 Chayes placed great emphasis on the advantages of allowing normal physiological movement of the tissues, including gum, alveoli, and periodontium, and he thus advocated fixed-movable designs. He observed that

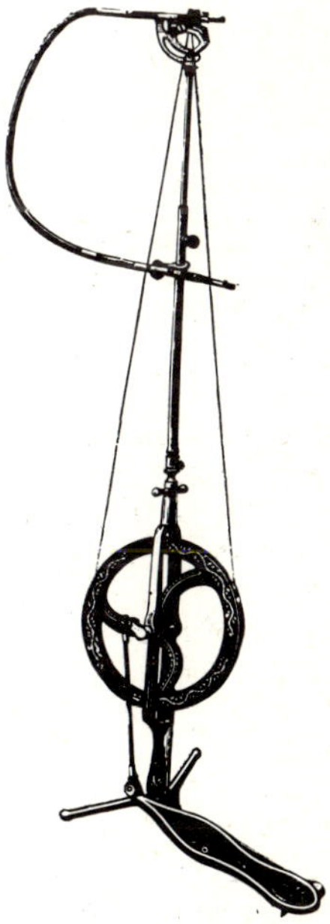

Fig. 1.10. *Dental foot engine. From Catalogue of Surgical Instruments by Arnold & Sons,* 1910.
(By courtesy of the Wellcome Museum.)

improvement in the drills and stones used, from the clockwork drill through to the foot engine, the low-speed and then high-speed electric engines, and finally the air turbines, has made the reduction of tooth tissue a relatively comfortable and effortless procedure.

The first of the elastic impression materials, the hydrocolloids, were discovered in 1925 and there have been continuous advances in this field ever since.

Although they were casting gold inlays relatively accurately in Ecuador at the end of the first century A.D. it is only in the last sixty to seventy years that this process has been scientifically investigated and perfected, using the lost wax technique.

The more recent advances in fixed bridge prostheses include the use of the aluminous and bonded porcelains which provide strength considerably in excess of anything available previously.

All the foregoing developments have greatly simplified bridge construction and have combined to enable one to be placed with the minimum of discomfort to the patient. It is this and the greatly increased living standards of the industrialized nations which have multiplied the demand for fixed bridge prostheses so much during the past ten to twenty years.

BIBLIOGRAPHY

Bremner M. D. K. (1954) *The Story of Dentistry*, 3rd rev. ed. Brooklyn, New York, Dental Items of Interest Publishing Co.

Brown L. P. (1934) The antiquities of dental prosthesis. *Dent. Cosmos* **76**, 826, 957, 1078, 1155.

Cohen R. A. (1959) Methods and materials used for artificial teeth [abridged]. *Proc. R. Soc. Med.* Sec. Odont. **52**, 775.

Galgono F. J. (1946) Dental prosthesis in antiquity. *Columbia Dent. Rev.* **18**, 11 (Jan.).

Rath G. (1959) History of prosthetic dentistry, 1 and 2. *Dent. Abstr., Chicago* **4**, 50 (June), 8 (Dec.).

Sanoff N. and Turner E. K. (1941) Dental bridges of the ancients. *Contact Pt* **18**, 226 (April).

Ward G. (1962) Some interesting examples of crown and bridge prosthesis. *Dent. Mag.* **79**, 96 (June).

Ward G. (1962) Origins of dental prosthesis. *Br. Dent. J.* **112**, 10.

Weinberger B. W. (1947) The dental art of ancient Egypt. *J. Am. Dent. Assoc.* **34**, 170.

Weinberger B. W. (1948) *An Introduction to the History of Dentistry*, Vols. I and II. St Louis, Mosby.

Williams G. L. (1967) A history of prosthetic dentistry. *Dent. Techn* **20**, 55 (June).

Woodforde J. (1968) *The Strange Story of False Teeth.* London, Routledge & Kegan Paul.

2

REPLACEMENT OF MISSING TEETH: REASONS AND METHODS

Effects of Tooth Loss
Prevention of Tooth Loss
Maintenance of Space
Reasons for Treating Tooth Loss
Methods of Treating Tooth Loss

Before commencing our discussion of bridges it is as well to consider why it is usually desirable to replace missing teeth and the various alternative methods which may be used for doing so.

EFFECTS OF TOOTH LOSS

If a tooth is congenitally absent, fails to erupt, or is lost, the effect may vary greatly depending upon such factors as which particular tooth is involved, whether any other teeth have been lost in the same arch, the articulation, local and general periodontal condition, and the skeletal and muscular patterns of the patient. However, any of the following may take place (*Fig.* 2.1):

■ A. Drift of Neighbouring Teeth

The extent to which this occurs depends mainly on the intercuspation of the teeth on either side of the space with those of the opposing arch. Thus if they are positively locked little tooth movement will occur. Other factors which will influence tooth drift are the age of the patient and the periodontal condition. The worse the latter, the greater the liability for tooth movement to take place.

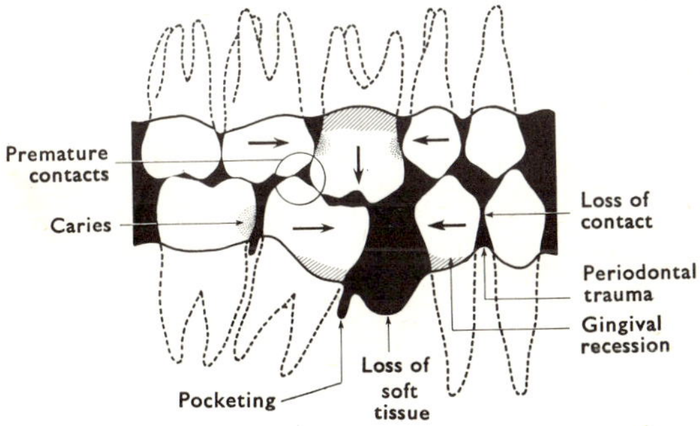

Fig. 2.1. *Effects of tooth loss: drift of neighbouring teeth, over-eruption of opposing teeth, loss of contacts, periodontal trauma, gingival recession, pocketing, caries and premature contacts.*

The way in which each tooth moves varies, depending largely upon its position in the arch. Thus in the posterior region, forward to about the first or second premolar, the anterior vector of force largely determines tooth drift. The lower molars usually tilt mesially, whereas the upper molars tend both to tilt mesially and to rotate around the palatal root. The premolars, particularly the lower first bicuspid, usually stay upright and move bodily into any space created by tooth loss. They may move either mesially or distally as also may the incisors and canines.

When a tooth moves there will be a derangement of the occlusion which can lead to premature contacts and periodontal trauma. A further problem will be loss of contacts causing food packing, periodontal breakdown, and interstitial caries.

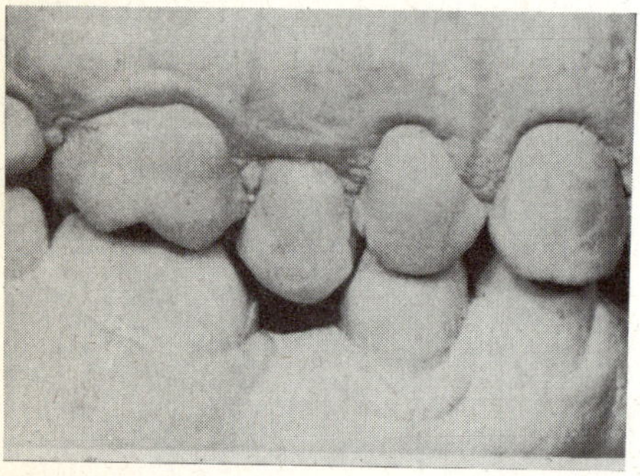

Fig. 2.2. *Over-eruption causing locking of the occlusion.*

■ B. Over-eruption of the Opposing Teeth

As the opposing tooth cannot occlude because of the edentulous space it will generally over-erupt, continuing to do so until it comes into contact with one of the teeth in the opposing arch, or, in extreme cases, the mucoperiosteum. The over-eruption of the tooth usually results in loss of bony support for that tooth, although sometimes the alveolus will follow the erupting tooth. It also frequently causes traumatic occlusion or locking of the occlusion which may sometimes be almost total and seriously limit masticatory function (*Fig*. 2.2).

Over-eruption can lead to the loss of normal contacts between the over-erupted tooth and its neighbours, resulting in food packing, periodontal breakdown, and subgingival caries. The latter, because of its position, is often very difficult to gain access to and treat.

■ C. General Effects

If tooth loss is left untreated then the effects mentioned previously may become more widespread. Thus generalized tooth movement can occur which might result in the relapse of a completed orthodontic case. This may be either a direct or an indirect result of the tooth loss. A direct result would be loss of a tooth adjacent to the one(s) which have been realigned, thus allowing them to relapse. An indirect effect would be the generalized collapse of the lower arch and subsequently the upper arch, which is liable to occur when the lower first molars are lost.

Another effect of the derangement of the articulation may be premature contacts causing deviations in the normal movements of the mandible. This may result in temporomandibular joint dysfunction and muscle spasm which will cause pain.

Because of reduced function due to the tooth loss there may be an increased liability to food stagnation and caries on the affected side with unilateral mastication on the opposite side of the mouth.

PREVENTION OF TOOTH LOSS

For all the foregoing reasons it is desirable to prevent tooth loss if at all possible. The preservation of teeth is particularly important in children as their replacement in this age group is far more difficult. All the teeth may not have erupted, either partially, completely, or at all. The crowns are very short (*Fig*. 2.3) and will give poor retention for whatever

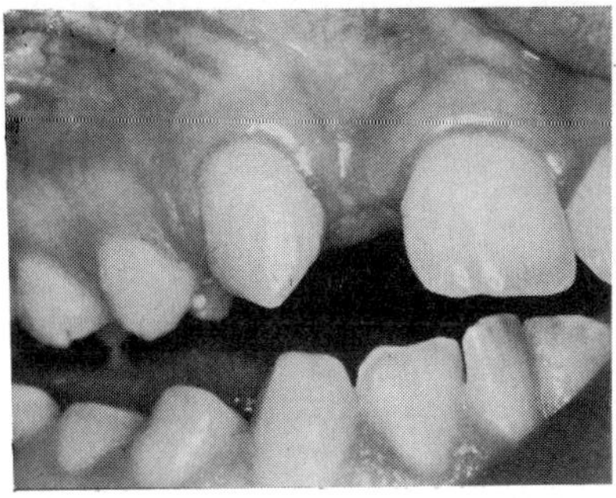

Fig. 2.3. *Short clinical crowns in the younger patient which will give poor retention for any prosthesis.*

prosthesis is placed. If a bridge is used, then apart from the liability of the retainers to become uncemented, as the teeth erupt their margins will become exposed and the high caries rate frequently present is likely to result in their failure, with possible further tooth loss.

No prosthesis can ever hope to be as satisfactory as the tooth it replaces. Functionally it is likely to be less effective and there is always the possibility, however well it is constructed, that it will have a deleterious effect on the teeth from which it gains its support, and sometimes on the mouth in general.

The time and expense involved in a difficult posterior root-canal therapy will

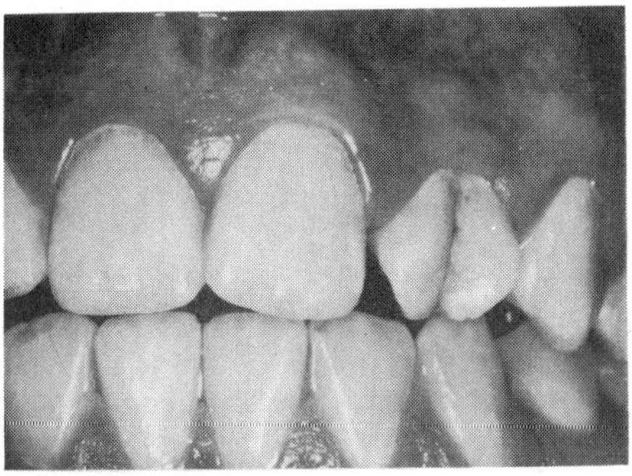

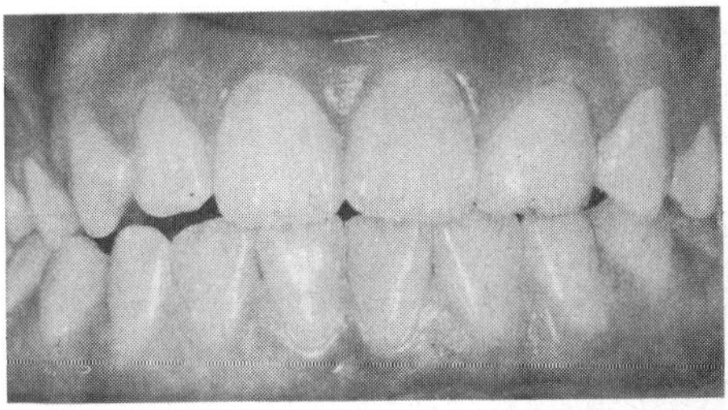

Fig. 2.4. *Dichotomy of the upper left lateral and its treatment by crowning.*

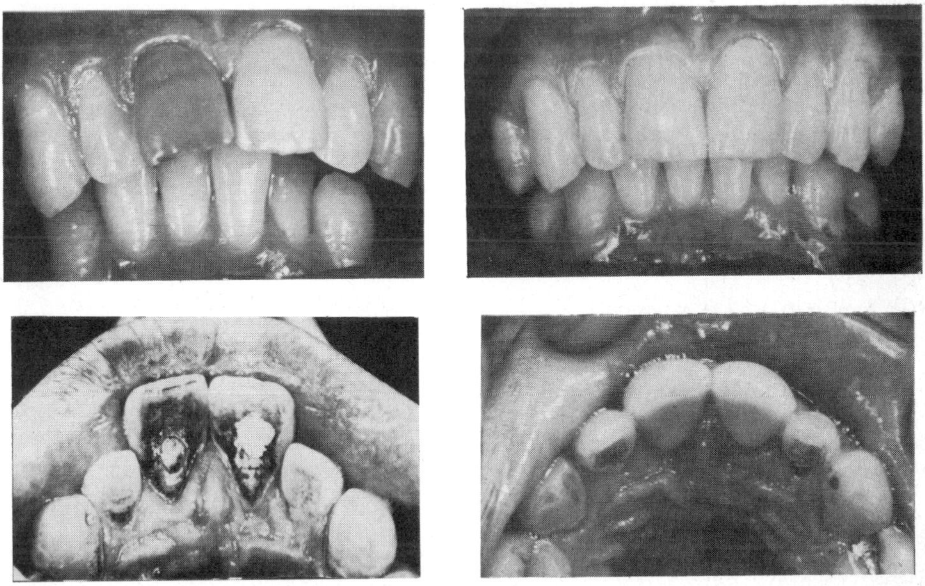

Fig. 2.5. *Protrusive and unsightly centrals treated by crowning.*

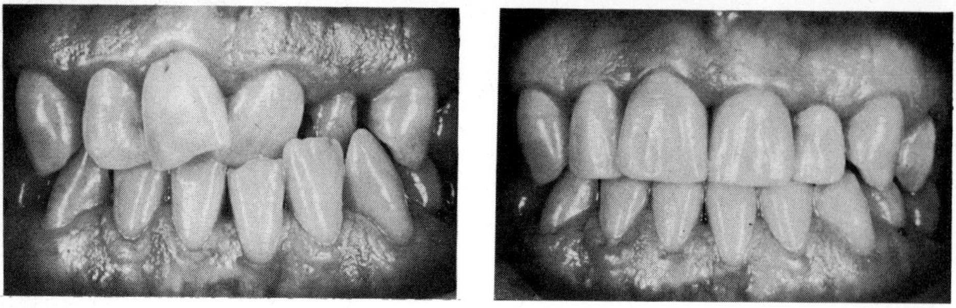

Fig. 2.6. *Instanding and imbricated teeth treated by post and jacket crowns.* (By courtesy of J. Lavis.)

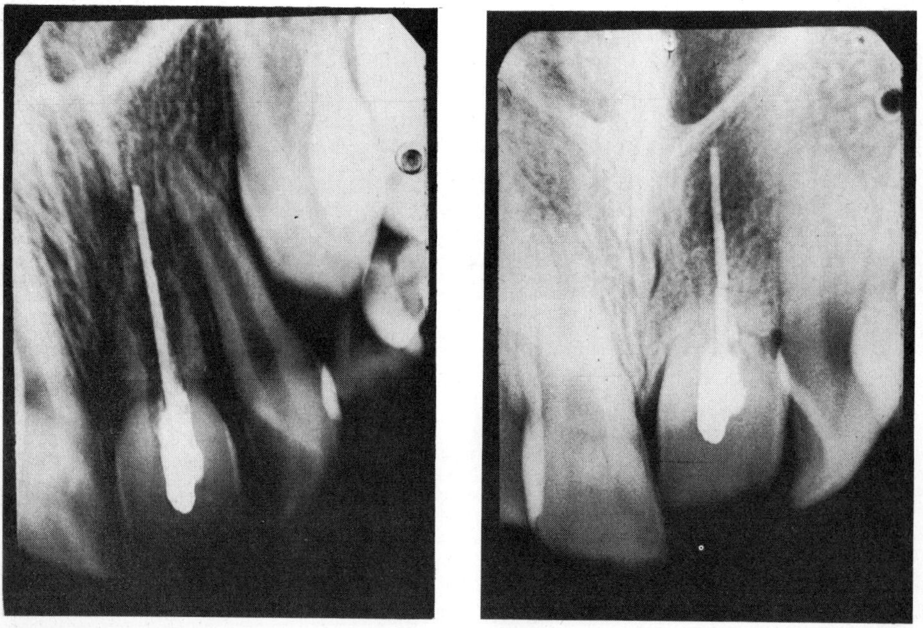

a *b*

Fig. 2.7. *Reimplantation of the upper left central in a patient of* 7. *a,* 4 *years later; b, At the age of* 16.

be amply repaid in the years to come if it is successful. Even if it fails after 7–8 years, if it has carried a patient through from childhood to early adult life it will have been well worth while. At this stage it will be infinitely easier for a satisfactory prosthesis to be fitted to replace the missing tooth. For this reason even when children's teeth are very badly broken down it is worth attempting their conservation and it is surprising how often this treatment is successful, possibly due to the lowering of the caries rate which frequently takes place.

In the case of malformed (*Fig*. 2.4) and malplaced teeth such as those shown in *Fig*. 2.5, although their crowning may prove difficult, it is nearly always to be preferred to extractions and a fixed or removable prosthesis. Similarly, instanding and imbricated teeth can often be realigned and moved over the bite by devitalization and post-crowning (*Fig.* 2.6).

Reimplantation of the teeth (*Fig.* 2.7), which is usually unsuccessful in the long run, is well worth carrying out on a child, as the tooth will frequently be retained for 7–8 years before the root is finally resorbed, by which time all the teeth will have erupted and a satisfactory prosthesis can be placed relatively easily.

MAINTENANCE OF SPACE

Where a gap exists in the younger patient it is desirable to obtain an orthodontic opinion to assess whether the space should be maintained or closed, either actively or passively. If it is desirable to maintain the space the way by which it is done will vary with the age of the patient.

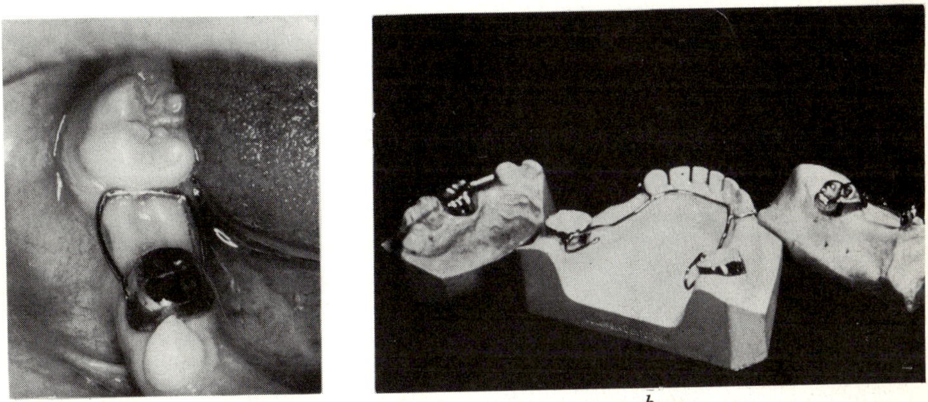

a *b*

Fig. 2.8. *Space maintainers.*
(By courtesy of Department of Children's Dentistry, Eastman Dental Hospital.)

Points to bear in mind when carrying out reimplantation are that the prognosis is improved if:

1. The tooth is replaced as quickly as possible and certainly if it is put back within an hour or so of having been lost.
2. It is not sterilized but only gently cleaned with gauze in an isotonic solution of saline and stored in this.
3. A root filling is not placed before reimplanting the tooth. It merely increases the amount it is handled and the length of time it is out of the mouth. Endodontic therapy may be carried out at a later date.
4. The tooth should not be splinted for longer than necessary; possibly 1–2 weeks, as this increases the likelihood of ankylosis and eventual root resorption.

Finally, an antitetanus injection should always be given unless this is contra-indicated for any reason.

The ideal method is a fixed partial prosthesis; however, this can usually only be carried out successfully on the older patient and thus other methods have to be resorted to until they reach adult life.

If a bridge is placed in the mouth of a child of 12–13 and this fails, as is very likely to happen because of the short clinical crowns and large pulps, then the resultant loss or mutilation of another tooth may cause irreparable harm to the mouth out of all relationship to the benefits to be gained.

There are two basic types of space maintainer, fixed and removable (*Fig.* 2.8). The former are the more desirable as they cannot be left out, which can rapidly prove disastrous because of tooth drift, and are not so liable to be broken. However, it will depend on many factors such as the length of time the space has to be maintained, whether it is unilateral or bilateral, if aesthetic considerations are involved, and the age of the patient, as to which method should be employed.

In the adolescent a removable partial denture, preferably of chrome-cobalt or gold, is often the best treatment, particularly if good aesthetics is required. However, this is usually only practical when all the permanent teeth, except the third molars, have erupted. In the younger patient an acrylic prosthesis is better as it is more easily adapted to allow for tooth movement and eruption.

In children, particularly in the posterior region, a simple fixed space maintainer can be made by cementing a full crown, usually of very thin stainless steel, to which is attached a strong loop which will maintain the space (*Fig.* 2.8*b*).

Experience has shown that the longer the construction of a bridge can be delayed the better its prognosis (*see Fig.* 3.4, p. 35) and that it is generally undesirable to place such a prosthesis before the patient is 21. Even at this age the case must be carefully chosen and all the details of design, in particular the provision of adequate retention, thoroughly analysed.

REASONS FOR TREATING TOOTH LOSS

■ 1. Aesthetics

Prostheses placed for this reason are usually at the patient's request and are confined to anterior teeth or the upper premolars. The psychological benefits to be gained by the restoration of the patient's appearance are often considerable and can make a very real difference to their whole outlook on life.

■ 2. Function

It is far less common for a patient to request a bridge on functional than on aesthetic grounds; indeed it is surprising how efficiently a patient can eat even with a grossly mutilated dentition. However, this factor is particularly important in cases where two or more neighbouring teeth are missing in one posterior quadrant, thus virtually rendering that side of the mouth non-functional.

■ 3. Pain due to Temporomandibular Joint Dysfunction (Pain-dysfunction syndrome)

Tooth loss and the associated tooth movements described earlier can result in pain from muscle spasm protecting the temporomandibular joint. This may be treated by spot grinding to relieve premature contacts, the correction of any other occlusal disharmony, and then the replacement of the missing tooth, together with the stabilization of those on either side.

■ 4. Maintenance of Dental Health

The unfavourable effects of tooth loss have already been enumerated and it is to prevent these occurring that a missing tooth should normally be replaced.

■ 5. Speech

The loss of a tooth, particularly a lower incisor, may occasionally give rise to a speech problem. However, the actual results will vary greatly from person to person, being dependent on the type of occlusion they possess, whether or not spacing is present, the muscular and skeletal patterns, and various other physiological and psychological considerations.

For all the foregoing reasons it is desirable to replace missing teeth as soon as possible after they have been lost. However, if the tooth has been absent for many years, the other teeth have assumed a stable position, and there are no obviously adverse effects then it may be best to leave the space untreated, although in practice this is seldom so.

This most commonly applies when the space ensuing after early tooth loss has partially or almost completely closed and any over-eruption of the teeth which is liable to occur has already taken place. It is likely that any prosthesis placed in such a case will do more harm than good. One often sees a small bridge replacing something less than one unit of space which, possibly because of the drift which has occurred, was difficult to construct, has subsequently failed and in doing so has caused further tooth loss. Obviously the patient would have been better off without a bridge in the first instance. In these cases the benefits to be gained in masticatory efficiency are so small as to be insignificant.

to increase the width of a space to that of the tooth which was present and thus allow a pontic of normal width to be fitted (*Fig.* 2.9). An example of this is the loss of an upper lateral. The canine will drift mesially towards the central incisor and will have to be repositioned before a satisfactory prosthesis can be placed.

2. The rotation of a tooth so as to improve its appearance and, if a fixed prosthesis is to be placed, simplify the provision of adequate retainers.

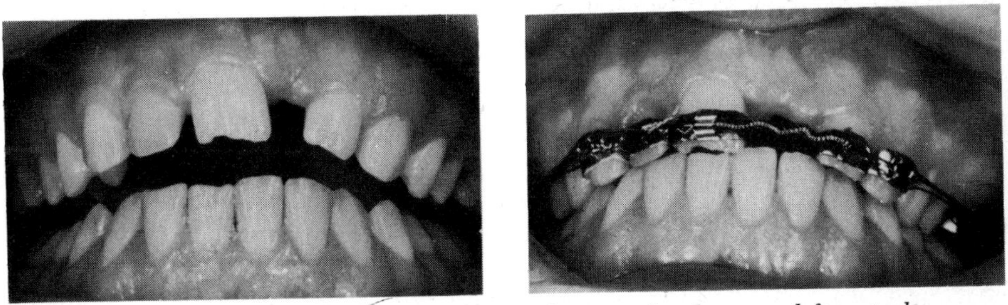

Fig. 2.9. *Orthodontic treatment used to recreate the space for the upper left central.*

METHODS OF TREATING TOOTH LOSS

There are four main ways of making good tooth loss:

A. Orthodontics.
B. Implants.
C. Removable prostheses.
D. Fixed prostheses.

■ A. Orthodontics

In the younger patient it is sometimes practical to make good tooth loss and entirely eliminate a space by orthodontic treatment and indeed on occasions the loss may be beneficial in preventing over-crowding. However, in these cases the patient must be fully assessed from an orthodontic viewpoint; it may then prove desirable to carry out other extractions and provide appliance therapy.

More commonly orthodontics is of value in repositioning the teeth prior to the placing of a prosthesis, particularly a fixed one. For instance in:

1. The moving of a tooth or teeth so as

3. The alteration of a tooth's angulation so as to eliminate undercuts and stagnation areas and allow a satisfactory artificial tooth to be placed. In the case of a bridge, the necessity for undue tooth tissue removal with possible pulp exposure and poor retention will be avoided. An example of this is the mesially inclined lower second molar following loss of the first molar.

4. The moving of a tooth over the bite to correct a cross-bite, enabling a reasonable aesthetic replacement to be placed and, with a fixed prosthesis, have both retainers on the same side of the opposing teeth.

■ B. Implants

In dentistry the term 'implant' is used to describe a foreign body which is inserted or implanted into the tissues to support or stabilize a prosthesis. There are four main types:

1. Mucosal inserts.
2. Subperiosteal implants.
3. Endosseous implants.
4. Endodontic implants.

1. Mucosal Inserts
These are usually in the form of studs attached to the prosthesis which are inserted into small pockets in the mucosa. These are created by making holes in the mucosa immediately prior to fitting the denture, complete with studs. The tissues then heal up and epithelize around the studs. They are most commonly used to assist in the retention of a full upper denture.

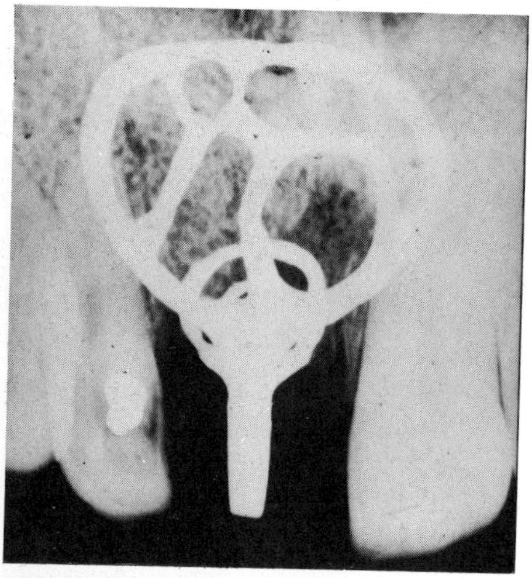

Fig. 2.10. *A single unit subperiosteal implant.*
(By courtesy of Professor A. O. Mack.)

2. Subperiosteal Implants
These are usually made of a chrome-cobalt framework which rests on the bone and is firmly bound down to it by the mucoperiosteum (*Figs*. 2.10, 2.11). To achieve a good result the casting must fit the bone very accurately and thus the mucoperiosteum has to be reflected twice, once to take an accurate impression of the bone and once to fit the subframe.

Posts extend upwards from this into the oral cavity and it is to these that the prosthesis is fitted. The theoretical disadvantage of this form of treatment is that infection could track down beside the posts to reach the underlying bone; however in practice, provided the framework is stable, this rarely occurs probably because of the epithelization which it is thought usually occurs around the implant, thus exteriorizing it. It is only when the epithelium breaks down that infection can track to deeper tissues. The mucoperiosteum seems to contract around the post and fits so firmly against it that it almost appears to form an attachment.

This type of implant is very valuable in stabilizing a difficult full lower prosthesis and is of assistance in the free end saddle case, where it may be used either alone or to provide the posterior abutment for a fixed-fixed bridge. Indeed when combined with a fixed prosthesis the

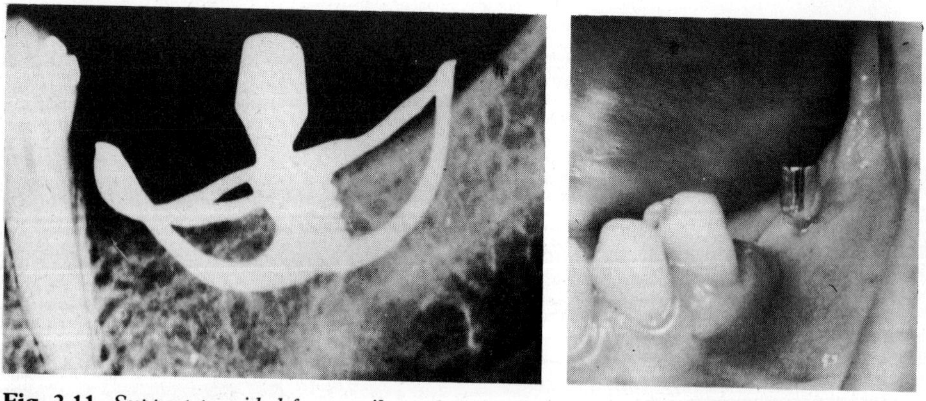

Fig. 2.11. *Support provided for a unilateral free-end saddle by means of a subperiosteal implant.*
(By courtesy of Professor A. O. Mack.)

prognosis for the implant is appreciably improved. In the maxilla the prognosis for the subperiosteal implant is far less favourable than in the mandible and although its application in cleft palate cases has theoretical advantages the high failure rate usually contraindicates its use.

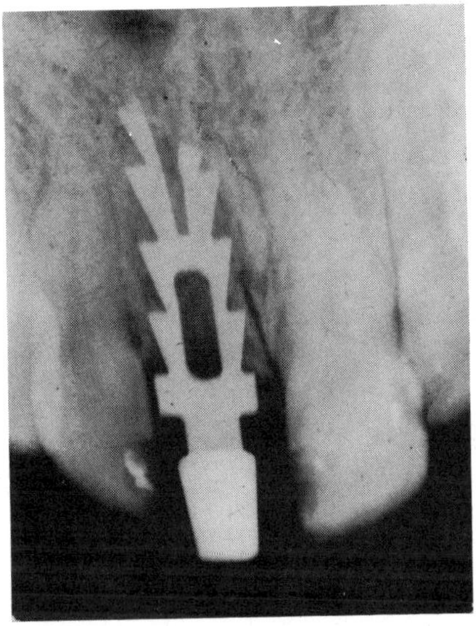

Fig. 2.12. *A single-unit endosseous implant.*
(By courtesy of Professor A. O. Mack.)

3. Endosseous Implants

In these types a pin, screw, blade or similar device is inserted into the bone and used to stabilize a prosthesis. Of

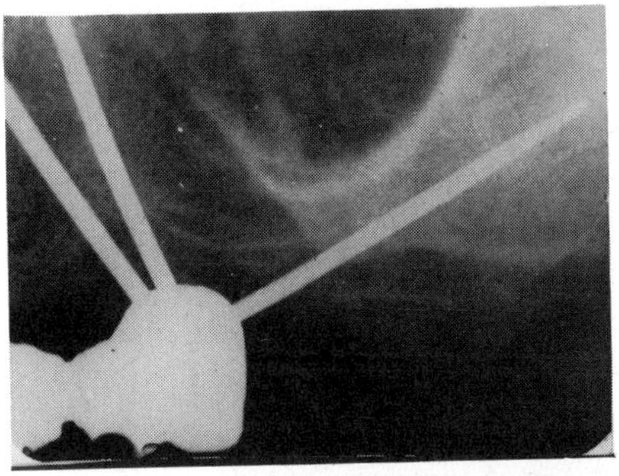

a

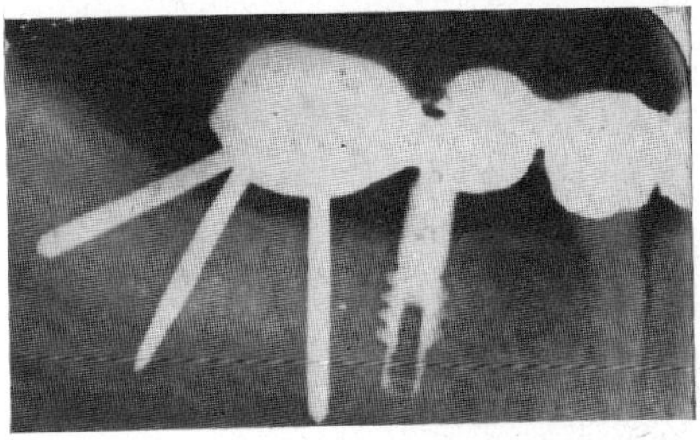

b

Fig. 2.13. *a, Endosseous pins circumventing the maxillary antrum. b, Endosseous pins and vent plant used in the lower arch.*
(By courtesy of Professor L. I. Linkow.)

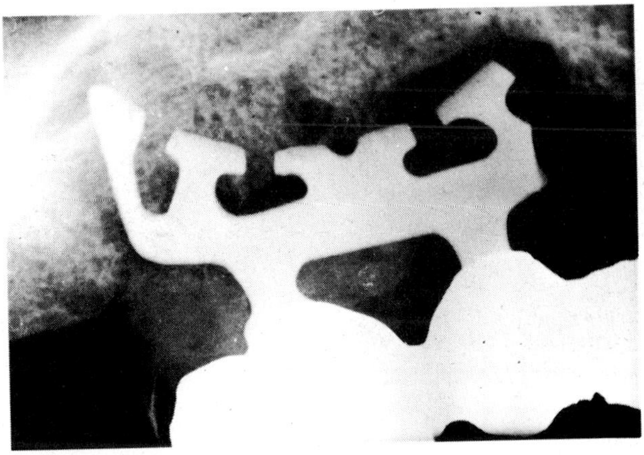

Fig. 2.14. *Extensive bone loss around a blade implant* 18 *months after insertion in the maxilla.*

these the pin would appear to have the worst prognosis, possibly because of its low surface area, and the blade the highest success rate. They have been used to replace just one tooth (*Fig.* 2.12) or several teeth, or to provide anchorage points by which to stabilize a full upper or lower denture. Great care must always be taken to avoid putting any implant into such structures as the antrum, nasal cavity, or inferior dental canal (*Fig.* 2.13).

The disadvantage of this type of implant is that if it does fail and infection occurs then there may be a considerable loss of bone (*Fig.* 2.14) which could affect the neighbouring teeth. Similarly, it may result in recession in the saddle area, thus preventing a fixed prosthesis being placed because an adequately self-cleansing pontic cannot be provided. This type of prosthesis may prove useful in the incisor region, particularly in the lower arch. It is here that most difficulty occurs in using other types of replacement.

The prognosis of the blade type of implant would appear to be best in the mandible. They are particularly useful in free-end saddle cases and in these instances can be successfully combined with fixed bridge prostheses (*Fig.* 2.15). Indeed they would seem to fare best when splinted to natural teeth or even to each other.

Polymer Tooth Implants

One of the most recent developments in implantology is the polymer tooth implant. This is still at an experimental stage but basically consists of the insertion into the socket of an exact polymethyl methacrylate replica of the tooth which has been extracted from it. Some authorities claim that a normal periodontium will form around the implanted tooth and that if channels are prepared in the roots bone will actually form in these. However, at the present time there is little clinical evidence to substantiate this claim.

For further information on this the reader is referred to the work of Hodosh et al. (1970).

Vitreous Carbon Endosteal Implants

Although vitreous carbon implants are still in a relatively early stage of development results so far obtained are reasonably encouraging: vitreous carbon appears to be well tolerated by the tissues (Hobkirk, 1975) and does not disintegrate. Moreover, bone lamellae seem to be laid down around the implant quite readily.

With this type of implant the shape employed is usually similar to that of the natural tooth it replaces with ridges and

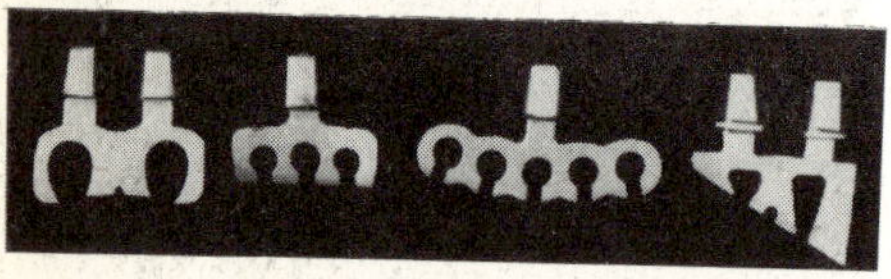

a

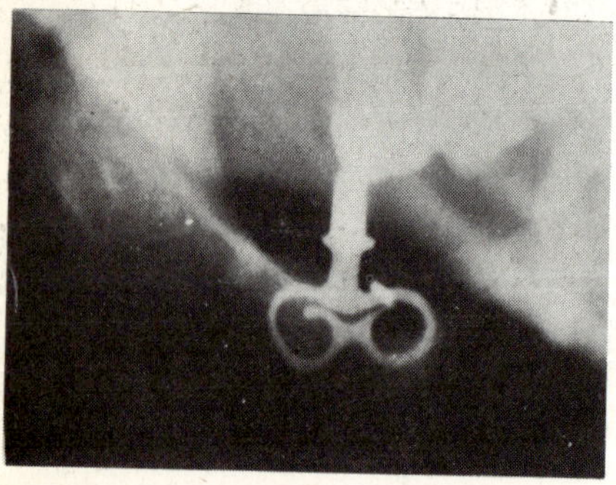

b

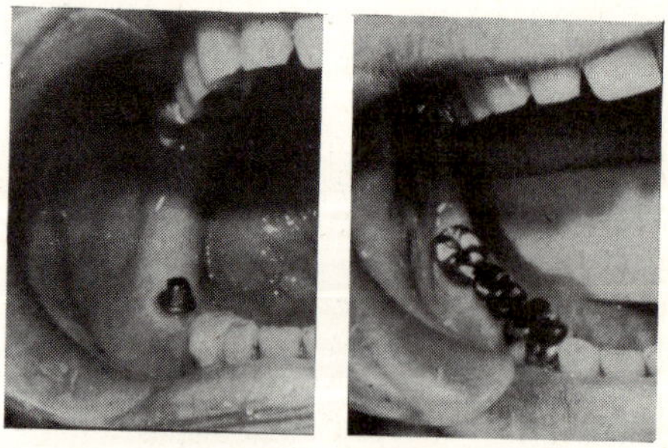

c *d*

Fig. 2.15. *a, Various types of blade implant. b–d, A unilateral free-end saddle treated by a blade implant and a fixed prosthesis.*
(By courtesy of Professor A. O. Mack.)

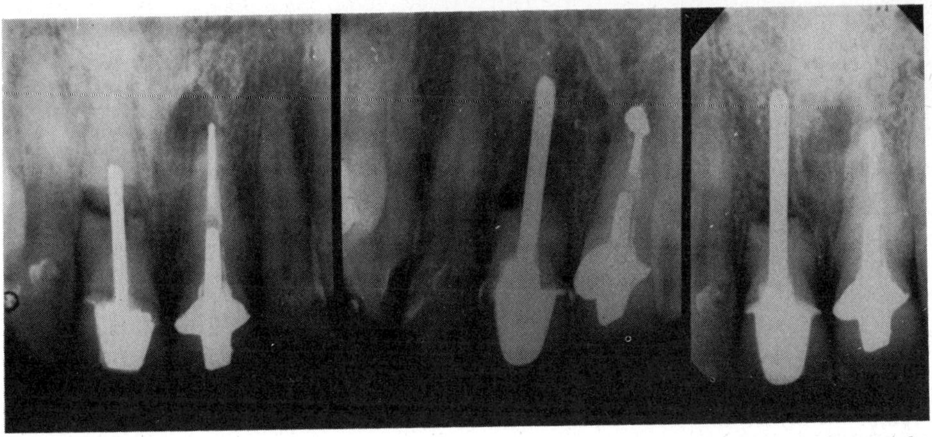

Fig. 2.16. (Left) *A tooth restored by a post crown the root of which subsequently fractured.* (Centre) *Treatment by endodontic implant.* (Right) 2 *years later showing bone regeneration around the post.*
(By courtesy of Mr F. J. Harty.)

grooves added to provide mechanical retention; tissue ingrowth occurring into the surface of the implant. In a report on their use (Grenoble and Voss, 1977) found that the gingival sulcus rapidly established itself and remained constant at 2–3 mm and no infection was observed.

4. Endodontic Implants

An endodontic implant may be described as the passing of a post through the root canal of a tooth and extending this into the underlying bone so as to increase the support for that tooth (*Fig.* 2.16).

The technique is of particular value in cases of root fracture where the removal of the broken segment, possibly half the root, leaves insufficient root surface area to support the crown. It may also be of value where periodontal breakdown has destroyed part of the bony support of the tooth, provided the periodontal condition has been stabilized.

The technique (Scopp et al., 1969) basically consists of using a matched drill and post system such as the 'Wiptam' technique (Harty and Leggett, 1972) so as to achieve a good seal as between the post and the top of the root, and extending the post for a predetermined distance beyond the apex; this being governed to some degree by the local anatomy. The advantage of this technique over other types of implant is that provided the periodontium is sound there is no

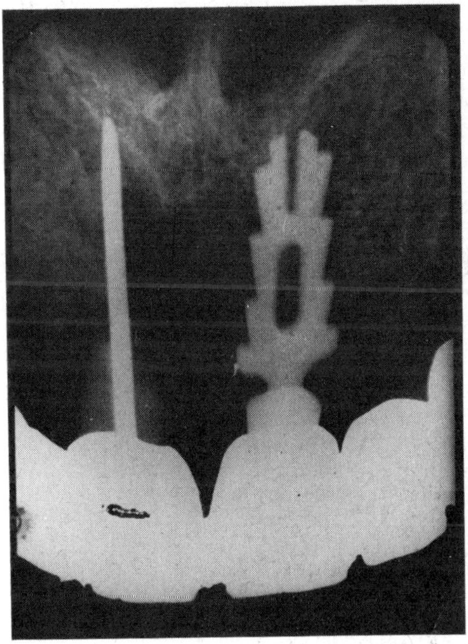

Fig. 2.17. *Extensive bone loss around an implant attempted in a case with advanced periodontal disease.*

continuity between the implant and the mouth and thus no chance of direct infection. If the periodontal condition is very poor endondotic implants should not be attempted (*Fig*. 2.17).

■ C. Removable Prostheses

The margin which exists between fixed and removable prostheses is a narrow one which has been rendered even less precise by the advent of precision retainers (attachments). Similarly, it is difficult to divide the various removable prostheses into definite groups, as each tends to overlap the other. However, removable prostheses may, for convenience, be separated into those which are entirely tissue-borne and those which are partially or fully tooth-borne.

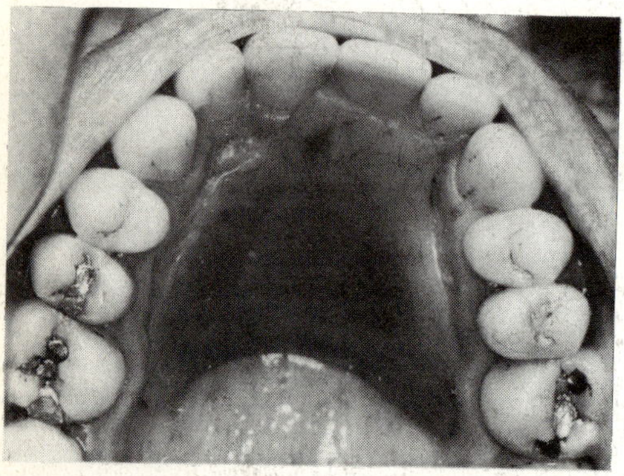

Fig. 2.18. *Spoon denture.*

Tissue-borne Prostheses

The two common types of tissue-borne partial prostheses are the spoon and the festooned acrylic denture.

Spoon Denture

This type of prosthesis is only applicable to the upper arch as it gains its support from an accurately fitting spoon-shaped section of plastic covering a large area of the centre of the palate (*Fig*. 2.18).

The fact that there is little or no tooth support for the prosthesis may in time result in overloading of the tissues in the saddle area with consequent bone loss and adverse effects on the adjacent teeth.

The design is of particular value where a single upper anterior tooth requires replacement as it is generally kept clear of the gingival margins and is thus unlikely to be detrimental to the periodontal tissues. It usually relies purely on close adaptation and the effects of surface tension for its retention, but this can be increased by passing acrylic collets around a single posterior tooth on either side and if necessary clasps may be added. However, this has the disadvantage that the tendency to gingival irritation is increased in this region. A little tooth support may sometimes be gained by covering a small part of the palatal surfaces of the teeth adjoining the gap. Labial gumwork is usually indicated and by covering as wide an area of soft

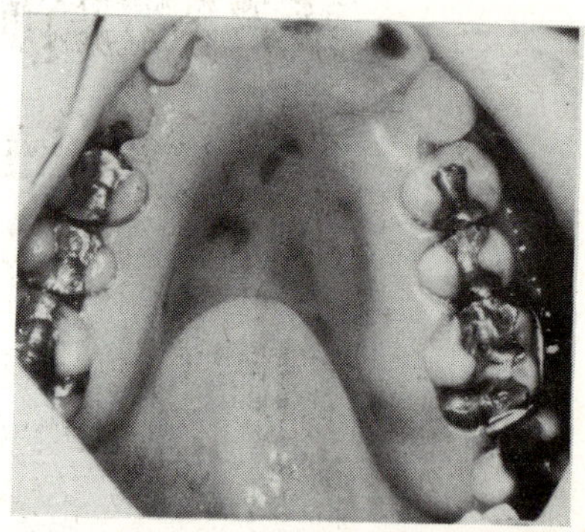

Fig. 2.19. *Tissue-borne acrylic denture festooned around the gingival margins.*

tissue as possible retention and stability will be greatly increased.

The main disadvantage of the spoon denture is its tendency to lack stability and retention which may be both a real and also a psychological embarrassment to the patient.

The Tissue-borne Festooned Acrylic Denture

This design (*Fig*. 2.19) probably has more detrimental effects on the mouth in general than any other, and these are greatly exacerbated if the patient's oral hygiene is poor or if he wears the denture at night. Unfortunately, however, patients often prefer this design, as it can be quite stable, does not usually incorporate clasps, and is relatively cheap to construct. As the prosthesis is entirely tissue-borne, resorption is liable to occur denture and ends up 7–8 years later with one carrying six teeth. The only justification for this design is where so few teeth are standing that no useful support can be gained from them and thus the prosthesis must be entirely tissue-borne.

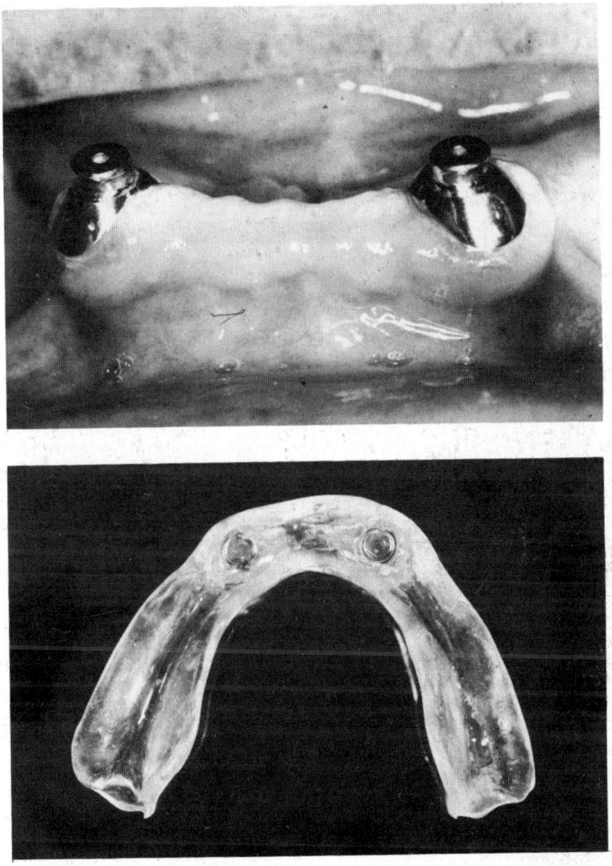

Fig. 2.20. *The Rotherman (eccentric) precision retainer used for stabilizing the full denture.*

in the saddle area. This results in the denture being forced up around the teeth and its acrylic collets stripping the gingivae from around them.

Because the prosthesis covers the gingival margins it is bound to have an adverse effect on the periodontal tissues and also greatly increases the liability to cervical and interstitial caries. All too often a patient starts off with a single-tooth replacement festooned acrylic

However, in these cases it is essential to instruct patients very carefully in their oral hygiene and where the caries rate is high consideration may be given to crowning the teeth before placing the prosthesis. This is particularly desirable in cleft palate cases where it is essential to retain as many of the teeth for as long as possible.

With the advent of the hybrid denture incorporating precision retainers such as the Rotherman (eccentric) (*Fig.* 2.20) and the bona, soldered to root caps, the necessity for placing a festooned acrylic denture has been further reduced. The advantage of precision retainers (attachments) such as those fitted to a root cap is that the liability to caries is greatly decreased and the abutment tooth is less likely to be overloaded because of the reduced leverage on it, the eccentric, for instance, being only 2·5 mm high.

The preservation of endodontically-treated roots retains alveolar height and even without precision retainers provides considerable stability for the full denture prostheses. Several cases have been seen in which there has been minimal bone loss over a 15–20-year period.

Partially and Fully Tooth-borne Removable Prostheses

The main types of removable, tooth-borne partial prostheses are—

1. The tooth-borne partial denture usually made of metal and incorporating clasps and rests.
2. The sectional partial denture.
3. The precision retained partial denture.

The Tooth-borne Partial Denture

This type of prosthesis is usually cast in chrome-cobalt or gold, thereby obtaining the most accurate fit (*Fig.* 2.21). However, on occasions it may be thought that acrylic will be sufficiently strong to be used for the base. Clasps with rests should be incorporated in the design and the outline made so that, as far as possible, the gingival margins remain uncovered. However, it is seldom possible to achieve with acrylic the fit and stability which is possible with a cast denture.

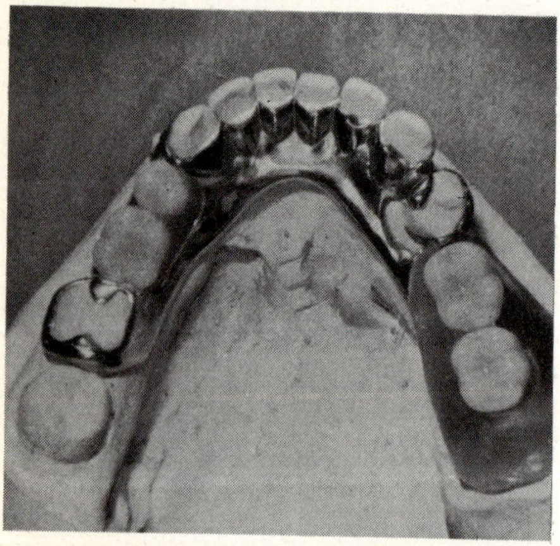

Fig. 2.21. *Precision partial denture constructed of chrome-cobalt.* (By courtesy of Mr P. L'Estrange.)

The metal base also has the advantage that it is unlikely to shrink, wear, warp or fracture during use. Further advantages are that it is simpler to design the base so that it avoids the gingival margins of the teeth. This is because its strength is far greater than acrylic and thus it can be used in thinner sections. There is the further fact that because of the thinness of the plate it is less noticeable to the patient and frequently in the upper jaw it is possible to avoid covering the palate.

Unfortunately, however, the incorporation of clasps, which is a necessity for the stability of nearly all metal partial dentures, affects the pattern of food shedding and this may result in direct trauma to the gingivae. Plaque formation is also likely to be increased.

When there is a choice of materials, gold is usually preferable to chrome-cobalt and similar alloys because there is less liability to caries beneath it, particularly when the oral hygiene is in the slightest degree suspect. However, a gold denture is considerably heavier and somewhat more expensive than one made of chrome-cobalt.

The Sectional Partial Denture

This type of prosthesis is of comparatively recent origin, having first been described by Professor Lee who developed it in conjunction with Mr Pullen-Warner at the Institute of Dental Surgery in 1964. Since this time quite a variety of sectional prostheses have been evolved. The basic principle of the design is that the denture consists of two or more components (*Fig.* 2.22), each having a different path of insertion. They are thus able to engage in different undercuts which, when the separate components are locked together, prevent displacement of the prosthesis.

Both soft- and hard-tissue undercuts are employed and, if necessary, restorations may be placed on the teeth to create these. The psychological benefit to the patient of knowing that the prosthesis cannot be displaced is probably as valuable to him as any strictly practical consideration.

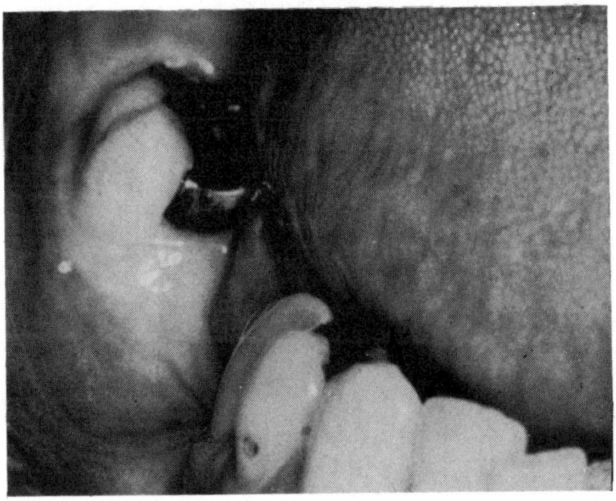

a

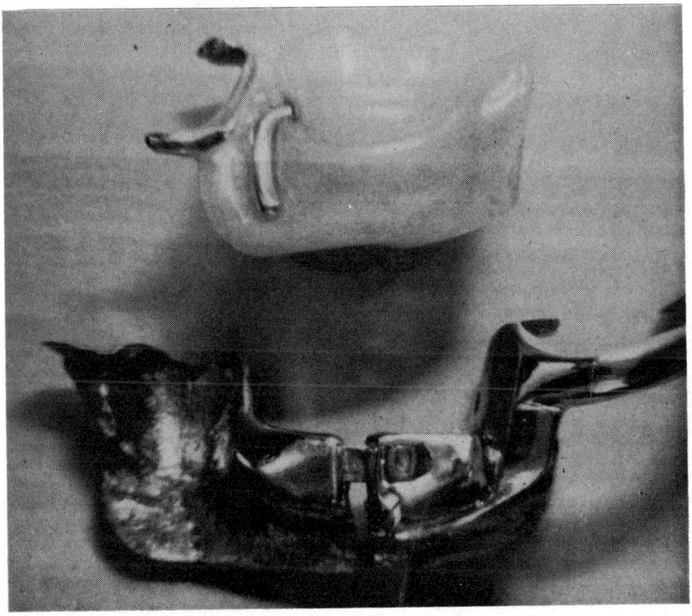

b

Fig. 2.22. *a, A suitable case for a two-part denture where there has been extensive soft-tissue loss and tooth drift. b, The separate components of the prosthesis which are locked together by a bolt.*
(By courtesy of Mr P. L'Estrange.)

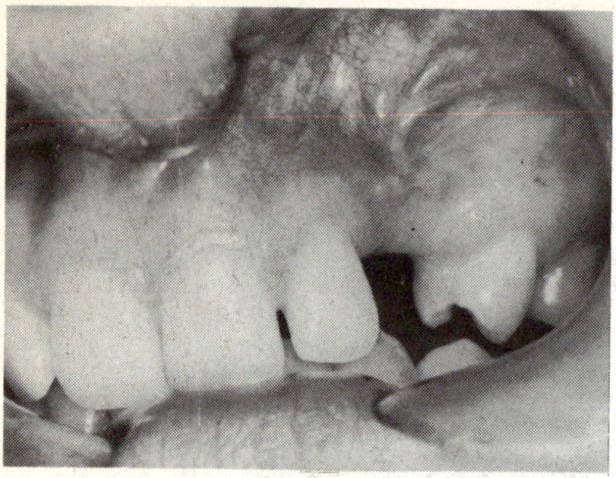

a

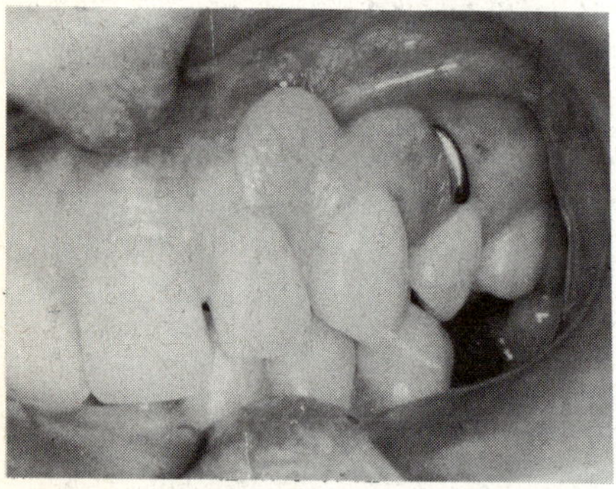

b

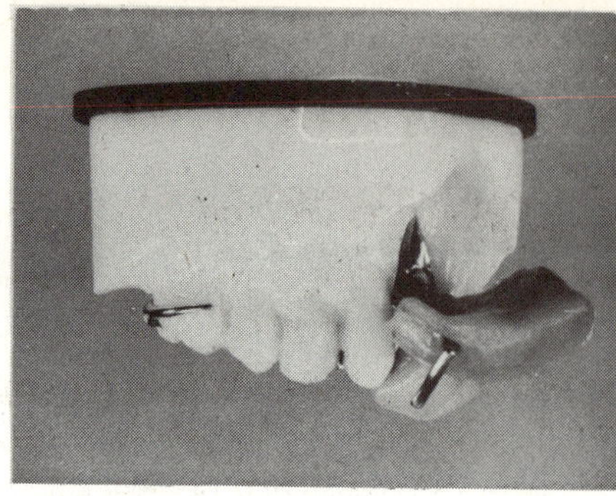

c

Fig. 2.23. *a, b, A sectional partial denture of the hinge type used to replace the upper left canine. Note how use has been made of the extensive undercuts. c, A sectional partial denture of the hinge type used in a case of extensive soft-tissue loss.*
(By courtesy of Mr P. L'Estrange.)

The individual parts of the prosthesis are, when fully seated, locked together by latches or bolts, a later development being that the different components of the prosthesis, instead of being entirely separate, are joined by hinges (*Fig.* 2.23). A variation developed by Messrs L'Estrange and Pullen-Warner incorporates the use of parallel pins in one part of the prosthesis engaging with tubes in the other, the two components again having different lines of insertion. The frictional fit between the different parts may be adjusted by fractionally bending one of the posts or by using a split post technique (*Fig.* 2.24). The retention achieved is usually excellent.

The advantage of a sectional denture is that undercuts can be engaged, which not only increases retention but also eliminates dead spaces which are liable to become food traps. Furthermore the aesthetic result achieved is usually excellent. Excess tissue loss in the saddle area generally contraindicates a fixed partial prosthesis but is often a positive indication for a sectional denture.

The Precision Retained Partial Denture
One of the main disadvantages of the conventional clasp-retained metal partial denture is that however carefully it is designed the clasps are usually visible.

Another disadvantage is that the clasp obtains its support and retention from the tooth extracoronally, whereas theoretically it is best to achieve this intracoronally. This is because there will be less displacement of the tooth on insertion and removal of the prosthesis. Similarly, unfavourable periodontal stresses will be minimized, as any force applied will be intracoronal and in the long axis of the tooth, which the periodontal membrane is best able to withstand.

This ideal can be obtained by the use of precision retainers (*Fig.* 2.25) which have the further advantage that they are aesthetically far more satisfactory than the clasp.

The precision retainer, as its name implies, is machined to very fine tolerances and thus the frictional retention which can be achieved as between the two components is far greater than that with a clasp; indeed it can often be too good and cause cementation failure of the casting on the abutment tooth.

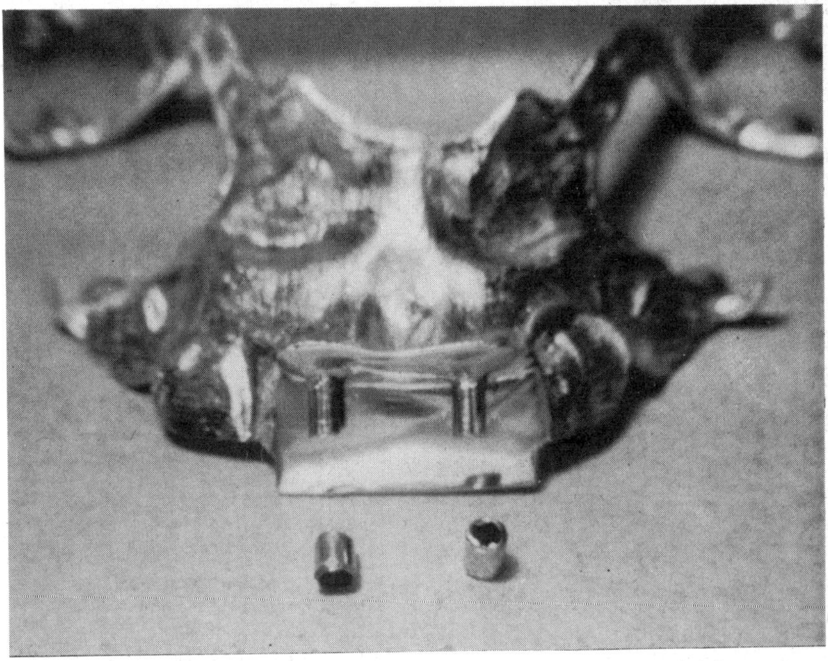

Fig. 2.24. *Frictional sleeves used for retaining a sectional partial denture.* (By courtesy of Mr P. L'Estrange.)

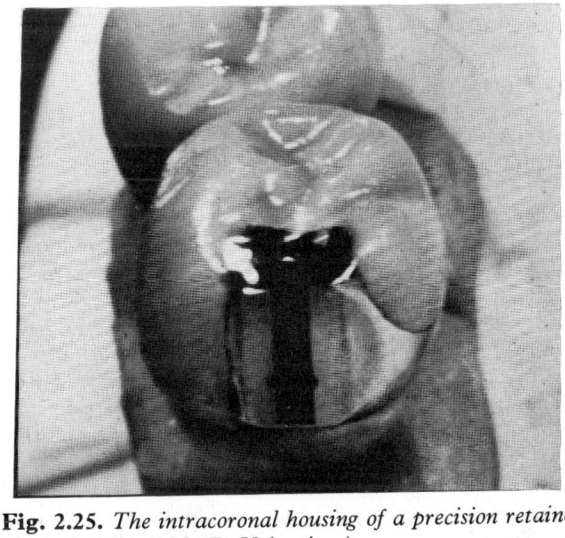

Fig. 2.25. *The intracoronal housing of a precision retainer.* (By courtesy of Mr R. Valentine.)

The time and expense involved in the construction of precision retained prostheses is far greater than with a conventional metal denture as the teeth used for housing the retainers require very accurate preparation. Similarly, the laboratory procedures are far more precise, necessitating the use of a parallelometer, milling and other devices.

The advantages, besides those already mentioned, are that greater stability is achieved than with a conventional prosthesis; frequently it can be considerably smaller, and often the midline need not be crossed in a unilateral case, as is normally necessary with a removable prosthesis.

The advantage of the precision retained over the conventional fixed bridge prosthesis is that extensive soft-tissue loss can be made good without the risk of creating food stagnation, as it is removable and thus easily cleaned.

The conventional bridge may be defined as a partial prosthesis rigidly cemented to one or more teeth and replacing one or more natural teeth. Its basic components are as illustrated in *Fig*. 2.26. With the use of precision retainers the pontic may still be rigidly connected to the retainers on the abutment teeth by means of screws or other devices. It is thus similar to a bridge, but does not meet our definition as the pontic is not rigidly cemented via the casting to the abutment teeth, but is additionally joined to it by some other means.

The advantage of this use of the precision retainer is that the replaced tooth or teeth may be detached, modified, and repaired as necessary without disturbing the casting on the abutment teeth. Precision retainers may also be employed where the splinting effect of a fixed-fixed bridge is required but it is impossible to align the various preparations on the abutment teeth.

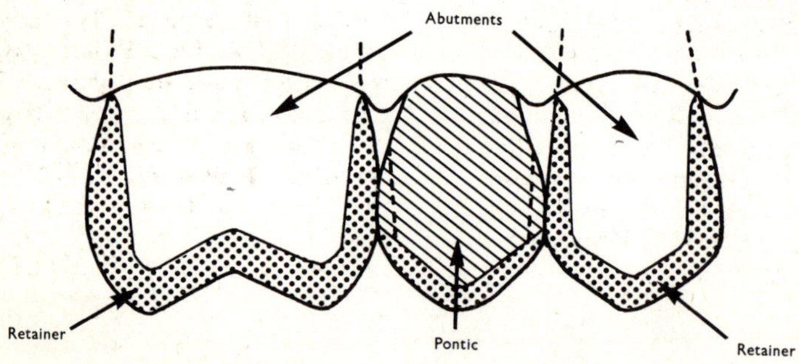

Fig. 2.26. *The basic components of a bridge.*

The fixed prosthesis is normally preferable to all other forms of replacement as its stability is excellent and it should not adversely affect the periodontal condition or the caries rate. Its advantages and disadvantages will be discussed in greater detail in the next chapter.

An example of a removable prosthesis incorporating precision retainers is shown in *Fig*. 12.7, p. 170. In this a milled bar is supported by full crowns and the prosthesis snaps on to this by means of a sleeve and small devices similar to ball catches. Further examples are given in the chapter on precision retainers.

■ D. Fixed Prostheses

Until comparatively recently a fixed partial prosthesis implied a bridge. However, with the advent of the precision retainer the margin between the fixed and the removable prosthesis has become far narrower.

Types of Bridge

In this textbook the word 'bridge' always implies a fixed prosthesis as opposed to a denture, which is considered to be removable. The terms 'fixed and removable bridge' and 'fixed and removable denture' will not be used as they tend to be confusing.

Bridges may be divided into five different types, as shown below, and two of these, fixed-fixed and fixed-movable, may be further divided into anterior and posterior. This subdivision is necessary because different design factors affect each type.

1. Fixed-fixed { Anterior / Posterior }
2. Fixed-movable { Anterior / Posterior }
3. Spring
4. Cantilever
5. Compound

The Fixed-fixed Bridge

In a fixed-fixed bridge all the components are rigidly joined (*Fig.* 2.27), either by soldering the individual units together or using a one-piece casting. Because of this all stresses imposed on the bridge will be relatively evenly distributed between the two or more abutment teeth. This is usually an advantage in long-span cases or where the periodontal condition is in doubt and the benefits to be derived from fixed splinting are required. However, it can be a disadvantage in short-span bridges because very good retention will be required from both retainers and if this is not achieved cementation failure will result. It must be remembered that if a patient bites on one abutment of a fixed-fixed bridge then, because all the components are rigidly joined together, the other abutment, although it will resist it, is forced via the pontics, to move also. This inevitably induces stresses in the bridge which can result in flexion of the castings and cementation failure or failure of the solder joint. This also explains why a 2-unit all-porcelain cantilever bridge, in which the components can move together freely if just one is bitten on, is relatively successful; whereas the 3-unit fixed-fixed all-porcelain bridge has a very high failure rate because of stresses induced in the porcelain when the patient bites on and displaces, albeit fractionally, just one of the abutments. The maximum strength of a chain is that of its weakest link and likewise the retentive power of a fixed-fixed bridge is only as good as its weakest retainer. Thus one is obliged to carry out relatively extensive preparations on all the abutment teeth.

Similar remarks apply if a precision retainer (attachment) is used to join the two parts of a bridge. These are partially or wholly machined devices consisting of male and female components. They are machined to such fine limits that they fit each other far more accurately than the conventional dovetail and slot made in the laboratory. Thus, when a bridge incorporating them is fully seated the different parts will be firmly locked together and the bridge is virtually fixed-fixed.

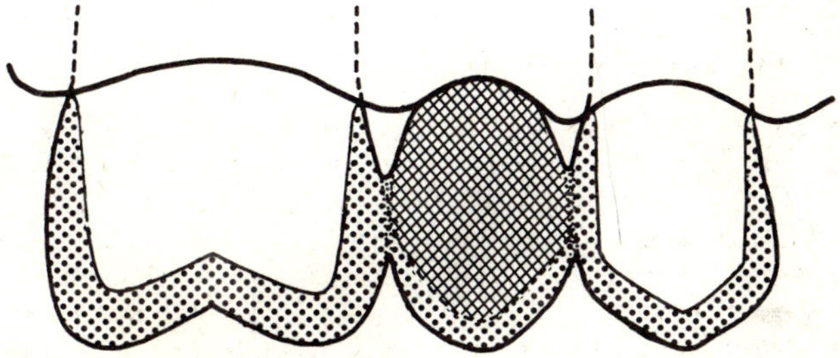

Fig. 2.27. *Fixed-fixed bridge. All components are rigidly joined together.*

The Fixed-movable Bridge

In the fixed-movable bridge a degree of stress breaking is introduced, by dividing the bridge into two sections using a

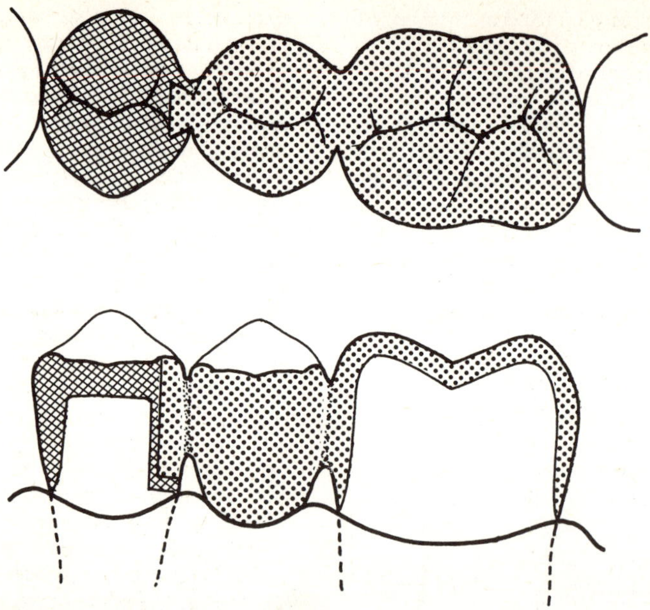

Fig. 2.28. *Fixed-movable bridge. The components are joined by a dovetail and slot.*

dovetail and slot (*Fig*. 2.28). The part to which the pontic is attached is designated the major retainer and that into which the dovetail slots is called the minor retainer. Similarly, one has major and minor abutment teeth. The components of the laboratory-made dovetail and slot do not fit each other nearly as accurately as do those of a precision retainer and thus permit some slight movement between the two parts, mainly in a vertical plane. This allows a far lighter preparation to be placed in the minor abutment, as is illustrated by the fact that a Class II inlay, which is useless as a major retainer in a fixed-fixed bridge, is adequate in some cases as a minor retainer. This emphasizes the far lower demands made on retention by a fixed-movable bridge. Even the major casting does not have to be so retentive.

For the foregoing reasons a fixed-movable design is to be preferred for the majority of short-span posterior bridges, as far less tooth tissue has to be destroyed and the aesthetic result achieved is usually better. Thus when replacing the upper first premolar only a relatively light and aesthetic restoration such as the Selberg modified three-quarter crown may be used as the minor retainer in the canine and any display of gold avoided.

Because the two retainers of a fixed-movable bridge do not have to have the same line of insertion, less tooth usually has to be removed and the preparations are far more retentive.

A halfway-house between the fixed-fixed and fixed-movable bridge is the fixed-semi-movable design. This allows of very limited movement as between the two components.

One method of achieving this is by a ball and socket joint; however, this has the disadvantage that it does not limit the movement to a vertical plane, as does the dovetail and slot. Other means are the covered dovetail, the 45° pin, and the Vale sliding bar, which will be discussed in more detail in Chapter 8.

The Spring Bridge

In the spring bridge the pontic is connected to the retainer by means of a relatively long, flexible palatal bar (*Fig*.

2.29). It is basically a tooth-retained and tissue-borne prosthesis, the forces of mastication applied to the pontic being absorbed by the palatal mucoperiosteum and completely dissipated before they reach the abutment tooth.

It is a somewhat controversial design and is unfortunately condemned out of hand by all too many dental surgeons with no practical experience of its use. However, it has several advantages, amongst which are the following:

1. Only one tooth, and that a posterior one, is usually required as the abutment.

2. It is the only bridge design in which it is possible to have a diastema on either side of the pontic.

3. The flexion of the palatal bar acts as a shock absorber and thus permits the use of a porcelain jacket type pontic, with little chance of its fracture.

The difficulty with the spring bridge is that the theoretical considerations involved in its construction have to be fully understood by both operator and technician, and this only comes after considerable experience with the design. However, once mastered this bridge is an extremely valuable addition to a dental surgeon's armamentarium and is always greatly appreciated by the patient. It overcomes difficulties which may be wellnigh insurmountable with a conventional bridge.

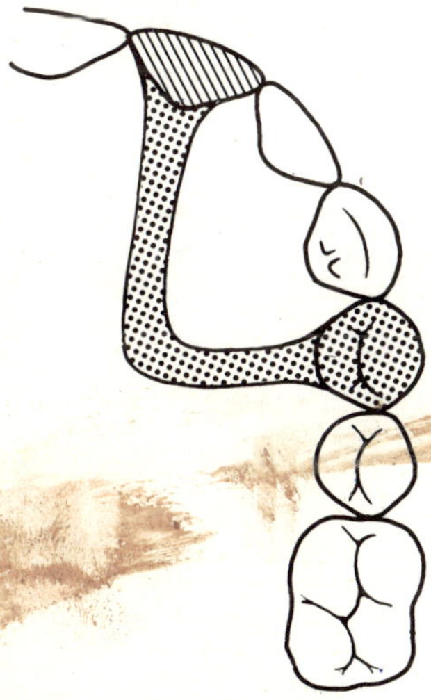

Fig. 2.29. *The spring bridge. In this design the pontic is connected to the retainer by means of a relatively long, flexible palatal bar and is largely tissue-borne.*

The Cantilever Bridge

This is the simplest of all bridge prostheses and, providing it is correctly designed, has a greater chance of success than any other type. The pontic is directly cantilevered off from one side of the abutment tooth (*Fig.* 2.30) and, because of this, the strain imposed on the periodontium is far greater than with a fixed-fixed or fixed-movable bridge. Thus the root surface area of the abutment tooth or teeth must usually be considerably more than that of the tooth being replaced.

Its main use is in the anterior region; the upper lateral, for instance, can nearly always be safely cantilevered off the canine. However, when replacing the canine both premolars must be used as abutments.

In the posterior region cantilevering must be approached with caution as a safe occlusal load may easily be exceeded, particularly if there are any faults in the occlusion. An exception to this rule is the lower first premolar which may usually be cantilevered off retainers on the second premolar and first molar soldered together, as its occlusal surface area is low and it can be made relatively caniniform. Likewise cantilevering

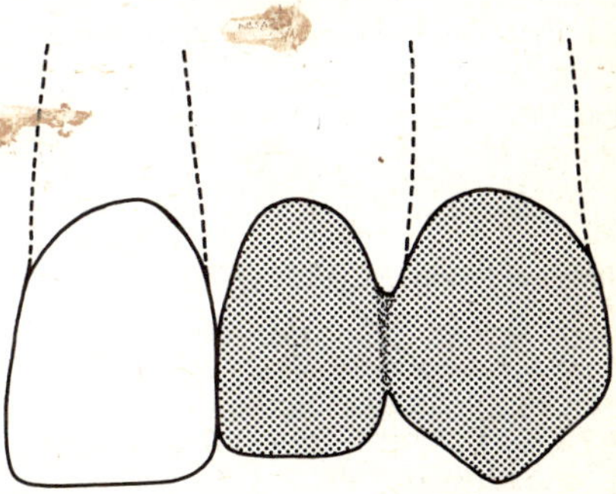

Fig. 2.30. *The cantilever bridge. In this design the pontic gains support from the tooth or teeth on one side of the gap only.*

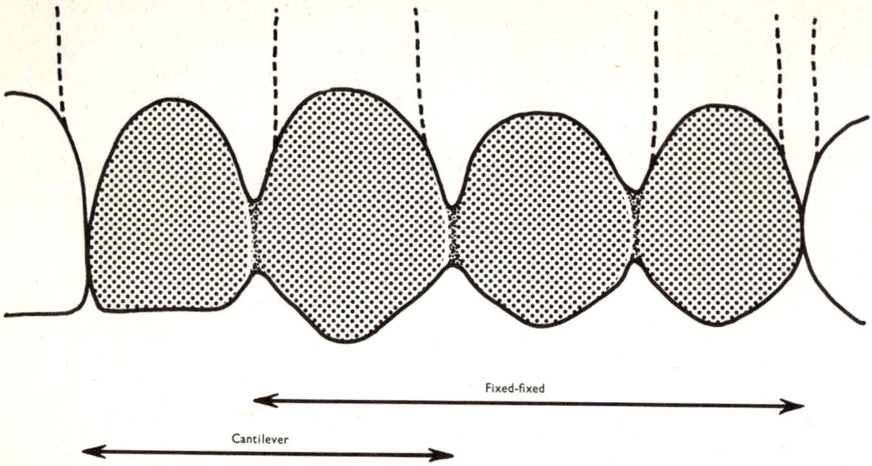

Fig. 2.31. *A compound bridge. Fixed-fixed* (|345) *and cantilever* (|23) *designs being combined.*

distally from the lower premolar or first molar may sometimes be justified in order to stabilize the occlusion, prevent over-eruption and avoid the construction of a difficult and often unsatisfactory free end saddle prosthesis.

The Compound Bridge

By this term is implied the combination of two or more of the types of bridge already mentioned. Thus, if a fixed-fixed bridge is required to replace the upper first premolar and the lateral is also missing, a fixed-fixed bridge may be constructed from the canine to the second premolar and the lateral cantilevered off the mesial aspect of the canine (*Fig.* 2.31).

Similarly, fixed-fixed and fixed-movable bridge designs may be combined and in this way the construction of a relatively complex bridge can be simplified. A further example is the combination of fixed-fixed and spring bridges.

All the foregoing bridge designs have their correct place in restorative dentistry. By selecting the right one for each individual case and on occasions combining more than one type most of the problems of fixed partial prostheses may be overcome.

BIBLIOGRAPHY

Sectional Partial Dentures

Lee J. H. (1964) A new design for removable partial dentures. *Dent. Practnr Dent. Rec.* **14**, 284.

Lee J. H. (1967) Sectional partial metal dentures incorporating an internal locking bolt. *J. Prosthet. Dent.* **13**, 1067.

L'Estrange P. R. and Pullen-Warner E. (1969) Sectional dentures. A simplified method of attachment. *Dent. Practnr. Dent. Rec.* **19**, 379.

L'Estrange P. R. and Pullen-Warner E. (1969) Sectional dentures. Aids to removal and adjustment. *Ibid.* **20**, 135.

Pullen-Warner E. and L'Estrange P. R. (1978) *Sectional Dentures. A Clinical and Laboratory Manual*. Bristol, Wright.

Implants

Bodine R. L. and Mohammed C. I. (1969) Histologic studies of a human mandible supporting an implant denture. *J. Prosthet. Dent.* **21**, 203.

Grenoble D. E., Melrose R. J. and Markle D. H. (1975) Histologic evaluation of vitreous carbon endosteal implants in occlusion in dogs. *Biomater. Med. Devices Artif. Organs* **3**, 245.

Grenoble D. E. and Voss R. (1977) Analysis of five years of study of vitreous carbon endosseous implants in humans. *Oral Implantol.* **6**, 509.

Harty F. J. and Leggett L. J. (1972) A post crown technique using a nickel-cobalt-chromium post. *Br. Dent. J.* **132**, 394.

Hill T. R. (1974) Surgical endodontics. In: Harty F. J. and Roberts D. H. (ed.) *Restorative Procedures for the Practising Dentist.* Bristol, Wright. p. 204.

Hobkirk J. A. (1975) The reaction of rabbit tissues to implanted vitreous carbon. *J. Dent.* **3**, 271.

Hodosh M., Shklar G. and Povar M. (1970) Current status of the polymer tooth implant concept. *Dent. Clin. North Am.* **14**, 103.

Linkow L. I. (1968) The blade vent. A new dimension in endosseous implantology. *Dent. Concepts* **II** (Spring), 3.

Linkow L. I. (1970) Endosseous oral implantology: a 7-year progress report. *Dent. Clin. North Am.* **14**, 185.

Mack A. O. (1960) Histological investigation of effects of subperiosteal dental implants in monkeys. *Br. Dent. J.* **108**, 217.

Mack A. O. (1968) Reactions of the oral tissues to subperiosteal appliances. *Int. Dent. J.* **18**, 779.

Mack A. O. (1971) The status of dental implants. *Dent. Pract.* **3** (3), 1.

Scopp I. W., Dictrow R. L. and Lichtenstein B. S. (1969) Endodontic endosseous implants—A conservative method for stabilisation in geriatric patients. *J. Periodontol.* **40**, 664.

3

INDICATIONS AND CONTRAINDICATIONS FOR BRIDGES

General Considerations. Indications
Contraindications to Bridge Prostheses

GENERAL CONSIDERATIONS

■ Attitude of Patient to Dentistry

Probably the most important factor in deciding whether or not a bridge should be placed for patients is their attitude to dentistry and the degree of enthusiasm which they exhibit for having the work carried out. It must always be remembered that the clinical procedures involved in the preparation of the teeth and the fitting of a bridge are relatively long and arduous, placing a considerable strain on both the operator and the patient. Thus, unless full cooperation is likely to be obtained it will be difficult to achieve a satisfactory result.

Furthermore, unless the patient is willing to attend for regular recall checks of the bridge and indeed the whole mouth, which can only be safely judged from his previous record, then it is unwise to proceed with a fixed prosthesis. If a partial denture fails then little untoward effect, other than minimal inconvenience to the patient, will result, but if, for instance, caries at the margin of one of the retainers is left untreated, not only may the bridge be lost, but one of the abutment teeth as well and a long and costly remake will be required.

■ Oral Hygiene

Poor oral hygiene (*Fig*. 3.1) is a positive contraindication to fixed bridge prostheses as not only is it likely to result in recurrent caries around one of the abutment teeth but it may also cause periodontal breakdown. A further factor is that poor oral hygiene usually indicates an indifferent attitude of the patient to dentistry. It is often better to get these patients to visit the hygienist regularly over a period of 1–2 years and make certain that their oral hygiene improves and their periodontal condition is good before proceeding with a bridge. Disclosing tablets are a considerable aid in this respect in convincing these patients that they are not cleaning their teeth adequately.

INDICATIONS

These may conveniently be divided into general and local.

■ General Indications

The main reasons for replacing a missing tooth have already been discussed in the previous chapter and the more specific indications for the placing of a fixed prosthesis will now be considered.

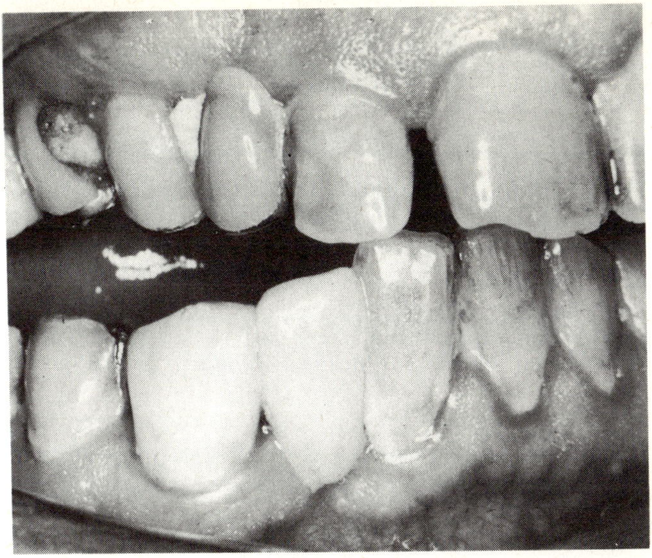

Fig. 3.1. *Poor oral hygiene contraindicating bridge work.*

Psychological
Many patients just will not tolerate a removable prosthesis as they feel that it is not 'part of them', but a fixed prosthesis is usually rapidly accepted as part of their natural dentition. Undoubtedly the wearing of a denture is felt by many to be a sign of declining virility and impending old age. The fitting of a bridge will bring benefits to these patients out of all proportion to the time and money involved and can be vastly more important than any aesthetic or functional improvement which may be achieved.

There is only one case on our records of a bridge having to be removed for psychological reasons. In this instance it was realized before placing it that the chances of success were poor as the patient had already rejected a denture and was at the time undergoing psychotherapy.

A further factor to be considered is that whereas a patient can leave out a partial denture rather than take the trouble to get used to it, a fate which befalls all too many, this is not possible with a bridge, the patient being virtually forced to become accustomed to it.

Systemic Disease
When a patient is likely to suffer from sudden bouts of unconsciousness, or fits, as in epilepsy, then any form of removable appliance is positively contraindicated for fear of its movement, fracture and inhalation during an attack. In these cases, where the replacement of one or more missing teeth is essential, a fixed prosthesis should be placed. However, experience indicates that a considerably higher failure rate is to be expected with this group of patients than with any other because of the increased liability to trauma. Thus, great care must be taken to ensure that adequate strength and retention are provided.

Orthodontic Considerations
The value of replacing a missing tooth for orthodontic reasons has already been mentioned. However, the fixed bridge prosthesis is of particular value in these cases as it provides a more positive location of the teeth than any other method.

A bridge may be of either direct or indirect use in the stabilization of an orthodontic result. An example of the former is the use of a fixed prosthesis to replace a missing lateral after the diastema between two centrals has been closed.

An example of the indirect use of a bridge to prevent the relapse of an orthondontic result is the replacement of a lower first molar which has had to be extracted some time after the completion of orthodontic treatment. If the lower molar is not replaced, drift and possible imbrication of the lower teeth may result and this in turn can affect the upper arch.

Where the patient is too young for a fixed prosthesis then a space maintainer, preferably of the fixed type, may be placed to stabilize the arch until a bridge can be fitted. Examples of these may be seen in *Fig*. 2.8, p. 11.

Periodontal Reasons

When teeth are somewhat mobile or tending to drift then the ideal way of achieving their stabilization is by placing a fixed splint or, if a tooth requires replacement, a fixed-fixed bridge. Both will join the teeth together with complete rigidity. This has several advantages. It prevents tooth movement or drift which may be undesirable both aesthetically and for the long-term prognosis of these teeth. Furthermore, the forces of mastication, when applied to any one periodontally weakened tooth, may be sufficient to overload it and contribute to its further breakdown, but if 4 or 5 teeth are joined together and particularly if any occlusal irregularities are corrected then their combined bony support will usually be sufficient to withstand normal occlusal loads and prevent the periodontium of the individual tooth from being damaged further. Theoretically the weak periodontium of a single tooth will be protected by its proprioceptive fibres but obviously there comes a stage at which the loads permissible without causing damage to the periodontium are so low that the tooth becomes functionally useless. Lastly, a fixed bridge or splint avoids over-eruption with resultant loss of bony support.

However, despite all the foregoing, it must be remembered that teeth which are mobile or tending to drift are poor bridge abutments. Thus, it must only be as part of the overall periodontal and occlusal therapy, which will of course include the elimination where possible, of the cause of the mobility, that a fixed bridge prosthesis should be placed. In the shorter term and particularly where the prognosis is suspect, simpler methods of splinting, such as acid-etch techniques, 'A' splints and removable prostheses may be resorted to. Should periodontal therapy prove successful then fixed splinting may be undertaken.

Immediate Replacement of Teeth

The sudden or even the planned loss of a tooth is often better dealt with by a bridge than a partial denture. A short-term temporary replacement can frequently be provided by employing acid-etch techniques or the use of threaded pins which may be inserted into the teeth on either side of the gap. Where more time is available the teeth on either side may be prepared, the restorations for these tried in and then the bridge constructed and fitted immediately after the extraction of the tooth (*see Figs*. 16.13–16.17, p. 226). The bridge may be made of either all acrylic or gold and acrylic, depending on the time it is intended to leave it in place. This will vary with the rate of healing and also what other treatment, for instance periodontal surgery, may be required.

The advantages of the immediate replacement bridge are that such problems as the close bite (*see Fig*. 16.12, p. 226) are overcome; the patient tolerates it far more readily than a denture and much less damage to the periodontium occurs. Furthermore, bone loss in the saddle area is reduced, thus simplifying the permanent replacement. Indeed it is quite usual to see immediate replacement bridges 2 years after insertion in which the pontic still has good soft-tissue contact.

Speech

Although the replacement of one or more missing teeth by any form of prosthesis may assist in the correction of a speech defect, the bulk of a removable prosthesis is often such that it may induce further difficulties in this respect. With a bridge and some forms of precision retained prostheses the size is usually very similar to that of the teeth it replaces and rarely causes any speech impediment. In cases where this does arise it is usually due to some fault in the morphology of the pontics or retainers fitted. Even with the spring bridge, which has a palatal bar, it is very unusual for any speech defect to occur. It is only when the bar is taken off the molars, particularly when the angulation of the palate is relatively steep, that it will occasionally impinge on the tongue and, generally only for a very short period after fitting, give rise to some slight difficulty with speech.

Function and Stability

Undoubtedly the greater stability imparted to a prosthesis by being positively fixed to the abutment teeth is of considerable benefit to the patient psychologically. It also provides him with better function than can be obtained from most removable prostheses. There are two main reasons for this: (i) Its complete stability during normal mastication; (ii) The fact that the forces of occlusion are being applied to the periodontium and thence the alveolar bone and the bone of the jaws as nature intended, whereas with a removable prosthesis this objective is rarely achieved, except with the aid of precision retainers which usually impart the load intra- instead of extracoronally. With a tissue-borne denture the load has to be transmitted to the underlying bone via the mucoperiosteum, which was never designed for this function and is ill able to withstand the stresses imposed.

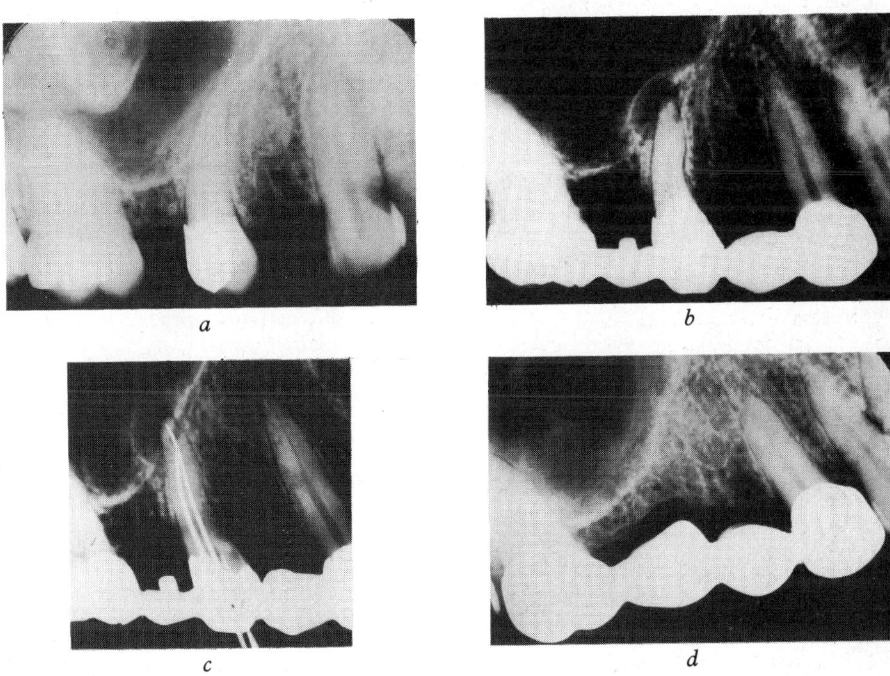

Fig. 3.2. *a, b, A bridge made at* 7 5 3| *shortly after a pulpotomy had been carried out on the second premolar. c, Some months later the tooth died, root-canal therapy proved unavailing, and eventually the tooth had to be extracted and d a new bridge made.*

■ Local Indications

Teeth Suitable for Abutments which require Restoration

Where teeth which would be suitable as bridge abutments require restoration, possibly by crowning, a bridge may be positively indicated, as little more chairside time will be involved in placing this than in just restoring the teeth. However, it is never wise to use teeth as bridge abutments just because they require restoration. They must also be the teeth most suitable for the purpose and there should be no doubts regarding their prognosis (*Fig*. 3.2). It is far better to use sound teeth as abutments rather than doubtful teeth and thus risk a bridge failure with the possibility of further tooth loss.

Lack of Space for a Suitable Replacement

If a tooth is not replaced immediately following its extraction there is often

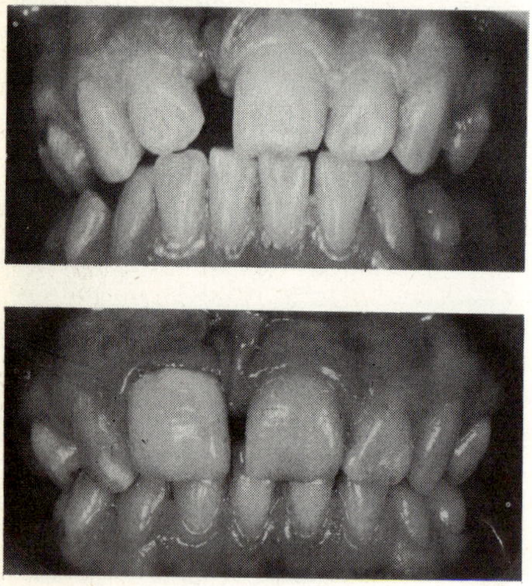

Fig. 3.3. *Crowning of* $\underline{2|}$ *to simulate a central in a patient with a cleft palate, thus eliminating the need for a bridge.*

some loss of space which may render the placing of an aesthetically satisfactory prosthesis extremely difficult. However, with a bridge, particularly if the abutment teeth are to be crowned, some space may be regained by reducing the size or altering the shape of the crowns of the abutments, and thus allowing more room for a satisfactory pontic. Occasionally the crowning of one or both of the teeth adjoining the space may eliminate the need for a bridge (*Fig*. 3.3).

The Morphology of the Abutment Teeth requires Changing

Where the morphology of teeth adjoining the one requiring replacement needs changing then a bridge is usually indicated. Examples of this are rotated or badly worn teeth which require crowning to make them aesthetically acceptable. With a bridge one constructs the retainers and pontic at the same time and this gives maximum flexibility in the laboratory and enables the best aesthetic results to be achieved.

Tilted Teeth

When teeth are tilted the occlusal forces applied to their periodontium tend to be unfavourable. However, by joining two tilted teeth together with a fixed prosthesis it has been shown that the occlusal forces applied will be in a far more favourable direction.

Unfavourable Angulation of the Teeth for a Removable Prosthesis

When teeth are badly tilted then a conventional chrome-cobalt denture may be contraindicated because it does not fill the resultant undercuts, which would give rise to food stagnation. This can sometimes be overcome by a sectional prosthesis but the best result will often be achieved with a bridge. However, severely tilted teeth can create a problem here too, and it may be necessary to use a fixed-movable design or resort to precision retainers to overcome these difficulties. This is dealt with more fully in Chapter 12. A sanitary pontic, providing that it is aesthetically acceptable, is often the best answer in these cases.

CONTRAINDICATIONS TO BRIDGE PROSTHESES

The contraindications to a bridge, like the indications, are nearly all relative and thus every factor has to be weighed carefully before deciding whether or not to go ahead with its construction.

■ General Contraindications

Some of these have already been mentioned at the beginning of the chapter. Probably the most important is an unfavourable attitude of the patient to dentistry in general and his teeth in particular. Another factor is the inability of patients to cooperate, often through no fault of their own.

Inability of Patient to Cooperate

There are two main reasons why a patient may be unable to withstand the prolonged operative procedures necessary to provide a bridge; they are psychological and medical.

The young and the old do not tolerate prolonged dental procedures well, neither do the highly strung and apprehensive patients. Their very apprehension is bound to have an adverse effect on the operator so that he will be more inclined to hurry his work and thus make mistakes. These will either lengthen the operative procedures or result in a lower standard of work and an increased chance of the bridge failing after a few years.

Certain illnesses make it impossible for the patient to cooperate however willing he may be. Examples of this group are the spastics and those who have had a cerebral thrombosis.

These difficulties may sometimes be overcome by premedication or general anaesthesia. However, the latter may be contraindicated because of the medical history and is, in any case, not often justified. Furthermore it is extremely difficult to carry out the operative procedures necessary for the construction of a bridge without the patient's cooperation, even the registering of centric relation becoming very much a matter of guesswork.

Age of Patient

Neither the young nor the very old are usually suitable for fixed bridge prostheses. In the case of the very old it is scarcely justifiable to inflict prolonged operative procedures on them unless the benefits to be gained are considerable. It is often wiser to accept an incomplete dentition providing the patient is symptom free. If necessary a removable prosthesis can be used, which will greatly reduce the chairside time. The elderly, although willing, are often physically

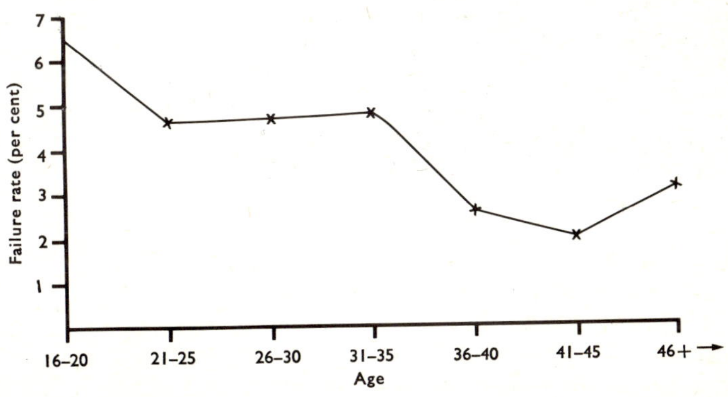

Fig. 3.4. *Relationship between the age of the patient when the bridge is cemented and the failure rate.*

incapable of giving the cooperation which is so necessary for the construction of a successful bridge.

Similar remarks apply to patients where the expectation of life is short and particularly if the operative procedures may adversely affect that expectation.

So far as the younger patient is concerned research at the Institute of Dental Surgery, based on over 1000 bridges, has shown that the younger the patient at the time a bridge is cemented the more likely it is to fail.

In analysing the results it was realized that it would be illogical to call a bridge a success just because it has been in place for a year or two and that it would be equally wrong to call it a failure if it has to be remade after 30 years. Thus the results of the research expressed in *Fig.* 3.4 are in the form of the failure rate per year each group of bridges has been in the mouth. Thus if one bridge in a group of ten cemented at the same time becomes uncemented after 1 year, then the failure rate will be 10 per cent per year. However, if only one bridge out of the same group fails in 10 years then the failure rate will be one-tenth of this, i.e. 1 per cent per year.

From the results, it will be seen that the failure rate of bridges in the under 20 age group was 6·41 per cent per year, an unacceptably high figure, whereas in the next three groups with ages ranging from 21 to 35 years it fell to between 4·73 per cent and 4·81 per cent. After 35 there is a further considerable improvement in the failure rate with a drop to 2·63 per cent in the 36–40 age group and to 2·00 per cent in those aged 41–45. In those over 45 years there is a slight reversal in the trend, the failure rate increasing to 3·08 per cent.

■ Discussion

It would seem likely that three factors affect the result during the various periods:

1. The length of the clinical crown.
2. The caries rate.
3. The periodontal condition.

1. Length of Clinical Crown

The length of the clinical crown is a major factor in determining the degree of retention which can be achieved on any tooth. Generally, the younger the patient the shorter the crown and therefore the greater the convergence angle between the sides of the conventional three-quarter or full crown preparation, i.e. the less closely the preparation can be made to approach the ideal of near parallel sides (*Figs.* 3.5, 3.6).

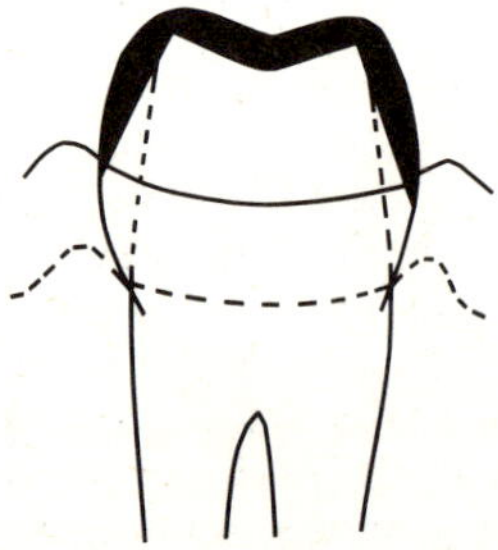

Fig. 3.5. *Three-quarter or full crowns compared on a young patient (shown in solid) and an older patient (shown in dotted outline). It will be seen that the former has more divergent sides, covers a lesser surface area, and is thinner—all factors which decrease retention. Some improvement in retention could have been achieved by employing a chamfer rather than a feather finishing margin.*

The inverse relationship between retention and convergence angle has been demonstrated by Jørgensen (1955). An experiment was conducted using cones of Galalith and brass caps, the bonding medium being oxyphosphate cement. The figures which Jørgensen obtained are given below:

Convergence (degrees)	*Retention (g per sq mm)*
5	81·3
10	41·4
15	35·3
20	25·7
25	17·3

crown because of the greatly reduced length of finishing margin which will be in apposition to the gingival tissues, particularly on the critical buccal aspect.

Advanced Periodontal Disease
When the general periodontal condition of the mouth is poor and drifting has started to occur, the time and trouble required for the construction of a bridge is generally not justified unless it is part of the overall periodontal therapy. The prognosis of the remaining teeth is obviously poor and it only needs one further tooth to be lost for the work undertaken to become pointless. However, in cases where the periodontal condition is somewhat more favourable a fixed bridge prosthesis with its beneficial splinting effect may well prolong the life of the teeth.

■ Local Factors Contraindicating a Bridge

Prognosis of the Abutment Teeth

One of the most important factors to be considered before deciding to construct a bridge is the prognosis of the possible abutment teeth. If there is any doubt on this score then it is far better to delay until the outcome of any treatment of these teeth is reasonably certain (*see Fig.* 3.2, p. 33).

The factors which contraindicate the use of a tooth as an abutment may be divided into those affecting the crown and those concerning the root.

Factors affecting the Crown

1. The strength of the crown, including the tooth tissue remaining after any necessary treatment such as the removal of caries and the preparation of the tooth for a retainer. Similarly, where the dentine is malformed and weak as in dentinogenesis imperfecta (*Fig.* 3.7), teeth cannot be used as bridge abutments.

2. The extent and position of any caries and whether this can be satisfactorily eliminated. Deep subgingival caries is a fairly positive contraindication to the use of a tooth as a bridge abutment because of the risk of recurrent caries at the margins of the retainers. In these instances it is, where possible, better to delay treatment for a few years until it can be seen that the caries rate is well under control.

3. Whether adequate retention can be obtained. This depends on the length, size, shape and surface area of the crown (*Fig.* 3.8). This is discussed in more detail in Chapter 6.

Factors concerning the Root

Three main factors are of concern when considering the root:

1. The apical condition. If any apical infection is present this must be treated and ideally that treatment must be seen to be effective before using the tooth as a bridge abutment. Similarly, if there is any doubt regarding the vitality of the tooth this must be resolved, usually with the aid of an electric pulp tester.

2. The effective root surface area. The root surface area of the tooth must be sufficient to bear any load that may be placed on it. This factor is gone into more thoroughly in Chapter 6.

3. The periodontal condition of the teeth. Obviously the periodontal condition bears a direct relationship to the effective root surface area. The worse the periodontal condition the lower the effective root surface area and bony support available for the bridge. However, of equal importance are the patient's oral hygiene and the stability of their existing periodontal condition. If further bone loss is likely to occur then this will adversely affect the prognosis of any bridge placed.

Length of Span

The longer the span the greater the load which will be placed on the abutment teeth and obviously there comes a stage where a removable prosthesis is indicated so as to obtain some degree of tissue support and thus avoid overloading of the abutments. However, providing the periodontal condition and oral hygiene are satisfactory and likely to remain so, the fixed prosthesis is well designed and its occlusion is correct it is surprising how great the additional load which well chosen abutment teeth can carry. Certainly Antes' law which states that the area of the periodontal membrane of the abutment teeth must be at least as great as that of the teeth being replaced, can often be safely exceeded, although this does depend to some extent on the individual design of each bridge. Thus the use of single unit abutments for cantilever bridges in the posterior region can frequently give rise to signs of overloading.

It must also be remembered that the longer the span of a bridge the greater will be the stress imposed on the abutment teeth and the larger the number of abutments which will have to be provided to prevent periodontal overloading. In the anterior region the curvature of

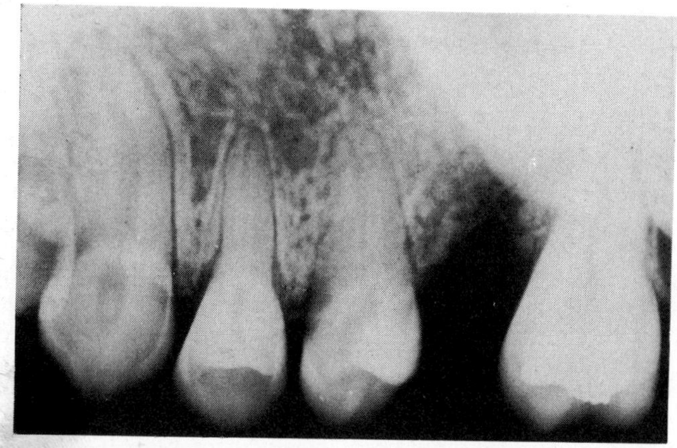

Fig. 3.7. *Dentinogenesis imperfecta resulting in weak teeth unsuitable as bridge abutments.*

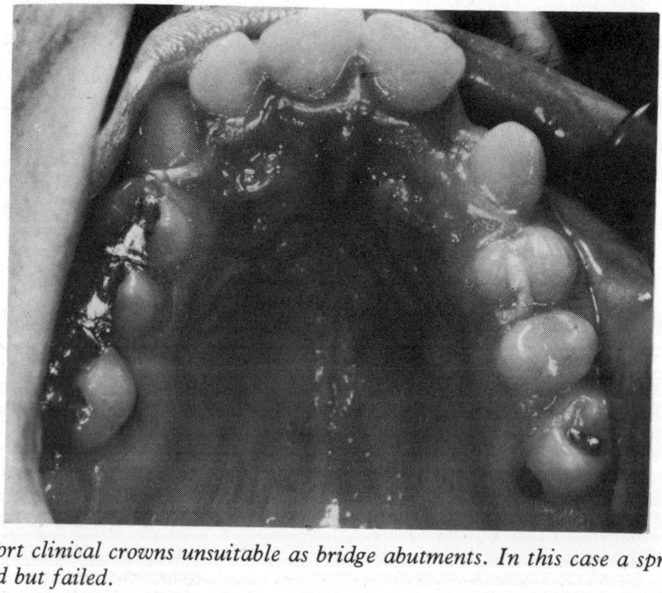

Fig. 3.8. *Short clinical crowns unsuitable as bridge abutments. In this case a spring bridge was attempted but failed.*

the arch imposes additional stresses and this must also be taken into consideration as the forces of mastication may well be applied outside the long axis of the teeth (*see Fig*. 6.5, p. 85).

Not only is a greater stress imposed on the abutments in a long-span bridge but also on the cement bond joining them to the retainer, and thus cementation failure is more liable to occur. Similarly, the longer the span the greater the stress which will be imposed on the solder joints, the occlusal gold, and the bridge structure in general. Thus these must be strengthened if a failure is to be avoided (*Fig*. 3.9).

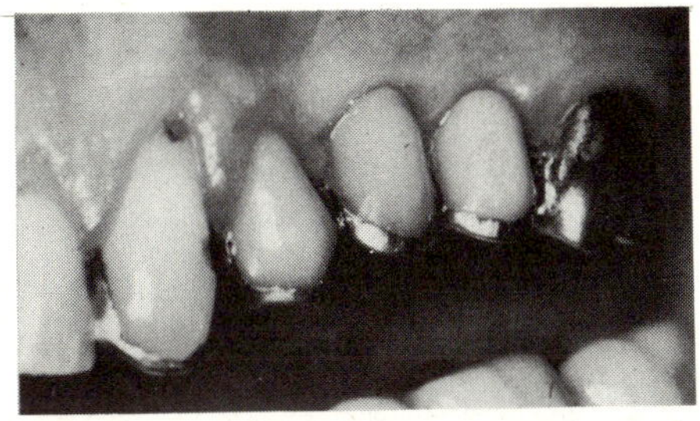

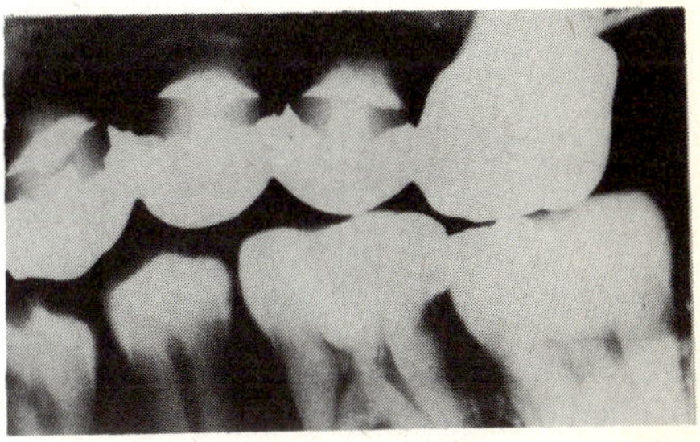

Fig. 3.9. *Flexion of a long-span bridge due to inadequate strength of the gold and the solder joints.*

Possibility of Further Loss in the Same Arch

Before considering a bridge the prognosis of all the teeth in the same arch should be ascertained and if there are any doubts these must be resolved before proceeding. If another tooth in the same arch is lost soon after the bridge is placed it often means that a removable prosthesis will be required, which will probably render the time expended on the fitting of a bridge worthless.

Ridge Form and Tissue Loss

Where tissue loss in the region of the missing tooth is so extensive that it requires replacement, normally by acrylic, a fixed prosthesis is generally contraindicated as it would become unhygienic because of the additional amount of soft tissue covered. Alternatively, a removable precision-retained prosthesis may sometimes be employed which will provide similar stability to a bridge but will still permit soft-tissue replacement.

Unfavourable Tilting or Rotation of the Teeth

Sometimes the teeth which one requires to use as abutments are so unfavourably angulated that their satisfactory preparation for a fixed bridge proves very difficult and devitalization may even have to be resorted to. However, this is a relative rather than an absolute contra-indication to a fixed prosthesis. The difficulties can nearly always be overcome with the aid of such devices as the dovetail and slot, precision retainers, and telescopic full crowns mentioned later in this book.

Maintenance and Repair

One of the biggest disadvantages of the bridge is that it is relatively complicated and if it fails replacement can be both expensive and time-consuming, whereas the repair of a removable prosthesis is relatively simple.

From the foregoing it can be seen that there are few absolute indications or contraindications to a bridge. Nearly all are relative and may even vary, depending on their degree of severity, as do the caries rate and the periodontal condition.

Every factor must be considered and the correct weight given to each before it is decided whether or not it is in the patient's best interests to have a bridge. All this adds up to good clinical judgement, which will obviously be related to the dental surgeon's experience.

However, it is hoped that this book, which is based on the experience of many operators over the past 25 years, will help in this respect.

Bibliography

Alexander A. G. (1968) Periodontal aspects of conservative dentistry. *Br. Dent. J.* **125**, 111.

Ericsson S. G. and Marken K. E. (1968) Effect of fixed partial dentures on surrounding tissues. *J. Prosthet. Dent.* **20**, 517.

Jørgensen K. D. (1955) The relationship between retention and convergence angles in cemented veneer crowns. *Acta Odontol. Scand.* **13**, 35.

Roberts D. H. (1967) Developmental defects of the teeth and their treatment by crowning. *Dent. Practnr Dent. Rec.* **17**, 431.

Roberts D. H. (1970) The relationship between age and the failure rate of bridge prostheses. *Br. Dent. J.* **128**, 175.

Roberts D. H. and Sowray J. S. (1979) *Local Analgesia in Dentistry,* 2nd ed., Bristol, Wright.

Silness J. (1970) Periodontal conditions in patients treated with bridges. *J. Periodont. Res.* **5**, 60, 219, 225.

4

MATERIALS

Materials used for Bridge Construction
Impression Materials. Die Materials. Dental Cements

In this chapter the materials used for the construction of a bridge will be considered. However, they will only be discussed from a relatively limited practical aspect, so as to give the reader some idea of the advantages and disadvantages of the various materials currently available and the indications for their use. For anyone who wishes to have a deeper understanding of the subject the specialist textbooks such as those listed at the end of the chapter are suggested.

The first part of this section will be devoted to the principal materials which may be used for constructing a bridge. In the second half, impression and die materials and the cementing media will be discussed.

MATERIALS USED FOR BRIDGE CONSTRUCTION

The principal properties required of a bridge are:

1. Accuracy of fit, to prevent gingival irritation and recurrent caries.
2. Strength, to resist the forces of mastication.
3. Rigidity, to avoid flexure and thus cementation failure.
4. Good aesthetics.
5. Colour stability.
6. A thermal coefficient which should approximate to that of tooth tissue.
7. Negligible water absorption.
8. That it should not attract plaque formation or calculus or become foul during use.
9. That it be non-irritant to the oral tissues.

There are four principal materials used in bridge construction: acrylic, porcelain, gold, and the base metals. Generally speaking no one of these can provide all the properties required of a bridge and thus they are used in combination. For instance, acrylic may be aesthetically pleasing but it lacks rigidity and this is normally provided by adding a gold substructure.

■ Acrylic

This material may produce a very satisfactory aesthetic result initially under normal lighting conditions although it can appear black under ultraviolet or fluorescent light. However, it has many disadvantages, amongst which are the following:

Lack of Rigidity

Acrylic is liable to flex when a load is applied to it and this will cause cementation failure of the retainers if the material is used on its own for this purpose.

Thermal Coefficients

There is a great disparity between the expansion and contraction of acrylic and tooth tissue, the former being seven times greater (*Fig.* 4.1). This is liable to lead to a breakdown of the cement bond between the two.

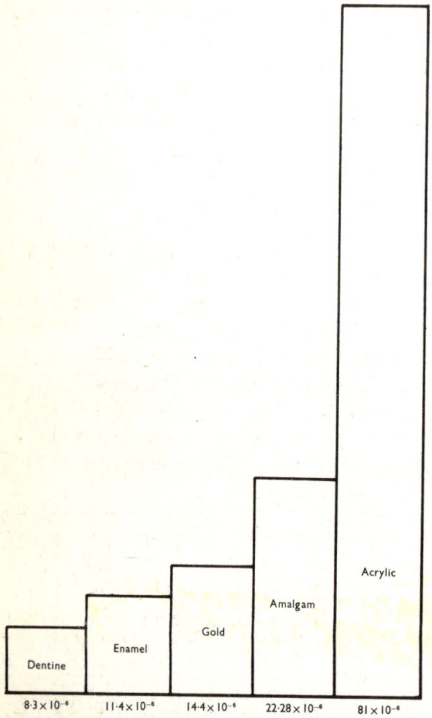

Fig. 4.1. *The thermal coefficients of expansion of dentine, enamel, gold, amalgam and acrylic.*
(Figures taken from Peyton F. A. 1968, *Restorative Dental Materials,* 3rd ed., p. 504. St Louis, Mosby.)

Wear

Acrylic is a fairly soft material and wears rapidly unless protected (*Fig.* 4.2). Thus, if a patient uses a toothpaste which is relatively abrasive then all the surface characterization may be lost in six months and the pontic will be a shapeless mass within five years.

Similarly, if acrylic is used alone on a biting surface it is likely to be worn through in a relatively short space of time (*Fig.* 4.3) and this will permit over-eruption of the opposing teeth until eventually they occlude with the underlying preparations, making a remake difficult.

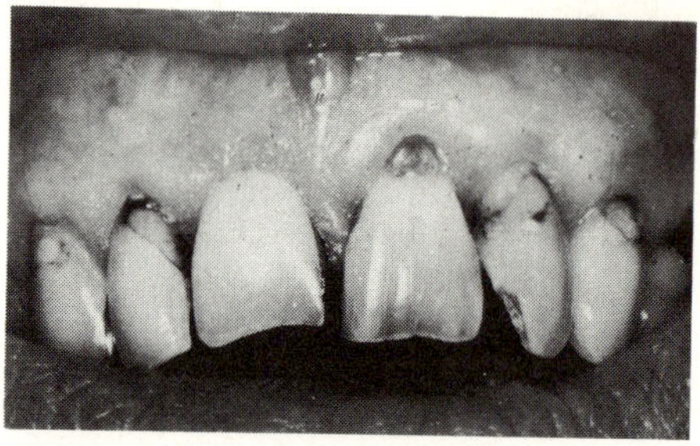

Fig. 4.2. *An acrylic pontic at* 1| *with complete loss of characterization.*

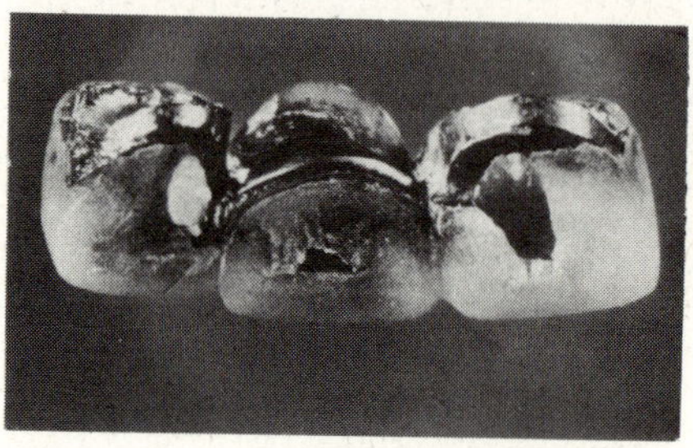

Fig. 4.3. *Wear of acrylic on the palatal aspects of an upper bridge which will allow over-eruption of the opposing teeth.*

Discoloration

Despite the continuous advances which are being made in the manufacture of the acrylic resins they still discolour in the mouth (*Fig.* 4.4). Thus an acrylic facing which is aesthetically excellent when first placed may be only fair after 2–3 years and will often be unacceptable, at least in the anterior region, after 5–7 years.

The rate at which acrylic discolours and wears varies greatly with the way in which it is manufactured and cured. Thus the cold or self-curing acrylic resins give a poor result and even a facing prepared in the laboratory by adding acrylic powders to monomer in the curing flask or by using a dough method will be markedly inferior to the teeth made by the manufacturers. Therefore, wherever possible when using acrylic it is best to use stock, i.e. manufactured, teeth or facings, grind these to a suitable shape, and then make the gold work to fit them.

Water Absorption
Acrylic is far more water absorbent than any of the other materials used in bridge work and because of this is dimensionally unstable and tends to become foul.

Gingival Irritation
A well finished and contoured acrylic pontic may initially cause little more soft tissue reaction than gold or porcelain. However, in the long term its use will result in more gingival irritation than any other material used in fixed bridge prostheses. The extent depends on the type of acrylic, the time it has been in the mouth, the form and size of the gingival contact, and the patient's oral hygiene. It is, of course, the plaque which causes the gingival irritation and not the acrylic. Plaque rarely adheres to porcelain but it does adhere to gold and especially acrylic due to the organic matrix of plaque interacting with the acrylic. Subsequently this plaque may become mineralized, as can be seen in *Fig*. 4.5.

For all the foregoing reasons acrylic used on its own can at best only be regarded as a material suitable for the construction of temporary or possibly semi-permanent bridges such as those fitted as an immediate replacement and designed to last, at most, 6–9 months. However, if the prosthesis is removable by the patient it is the ideal method of soft tissue replacement.

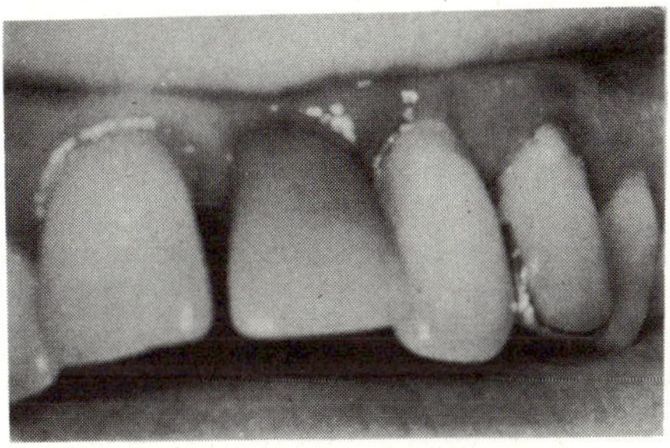

Fig. 4.4. *Discoloured acrylic facing of a spring bridge replacing* |1.

■ **Porcelain**
The construction of a bridge made entirely of porcelain has many advantages. It is well tolerated by the

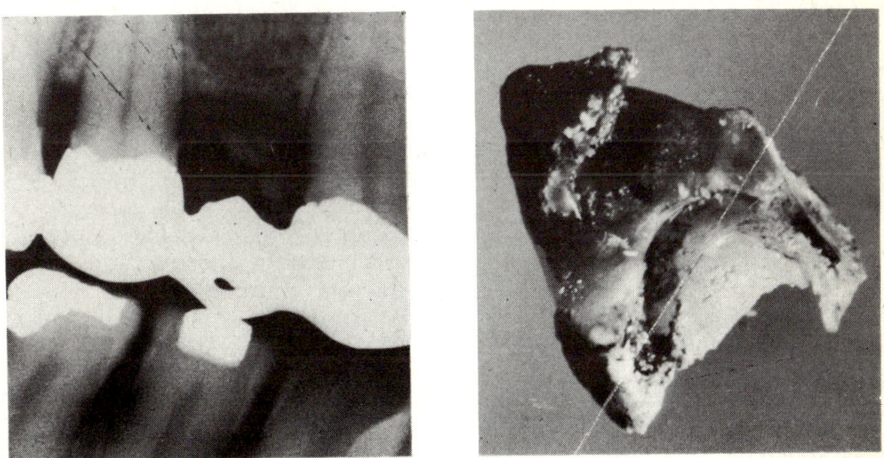

a *b*

Fig. 4.5. *a, Radiograph showing calculus formation beneath an acrylic pontic. b, Fit surface of facing.*

tissues, is not water absorbent and is aesthetically very satisfactory. It is also good in ultraviolet light and has complete colour stability, which generally gives it a big advantage over acrylic. However, this can be a disadvantage in that sometimes a porcelain crown or bridge may appear too light after it has been in the mouth 10–20 years, because of the darkening of the neighbouring teeth.

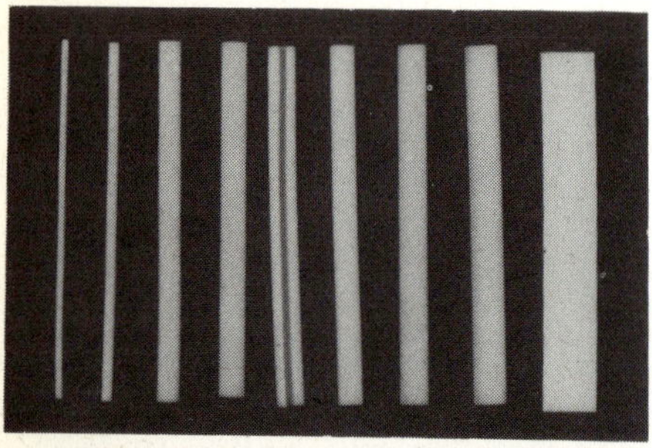

Fig. 4.6. *Rods, tubes and strips of pure alumina used for reinforcing all porcelain crowns and bridges.*

The only disadvanatges of the material are that the fit of a porcelain crown is inferior to one made of gold and that it is far more likely to fracture.

The conventional porcelains are normally adequate for the construction of a simple two-unit cantilever bridge such as that replacing a lateral with a full crown on the canine (*see Fig*. 9.1, p. 147) providing the occlusion is favourable. However, if the bite is fairly heavy the aluminous porcelains should be used and if very heavy, resort may be made to a metal-ceramic bridge.

The stress imposed on the porcelain when the material is used for a fixed-fixed bridge of three or more units is far greater and ordinary porcelain is generally inadequate. To try to overcome this, reinforcement of the material with platinum wire or mesh has in the past been attempted, but has not proved entirely successful. It is only with the advent of the aluminous porcelains that this problem has come nearer to a satisfactory solution.

Aluminous porcelains may be employed in several ways. The core mass and palatal aspects of the crowns may be built up in porcelain with a high alumina content, as aesthetics is of no importance in this region. Likewise discs or rods of pure alumina (*Fig*. 4.6), which is eight to nine times stronger than ordinary dental porcelains, may be used to reinforce the abutments, pontics, and in particular the joints between them. A more recent advance is the use of bonded alumina crowns as abutments in which aluminous porcelain is bonded to the oxidized tin plated surface of a platinum foil. In this way the likelihood of crack propagation in the porcelain is reduced, possibly by between 20 to 30 per cent and at the same time the thickness of the metal is reduced to only 0·05 mm (McLean and Sced, 1976; McLean et al., 1976). This technique is of most value for the construction of simple 2-unit anterior all-porcelain bridges.

■ Gold

Gold in the form of its various alloys has most of the properties required for a fixed bridge prosthesis. Retainers can be constructed from it which fit the abutment teeth very accurately and they can be made sufficiently rigid to avoid cementation failure.

It does not absorb moisture and pure gold itself will not corrode. However, under certain conditions gold-copper and some other alloys do corrode, although usually not significantly. The response varies appreciably from patient to patient, but at most usually only manifests itself as tarnish. Gold is relatively compatible with the oral tissues, although it may give rise to a little more gingival irritation than porcelain because of a greater tendency for plaque to form on its surface. The most serious disadvantage of gold is that it is impossible to provide adequate aesthetics. This may be of little consequence when replacing a lower molar but is of paramount importance in the upper anterior region. The only way in which this may be overcome is by providing a facing made either of acrylic or porcelain.

The Heat Treatment of Golds

Before going on to discuss the use of gold in combination with acrylic and porcelain it is as well to consider the heat treatment of the metal. This is a complex matter and it is not proposed in this book to go into it in any detail. However, there are two main reasons for carrying this out: either to anneal the metal or to harden it. The former may be required to make it more easily workable and is usually performed prior to manipulating it.

Most dental golds may be annealed by heating to a dull red and then plunging them in cold water. A more precise technique is to heat soak the gold in an oven at 650–700°C for 5 min, which results in homogenization of its alloying constituents, and then quenching it in water.

It is obviously desirable that the gold should be at its strongest when the bridge is cemented and this will generally not be the case if no heat treatment is carried out or if it is performed incorrectly. Indeed, after casting and quenching the strength of the gold may well be 30–40 per cent below its optimum (*Fig.* 4.7). If used in this state the restoration will be only equivalent in strength to a heat-treated casting of two-thirds its thickness and such a casting, when fitted on a conservative tooth preparation could fail.

The omission of heat treatment to strengthen a gold may to some extent be compensated by the work hardening of the material which takes place during polishing, and this process may be continued by the normal stresses of mastication. However, this probably just affects the surface of the casting. The only certain way of obtaining the optimal desirable properties of the material is by heat treatment. The technique required for this will vary considerably, depending on the alloys being employed, and thus each manufacturer's instructions need to be carefully followed if consistent results are to be achieved. It must also be remembered that some alloys, mostly the softer ones with a low copper content and no platinum, are little affected by heat treatment.

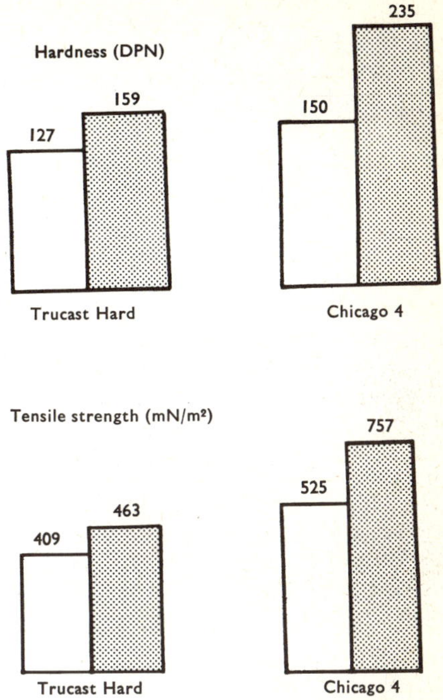

Fig. 4.7. *The hardness and tensile strength of golds before (on the left) and after heat treatment.*

Before hardening any gold it must first be annealed to homogenize the structure. A hardening technique applicable to most of the golds used in bridge work is to keep them at 400°C in a thermostatically controlled oven for approximately 10 min, then allow them to cool slowly to 200°C, and finally quench them. It is important that the correct time of heat treatment is not exceeded otherwise the material will gradually lose its optimum hardness and in time become softer.

A more arbitrary method of heat treatment which may be used when a thermostatically controlled oven is not available is to bring the gold up to a dull red and then allow it to cool very slowly over a period of approximately 20 minutes. This can be achieved by covering it with a refractory crucible, thus reducing the rate of heat loss.

Alternative Alloys to Type III Gold
Largely because of the increase in the cost of noble metals Nitkin and Asgar (1976) investigated the fit of castings made of nickel-chrome, silver-palladium, low (50 per cent) gold, and type III gold. It is interesting to note that the fit of castings made with a low (50 per cent) gold were fully comparable in fit and marginal completeness with those made of type III gold.

The gold-silver-palladium alloys yielded castings almost comparable in accuracy and completeness of fit to the type III gold. Silver-palladium alloys yielded castings that might be acceptable to some clinicians but were not comparable to those obtained with class III gold in terms of fit and completeness.

The problems associated with accuracy of fit are largely due to the difficulty in obtaining adequate expansion of the phosphate-bonded investments for alloys which melt at high temperatures. Even by using undiluted silica sol with the investment and allowing it to set in a 37°C water bath, expansion still tends to be inadequate particularly for the base metal alloys. Thus until an investment can be developed capable of higher expansion than is at present the case it would seem that base metal alloys are unsuitable for most dental restorations.

■ The Base Metal Alloys
Despite many advances in the development of non-precious metals such as the nickel-chrome and cobalt-chromium alloys, to try to achieve one with properties suitable for use in fixed bridge prostheses, none is yet as good as gold. Their advantages are generally also their disadvantages. Thus the greater strength of these materials is more than offset by the difficulties in handling them both at the chairside and in the laboratory. Furthermore because of their hardness their rate of wear is less than that of tooth tissue, which is undesirable.

The fits obtainable are not usually acceptable, except possibly in the case of full crowns with shoulder preparations where the model can be built up by foil or varnish beforehand to compensate for the shrinkage of the casting on cooling which will normally exceed the expansion of the investment. The maximum expansion obtainable from the investment is usually of the order of 1·7 per cent, whereas the contraction of nickel-chromium on cooling is 2·5 per cent.

Their relatively low cost is offset by the handling difficulties introduced in the laboratory because of their higher melting points and the fact that they work harden very rapidly which severely limits the amount of post-casting adjustments that can be made. The high surface hardness means that they are difficult to polish but that once a high finish has been obtained it is retained far better. It is important to remember that the heat treatment of these metals is entirely different from that used for the gold alloys.

■ Gold and Porcelain
The combination of porcelain and gold is capable, in the majority of cases, of producing bridges which fulfil more of our requirements than any other. One has the strength and accuracy of fit of gold combined with the excellent aesthetics which can be achieved with porcelain. Porcelain should always be used where the pontic touches the tissues, as it is better tolerated than any other material.

There are two main ways in which porcelain may be combined with gold:

a. By cementing the porcelain facing to the gold work.

b. By using a gold alloy and porcelain of similar thermal coefficients of expansion so that the porcelain can be bonded directly on to the metal.

The disadvantage of the former method is that the porcelain facing contributes little if anything to the strength of the pontic as a whole. Because of this the gold has to be made relatively thick and rigid. Should it flex then the cement bond between it and the facing will be broken and thus will then come out (*Fig.* 5.1, p. 68).

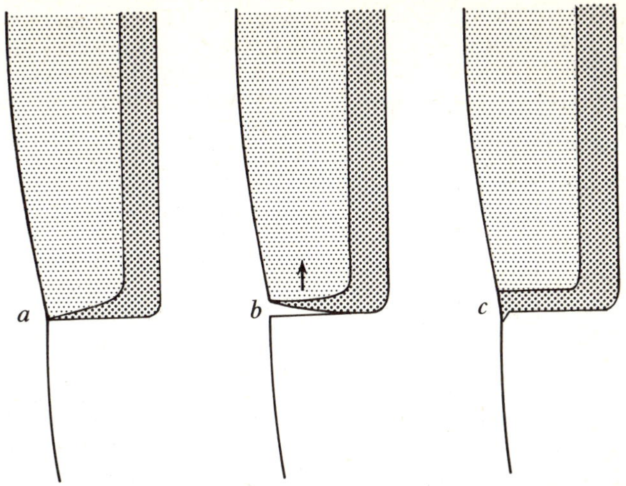

Fig. 4.8. *Although the casting may fit accurately (a) the sintering shrinkage of the porcelain when it is added and adheres to it may result in distortion of the margin (b) and a poor fit. To avoid this either a porcelain finishing margin should be employed (see Fig. 6.57d, p. 113) or a thickness of gold of at least 0.5 mm provided (c) which will be sufficiently strong to resist distortion by the porcelain.*

A further disadvantage is that it is not always easy to accommodate a manufactured porcelain facing in the space required, whereas a bonded pontic is far more adaptable.

This latter method has proved a near ideal combination for constructing bridges. It gives the aesthetic advantages of porcelain, although this is not quite so good as porcelain when used alone, and at the same time it obviates the brittleness of the material. As the porcelain is bonded to the metal it imparts rigidity to it, the combination of the two being mutually beneficial and stronger than gold on its own. Thus whereas the gold alloy 'Degudent'* on its own has a modulus of rigidity of 60 000 mN/mm^2 when porcelain is bonded to it this figure increases to 500 000 mN/mm^2.

The fit of a bonded crown in which the porcelain is allowed to extend to the margin of the preparation is usually adequate but not as good as gold. Thus if a finishing margin can be provided in gold this is best. However, it is essential that the gold is of sufficient thickness to resist distortion by the porcelain which has adhered to it during firing and will subsequently shrink (*Fig.* 4.8).

A greater reduction of tooth tissue is required on the labial or buccal aspect than with a porcelain jacket crown if reasonable aesthetics is to be achieved, as both the gold and the porcelain have to be accommodated. However, on the palatal aspect a saving of tooth tissue is achieved as usually only sufficient thickness for the gold has to be removed.

■ Gold and Acrylic

The combination of gold and acrylic retains most of the desirable properties of the former material and also provides good initial aesthetics. However, one still has the disadvantage that the acrylic will discolour and wear, although this latter may be greatly reduced by providing a gold occlusal or palatal surface which will prevent undue wear and over-eruption of the opposing teeth.

*Degussa Dental Postfach 2644, D-6000 Frankfurt 1, West Germany.

To keep gingival irritation to a minimum the whole of the fit surface of the pontic should be of gold.

One additional disadvantage of the combination of gold and acrylic is that the metal sub-structure will tend to shadow through the plastic and give it a greyish hue.

■ The Base Metal Alloys and Porcelain

The gold alloys used for bonded porcelains are very expensive and if these could be replaced by a non-precious metal the savings would be appreciable. Moreover, the fits obtained would probably be adequate for the full crowns employed in at least some of these cases, particularly if a full shoulder is employed so that the die can be relieved without fear of affecting the fit. However, until recently no porcelain and non-precious metal have been prepared so that their thermal coefficients exactly match, neither has any true bond been demonstrated between them. Thus the results have not been entirely satisfactory. It is only in the last few years that the bond of base metal alloy-porcelain systems has been given serious attention. (McLean and Sced, 1973; Trifunovic et al., 1976) and such variables as the alloy systems, metal pretreatment procedures, firing cycle and porcelain composition have been investigated.

With some of the base metal alloys used the high bond strengths obtained would seem to arise purely from the compression of the substrate metal by the porcelain and failure will occur (*Fig.* 4.9 *right*) if there is some fairly slight flexion of the metal which will release the compressional effect of the porcelain.

With the gold alloy/porcelain bond a surface oxide film is formed which reacts with the porcelain and results in interdiffusion between the oxide and the porcelain; furthermore wetting of the gold alloy by the porcelain is excellent and thus a very satisfactory bond is obtained. Unfortunately, however, whereas the oxides formed with gold alloys have little adverse effect on the expansion of porcelain coming in contact with them, with the base alloys quite a small amount of Cr_2O_3 in solution in the porcelain can have a marked effect on the coefficient of expansion of the porcelain and induce stresses which may result in failure. Thus it would seem that it is best to avoid using alloys with substantial amounts of chromium because of the marked lowering of the expansion coefficient of the porcelain which results.

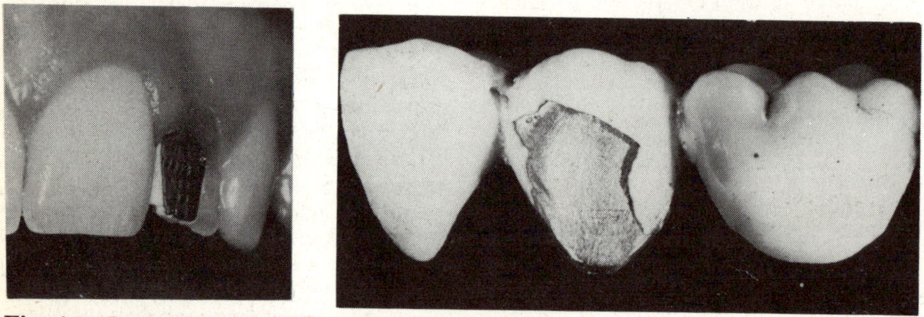

Fig. 4.9. *Bridges in which the porcelain has been fired directly on to a non-precious metal alloy and has subsequently failed. Note that the porcelain has come away from the metal completely cleanly with no sign of a bond between the two.*

Whereas some degree of oxidation is desirable since it will contribute to the bonding process it is important that the coefficient of expansion of the oxide must be similiar to the alloy and the opaque porcelain. Furthermore it must adhere to the alloy and react with the porcelain but not adversely affect it in any way.

With gold alloys indium and tin oxides

are formed which fulfil most of the foregoing requirements. With most of the base metal alloys in use the formation of too much Cr_2O_3 has an adverse effect on the bond. However this problem is coming nearer to solution with the development of complex base metal alloys containing elements which form stable oxides which improve the bond between the metal and the porcelain without adversely affecting the expansion or colour of the latter.

In conclusion it can be stated that whereas the base metal alloys are inferior to gold alloys for bonding to porcelain continuing improvements are being introduced. Probably the biggest difficulty now is the relatively poor fits obtained because of the problem of finding an investment which will expand sufficiently to compensate for their marked shrinkage on cooling.

From all the foregoing it will be seen that in the majority of cases the best materials to use in fixed bridge prostheses are porcelain and gold combined and preferably bonded although cost or the lack of suitable laboratory facilities may sometimes indicate the use of porcelain facings cemented to gold.

IMPRESSION MATERIALS

In this chapter only indirect impression materials will be discussed as it is seldom that a direct impression is of value when constructing a bridge. However, the use of waxes and acrylic resins will be briefly mentioned as they have certain specific applications in bridge work and the former are invariably employed in the construction of the casting in the laboratory.

There are three main reasons why an impression is taken and it will help if we enumerate these before going on to discuss the various materials we may use:

1. Reproduction of the prepared teeth. This makes the highest demands on the impression material as extreme accuracy in the fit of any restoration is always required, particularly at the margins.

2. Reproduction of the occlusal surfaces of all the teeth. In bridge work it is usually advisable to take an impression of the occlusal surfaces of all the teeth in the arch being treated and also those of the opposing arch so as to be able to assess the articulation as accurately as possible.

3. Reproduction of the general morphology of the teeth. This applies particularly to those adjoining the bridge and the corresponding teeth on the opposite side of the mouth so as to produce a bridge which will blend in with the rest of the patient's dentition.

The main properties which we require from an impression material are:

1. *Accuracy*. It must be capable of reproducing detail and contour of the prepared surfaces of the teeth with extreme accuracy, i.e. to within a tolerance of ±20 μm.

2. *Elasticity, strength and freedom from distortion*. The impression material must be sufficiently elastic to reproduce any undercut areas accurately and for this reason must not tear or suffer permanent distortion on removal from the mouth, i.e. good elastic properties are required.

3. *Dimensional stability*. After the impression is removed from the mouth it should be stable and exhibit no signs of distortion prior to casting. To achieve this it is essential that the correct storage technique for each different impression material is employed (Bell et al., 1975).

4. *Flow*. The material must have a low viscosity so as to flow readily when inserted into the mouth and thus penetrate the finest crevices and reproduce the smallest details.

5. *Favourable setting characteristics*. A good working time is an essential property of an impression material used for crowns and bridges. Ideally there should be an adequate mixing time and a relatively long working time followed by a rapid (snap) set which should be achieved within 5 minutes of insertion of the material in the mouth. This is difficult to obtain with the elastomers. The shrinkage on setting should be minimal.

6. *Shelf life.* It should be capable of storage in the unset condition in the dental surgery for at least 1 year without sign of deterioration.

7. *Compatibility with die materials.* It must be compatible with the materials and techniques used for producing a working model in the laboratory.

8. *Acceptable to patient.* The use of the material must be acceptable to the patient and not cause him any undue discomfort or irritate the tissues.

9. *Economic.* The material should be as simple and cheap to use as is compatible with the other properties required. However, the cost, for instance, of a final bridge impression is relatively unimportant when related to the expense and inconvenience caused by an inaccurate impression.

There are many impression materials which may be used for constructing crown and bridge prostheses and more are constantly coming on to the market. The commoner ones which may be employed are wax, acrylic resins, impression compound, reversible hydrocolloids, irreversible hydrocolloids, polysulphides, silicones, polysiloxane and polyether rubber.

With all of these it is essential that they are handled correctly if the best results are to be achieved. This is discussed in more detail in Chapter 16.

■ Wax

The use of this material is normally confined to taking direct impressions of simple intracoronal restorations, such as may be used for the minor retainer of a bridge. It has the disadvantage that the casting has to be tried in and then a further impression taken to locate this to the neighbouring and occluding teeth. However, it is invariably used in the laboratory, as all dental castings are still produced by the lost wax technique.

The one occasion when wax is of particular value is where an inlay or crown has to be fitted below a prosthesis. In this case the casting must be made to fit not only the tooth but the denture as well. The simplest way of doing this is to employ what is known as the direct-indirect technique. An indirect impression is taken and the crown is waxed up in the laboratory, forming the external surface as nearly correctly as possible. Sometimes a base of acrylic is used to reinforce this. The wax crown is then tried in the mouth and final adjustments are made to its external surface by trying the denture in and out, before it is invested and cast.

The principal difficulty with wax as an impression material is that there is considerable thermal expansion and contraction, which in clinical practice is likely to be of the order of $\pm 0{\cdot}5$ per cent. This has to be compensated for in the casting technique. The time required to manipulate the wax is relatively limited as it is thermoplastic and it has to be so compounded that it sets at mouth temperature but must flow only a few degrees above this. It has virtually no elasticity and thus if subjected to even minor stresses wax is liable to distort.

Wax has a 'memory' and after removal from the mouth tends to warp because of the release of internal stresses (thermal relaxation). The higher the temperature of the wax when the pattern is being made the lower the stresses which will be induced in it. The higher the room temperatures to which the wax is subjected after removal from the mouth the greater the chance of distortion.

For all the above reasons it is essential that a wax pattern be cast as soon as possible after its removal from the tooth or die.

■ Acrylic Resin

Acrylic resins such as Duralay* are being used increasingly for such purposes as occlusal records, the fabrication of patterns for castings and transfer copings.

The advantages of these materials are their strength and stability when cured relative to wax, their ease of handling and the fact that they are inexpensive,

* Duralay and Duralay Lubricant. Reliance Dental Mfg Co., Worth, Illinois, USA.

particularly, for instance, in relation to cast transfer copings.

Inter-occlusal Relationships
Acrylic resin is of particular value for recording jaw relationships (Crispin, 1978). When the teeth have been prepared for full crowns copings are placed on them which are kept clear of occlusion with the opposing teeth. Small pyramids of acrylic are then built up on these to establish contact with an opposing cusp tip or fossa. The contact area should be low to minimize any inaccuracies during mounting. The covering of all the prepared teeth by a continuous layer of acrylic which contacts the opposing teeth is very likely to result in errors during the seating and mounting of the casts.

If copings are not made then acrylic resin may be built up directly on top of the prepared teeth, however, a lubricant and separating medium* must be employed to prevent the acrylic sticking to the teeth or causing any pulpal irritation.

Direct Patterns
Acrylic resin may be used for direct patterns and it is of particular value when greater strength may be required than can be obtained with wax. It is important to always use a slow build-up of the acrylic to minimize the effect of its shrinking on polymerization. Thus the pattern is built up by dipping a brush first in the liquid and then in the powder and applying it to the margins of the die and gradually extending this until a complete pattern is obtained. It is advisable to remove the pattern occasionally during its build up to check the fit and simplify its final removal from the die.

Acrylic resin is particularly useful for the fabrication of direct patterns for post/core units in the mouth. Its strength is an advantage here as it can be removed from the tooth and added to or reduced as many times as necessary until both its morphology and fit are exactly what is required.

A similar use is in the fabrication of a pattern which not only has to fit the tooth but also the chrome denture which surrounds it. Here the pattern can be made and tried on the tooth and subsequently its external surface may be modified to allow the denture to fit around it. The only disadvantage of using acrylic resin as a direct pattern is that the marginal fit is probably not so good as with wax and that the surface of the casting is rougher. The accuracy of fit may be improved by laying down a thin layer of wax first and then building up the acrylic on this.

Location
Acrylic resin is of particular value for locating bridge retainers and may be employed either by moulding it over the occlusal surfaces, removing the acrylic 'impression' and then relocating them, or, if their line of withdrawal permits it, joining the bridge retainers (or acrylic copings) together in the mouth.

Acrylic may also be of value for locating pins either in the mouth or directly as in the Ney technique.

Strengthening Wax Patterns or Models
Acrylic resins may be used for increasing the strength of any wax pattern. Examples of this include its incorporation in the underlying pattern when a wax-additive technique is being employed and its use around a porcelain facing prior to the wax up of the rest of the pontic. Where a model is likely to be subjected to particular stress in one area or if it will be especially weak at one point then this portion of the model can be built up in acrylic.

Copings
Acrylic is particularly useful for making up acrylic copings. It is quicker and simpler to use than a casting and is less likely to damage the model. Acrylic

* Duralay and Duralay Lubricant. Reliance Dental Mfg Co., Worth, Illinois, USA.

copings can be used to check the accuracy of the dies and their marginal extension and fit. Complete seating can also be checked by cutting a hole in the top of the copings so as to be able to see the tooth tissue. Occlusal clearance may also be noted and where necessary modified by reducing the tooth by grinding it with the coping on it. When the coping is transferred to the die the part of this which requires removing will be protruding through the acrylic.

Crown Removal

Acrylic may be used to simplify the removal of crowns which have been either temporarily or permanently cemented into place (Garver and Wisser, 1978). This is achieved by painting a layer of autopolymerizing resin onto the labial and palatal surfaces of the crown, joining these together and building the acrylic out on the labial surface so that a crown remover may be applied to it. In this way any risk of damage to the crown is reduced to a minimum. However, this technique should only be employed when the underlying crown of the tooth is sound and there is no risk of damaging or fracturing it.

■ Impression Compound

This material is compounded of synthetic and natural resins, waxes and fillers. It is thermoplastic, being quite hard at mouth temperature but becoming usable, i.e. malleable, only a little above this. The thermal contraction on setting is of the order of 0·3 per cent. It has good flow characteristics but only a very limited working time. The thermal conductivity is low and thus plenty of time must be allowed for it to be thoroughly softened before use and also for it to set before removing it. The die should be made as soon after this as possible so as to avoid warpage from stress release, particularly if room temperatures are high. However, when contained within a rigid copper ring it is relatively stable.

One of the main advantages of impression compound is that it can be readily electroplated. This produces a hard model which is of considerable value when, for instance, copings are to be used or a platinum matrix has to be burnished on to the model.

Its most serious disadvantage is its lack of elasticity. On cooling it sets to a rigid mass and if any undercuts are present distortion is bound to occur on removal. As all indirect impressions must extend at least a little beyond the margin of the preparation, which is nearly always into an undercut area, some distortion on removal is almost inevitable. A further factor is that undercuts may occur as between the prepared and the external surfaces, if the preparation is taken below the greatest diameter of the tooth.

If carefully used and if no undercut areas are involved in the impression, compound can produce a reasonably accurate impression. However, it has the further disadvantage that the die can only be located to the neighbouring teeth by means of an overall impression. This immediately introduces an additional stage in the production of the model when an error can occur, which may result in either poor contact points or a faulty occlusion.

For all the above reasons compound cannot be considered as a suitable impression material for a bridge. However, it may be adequate for the simple crown and has the advantage that, being usually enclosed in a copper ring, the production of a copper die is facilitated.

It is also of value for making accurate custom-made trays for a more precise impression material. However, care must be taken to ensure that they and also any adhesive used are compatible.

■ Reversible Hydrocolloids

Reversible hydrocolloids were the first of the elastic impression materials. They were introduced to the profession in the mid 1920s and by 1937 were sufficiently far advanced to be used in the production of fixed bridge prostheses.

As with most of the impression materials used in crown and bridgework they are available in different grades;

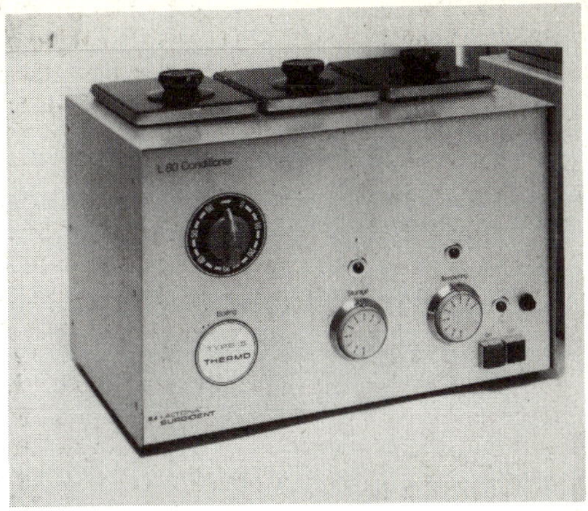

a

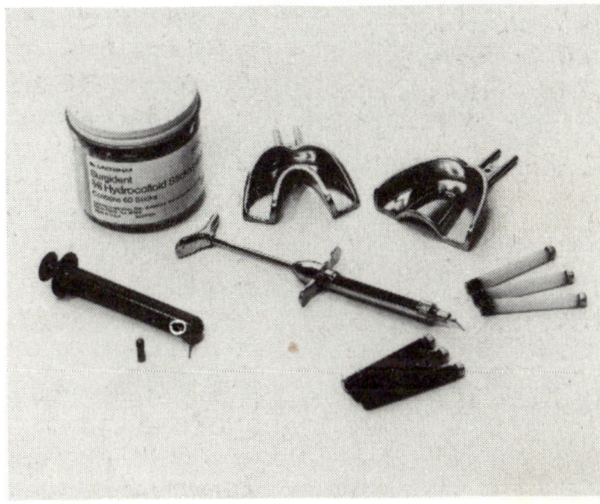

b

Fig. 4.10. *a, A Surgident hydrocolloid conditioning bath with liquefying, storing and tempering compartments. b, Surgident hydrocolloid sticks and cartridges and their respective syringes. The water-cooled trays are also shown.*
(By courtesy of Lactona Corporation.)

Lactona*, for instance marketing 3 different consistencies of both tray and syringe material. Those used in the syringe are thinnest whereas those employed in the tray range from heavy to relatively light bodied. The heavier bodied the material the less likely it is to tear.

The hydrocolloid changes from a gel to a sol when heated, and the phases are reversed on cooling. The technique required is relatively precise, and necessitates fairly expensive apparatus.

* Lactona Corporation, Brouwenjbaan 10, 4600 AH Bergen-op-Zoom, Holland.

This consists of a special bath (*Fig.* 4.10*a*) with three sections, one for softening the material in boiling water, a second which is kept at 46°C for tempering it, and a third for storing it at 62°C. When the material is in frequent use then the bath is normally coupled up to a time switch which makes certain that the bath is always on and at the correct temperature during normal working hours. Indeed some operators prefer to leave the bath on continuously, 24 hours a day. However, it should be borne in mind that the manufacturers recommend that the material should not be kept in the storage bath for more than 48 hours at a time.

The hydrocolloid will liquefy at 60–70°C but to speed this process it is generally immersed in boiling water for about 10 min. After this it is transferred to the storage bath and kept there until required. Prior to insertion of the tray material in the mouth it is placed in the tempering bath at 46°C for 5–10 min, to give it some degree of body.

When in the mouth it should be cooled at approximately 13°C for 5 min. If the cooling medium goes below 13 °C then the rate of cooling can be too rapid and distortion may occur. Reversible hydrocolloid should really only be used once as it is impossible to sterilize it and on no account should it be reused more than 3–4 times as its physical properties are altered by repeated heating and cooling.

Technique

The technique to be employed, assuming the baths to be switched on and at the correct temperatures, would be as follows:

a. Place a sufficient number of tubes of the tray material of the consistency you require in the boiling water compartment and leave it there to liquefy and homogenize.

b. Load the syringe with a stick of the thinner impression material, screw the cap onto the end of the syringe nozzle and place the syringe into the bath of boiling water also.

c. After 10 min transfer the loaded syringe and the tubes of tray material to the storage bath and leave them there for a minimum of 10 min.

d. Transfer the tubes of tray material to the tempering bath and leave them in this for 5–10 min to give them some degree of body. Some operators prefer to load the tray direct from the storage bath and then place this in the tempering bath prior to use. The disadvantage of this technique is that the surface of the impression material becomes wet and has to be dried off before inserting it in the mouth.

e. The loaded syringe is used direct from the storage bath to improve the fluidity of the hydrocolloid and give maximum working time. It should never be tempered.

Some authorities prefer to inject an appreciable quantity of the hydrocolloid into the tissues in the region of the preparations and leave it there for at least 10 min before proceeding with the impression as the hydrocolloid appears to have a beneficial 'tissue-conditioning' effect. This is possibly because of the various salts which are added to the hydrocolloid to improve its handling and other properties.

f. Any material which may have been injected around the teeth as a conditioning agent is now removed. It is assumed that gingival retraction, where necessary, has been carried out beforehand. The syringe material is now injected around the teeth, a relatively large amount being used to prevent its solidifying before the heavy bodied material is inserted otherwise the two would not bond.

g. The rim-lock tray, connected to the water tubing, is placed in the mouth and seated into position. 'Stops' should have been placed in the tray to prevent overseating and a post dam provided. Water is passed through the tray and after approximately 5 min it may be removed using a 'snap' technique. The impression should then either be cast immediately or placed in a control solution or 100 per cent humidifier from which it should be removed and cast within a couple of hours.

Advantages

When used correctly the material is capable of producing a very accurate die, is sufficiently elastic to reproduce most undercut areas satisfactorily, and has a good recovery after distortion. It is not hydrophobic as are some of the other impression materials and thus a better model surface results. It is reasonably palatable and well tolerated by the patient and acts as a tissue-conditioning agent.

Disadvantages

The flow of the reversible hydrocolloids,

although satisfactory, is not quite as good as some of the more recent impression materials; its ability, for instance, to flow into the gingival crevice and record the margin of a subgingival preparation is slightly less. Further disadvantages are that it cannot be electroplated and that its temperature on insertion or when being cooled may cause pain if local analgesia is not being used. Hydrocolloid does tear fairly easily on removal and this can give rise to problems with subgingival preparations, particularly if they are deep.

Rather more extensive gingival retraction is required than for instance, with polysulphides so as to increase the width of the gingival crevice and permit an adequate thickness of the relatively weak impression material. The depth of the crevice should not, of course, be altered. Only one model can be poured from each impression and therefore there is little scope for error in the laboratory; however, it is quite practical to take 2 impressions at the same visit as the technique is fairly quick and no special tray is needed.

Relatively complex equipment is required to take a reversible hydrocolloid impression and thus the initial cost is high; however, once a surgery is equipped to use this material the cost per impression is appreciably less than that of the other impression materials used in crown and bridgework.

■ Irreversible Hydrocolloids (Alginates)

The irreversible hydrocolloids were introduced more than 30 years ago and have become widely accepted because of their low cost and simplicity of use. They are similar to the agar hydrocolloids in that the material is inserted into the mouth as a sol which then changes to a gel; however, this process combines both a physical and a chemical change. The sol is prepared by mixing the alginate in powder form with water and the setting time may be varied by altering the water temperature.

Technique

It is important that the material is used in a well perforated tray to prevent distortion on removal, which should be by the 'snap' technique. Casting must be carried out immediately after this as it is even less stable than the reversible hydrocolloids. If it is essential that it be kept for a short while prior to casting then this may be done either by storing it in a humidifier or by wrapping it in moist gauze and placing it in a sealed plastic bag. Alternatively the impression may be immersed in liquid paraffin.

Advantages and Disadvantages

This material can prove very accurate if carefully used and if attention is paid to its retention in the tray. However, its elasticity and flow characteristics are not as good as the reversible hydrocolloids and it is liable to tear on removal if in thin section, for instance interstitially or subgingivally.

It is simpler to use than the reversible hydrocolloids and is much cheaper than the thiokols and silicones. However, these factors are more than offset by its disadvantages and its use in bridge work is now largely confined to taking impressions of the opposing arch, making study casts, or in the fabrication of temporary bridges.

■ Polysulphide Rubbers

The polysulphide rubber impression materials such as Permlastic* and Coe-flex† were first marketed in 1953 and have been progressively developed since then. Probably the main reason for their introduction and ready acceptance was that they are far more stable after removal from the mouth than the hydrocolloids.

They are converted from a paste to a solid by oxidative cross-linkage, lead dioxide being commonly employed for this purpose in the past; however,

---

* Kerr Europe, 1–84018, Scafari, Italy.
†Coe Laboratories, Chicago, Illinois, 60658, USA.

because of the concern about lead toxicity cupric salts are now being used increasingly which have the additional advantage that they are cleaner. When set the polysulphides are very resistant to solvents and will withstand temperatures in the range −57°C to +150°C.

The material is usually employed in two different viscosities for bridge work: one which is thin enough for injection through a syringe (light bodied) and another (heavy bodied) for the overall impression which is thick enough to force the light bodied material home and may possibly provide some degree of tissue compression. Manufacturers vary in the way in which they market the product. Some sell it in two or three different consistencies whereas others supply it in one consistency but also provide a thinner to reduce its viscosity to the degree required.

The mixing time of this material is critical and the manufacturer's instructions must be strictly observed otherwise its properties will be altered. The simplest method of mixing it is on a disposable paper slab. There are wide deviations in the mixing and setting times depending on the particular product being used. Temperature and humidity both markedly affect the setting time (Bell et al., 1975) and thus during hot humid weather it is best to keep the material in a cool place. However, it is necessary to avoid cooling the material below the dew point, otherwise condensation will occur on the rubber and again speed the set.

The extent of the variations produced by humidity and temperature are illustrated by *Fig.* 4.11, where it can be seen that a reduction in humidity from 51 per cent to 24 per cent increases the time to initial set by approximately 50 per cent. A fall in temperature of 6°C has a similar effect. Thus a combination of the two more than doubles the working time.

On mixing the material it initially thickens, and then becomes elastic.

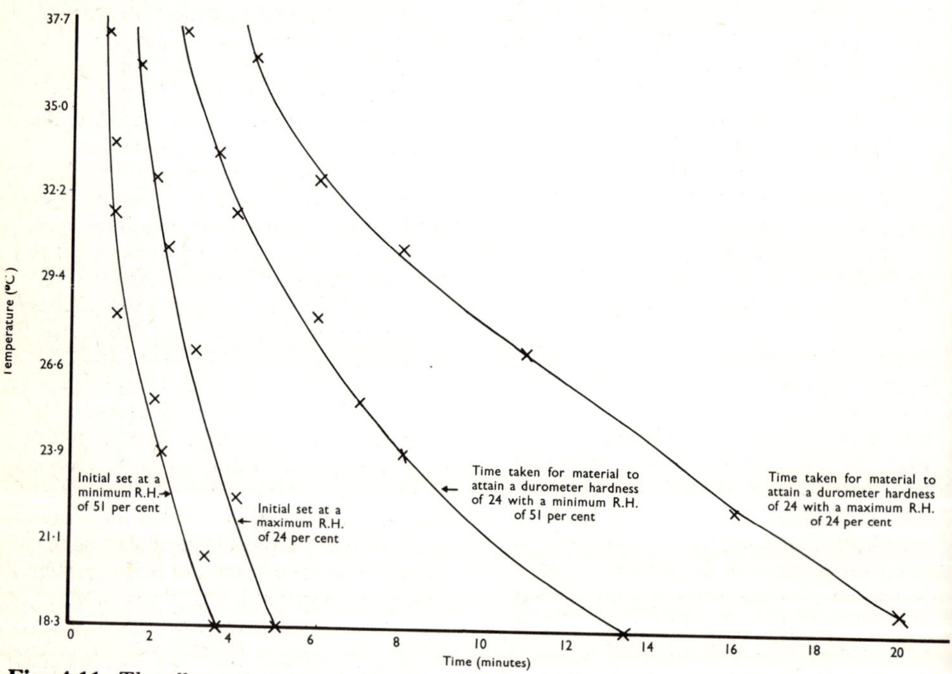

Fig. 4.11. *The effects of temperature and humidity on the setting time of polysulphide (Permlastic).*
(By courtesy of Dr Talbot of the Kerr Mfg Co.)

Obviously it must be inserted before this second stage is reached.

To ensure an even and adequate thickness of the rubber which ideally should be around 2–3 mm, a rigid special tray should be used and the material firmly retained in this by means of the correct adhesive. This usually consists of a rubber solution in a volatile organic solvent. The time that the impression must be left in the mouth is about 6–8 min, but this varies appreciably both with the weather and the particular material being employed. Although this material may be used with a reline technique there appears to be little advantage and thus a double mix is usually to be recommended.

Advantages and Disadvantages

The only disadvantages of the polysulphides are that they are relatively messy to handle in the unmixed state, have a somewhat unpleasant taste and smell, which has been partially overcome by the manufacturers, and are more expensive than most of the other impression materials. One further factor to be borne in mind is that they are almost completely insoluble in the set state and, should they be dropped on clothing, are impossible to remove.

The main advantages of the polysulphides are their extreme accuracy (*Fig.* 4.12) and their stability. Unrestrained shrinkage in the first 24 hours is of the order of 0·19–0·39 per cent and in the second 24 hours only 0·02 per cent. If restrained, as for instance in a special tray, then the figures are far less. This material when used in the less viscous form has excellent flow characteristics and will consistently reproduce fine details of deep subgingival preparations.

Its recovery from distortion is good but it takes longer to recover completely than, for example, the silicones and it is thus best to wait ½–1 hour before pouring the model.

The polysulphides are compatible with all the die materials in common use and can be silver plated.

■ Silicone Impression Materials

The first generation of silicones, such as Lastic 55,* Xantopren and Optosil† and Citricon‡ consist of partially polymerized polydimethyl silicone mixed with a zinc oxide filler to form a paste, to which is added a liquid catalyst of ethyl silicate containing an accelerator such as dibutyl tin dilaurate. As the paste is only partially polymerized this process will slowly continue during storage and thus it has a relatively short shelf life. To overcome this defect as far as possible the material should be stored in a cool place.

When first used the silicones were a considerable advance on the irreversible hydrocolloids. They have far greater stability and their ability to reproduce undercut areas without distortion is much better. However, like all materials they still require correct handling if optimum results are to be achieved. Thus to minimize distortion a perforated tray should be used to exercise restraint on the silicone and minimize any warpage. Ideally the thickness of the material should be about 4·0 mm. They are relatively stable dimensionally but polymerization of the material is by no means complete on removal and thus the model should be cast fairly quickly. Although its rate of recovery from distortion is far more rapid than the polysulphides, some time, possibly 15 min, should be allowed to permit it to recover after removal from undercut areas in the mouth. The accuracy of these materials, although satisfactory, is inferior to the polysulphides (*Fig.* 4.12). However, this has been improved in recent years in 2 ways: (*a*) By using a reline technique the dimensional stability of the material is improved as the silicone putty has a higher content of filler than the impression material and is therefore more stable. Moreover the thickness of actual impression material used, i.e. the 'wash' is greatly reduced. (*b*) A new generation of silicones, sometimes called

* A Kettenbach –6345, Eschenburg-Eibelshausen/Hessen, Germany.
† Bayer Leverkusen, Germany.
‡ Kerr Europe, 1–84018, Scafari, Italy.

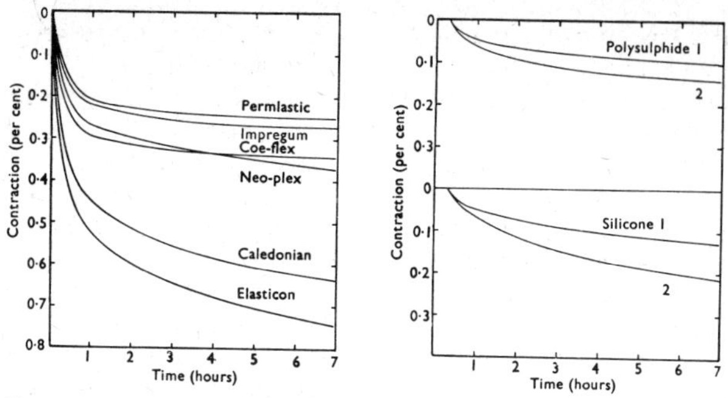

Fig. 4.12. *The dimensional stability of polysulphides (Permlastic, Coe-flex, and Neo-plex), polyether (Impregum), and silicone (Caledonian and Elasticon) impressions.* (Reproduced with permission from Chong M. P. and Docking A. R. (1969) *Aust. Dent. J.* **14**, 300.)

polysiloxanes such as President* and Permagum† have been produced which are catalysed by an addition reaction using chloroplatinic acid as opposed to the condensation reaction employed with the earlier silicones. This has resulted in the best dimensional stability of all the elastomeric impression materials (McLean, Monograph IV, 1976).

Advantages and Disadvantages

The flow of the silicones into small areas such as the gingival crevice is fair but not as good as that of the polysulphides and the working time for complex bridge work is somewhat limited with most of those on the market.

The material is relatively easy to mix as drops of coloured catalyst are added to the silicone and complete homogeneity is easier to obtain than with the polysulphides as it is far less viscous.

The fact that the material is relatively odourless and tasteless is appreciated by patients and the rapid set may sometimes be an advantage, as is the fact that it may be used in a stock perforated tray.

Gas production on polymerization particularly with the earlier silicones can cause a poor model, although this has now been largely overcome. The same factor can give rise to difficulties with electroplating, although the manufacturers of 'President', a polysiloxane, claim that it can be electroplated entirely satisfactorily.

Uses

The earlier silicones such as 'Lastic 55' are of particular value where extreme accuracy is not required and it is necessary to store the impression for some time before reusing it, for example in the construction of temporary bridges as described in Chapter 16. A further example is the use of the material for an overall impression for instance to locate several copper rings and enable their repositioning after they have been plated.

Silicones are also of value for impression techniques in periodontal cases with loose teeth or where large interproximal embrasures or gross undercuts are present which cannot be eliminated before taking the impression. In these cases the use of the harder setting polysulphides or more particularly the polyether rubbers would make removal of an impression extremely difficult.

Technique

There are two basic methods of taking an impression in silicone, either the double mix which is described in Chapter 16 or a reline procedure which involves taking a preliminary impression before the teeth

* Coltene Inc., CH-9450 Altstatten, Switzerland.
† Kerr Europe, 1–84108, Scarfari, Italy.

are prepared and then reintroducing this after the completed preparations have been covered with a second thin mix of the material. The advantage of the latter is that, in effect, a special tray is rapidly produced which reduces the thickness of the wash of impression material to a minimum and thus improves its dimensional stability. However, it is important that the initial impression is adequately relieved and has satisfactory spillways. If this is not done, or undue pressure is exerted when seating the impression for the second time, then distortion of what is, in effect, a rubber special tray will result and movement of the impression will occur on removal. This problem has been reduced by the advent of the silicone putties which are relatively inelastic when set. To increase the accuracy of the technique some operators prefer to use polysulphides as the reline material.

■ Polyether Rubber Impression Materials

This material marketed under the names of Impregum* and Polygel† is a polymer, mainly of tetramethylene-glycol with terminal aziridino groups. The catalyst contains a sulphonic acid ester which, by reacting with the aziridino groups, causes cross-linking which sets the paste to a stable elastomer.

It differs from the other materials mentioned in several ways. Thus when set it is far harder than the silicones and polysulphides, its elastic modulus being twice that of a heavy-bodied polysulphide. This may or may not be an advantage, as very serious difficulties can be experienced when trying to remove a full arch impression, particularly if the inter-proximal embrasures are wide. The hardness of the material can be reduced to some extent by using thinners, but this increases water absorption.

It is more hydrophilic than the polysulphides or silicones and for this reason must not be stored in water but in open air.

In practice the water-absorbent nature of the material does not affect its accuracy, provided that it is kept dry until cast. Similarly, more than one model can be reasonably satisfactorily taken from a single impression.

Electroplating may be carried out but it is advisable to switch on the current as soon as the impression is put in the plating bath. Because the material is hydrophilic its accuracy is probably affected by this method of model production.

Advantages and Disadvantages

The material is easy to mix, clean and odourless. The set is more sharply defined than with the polysulphides and this allows an adequate working time and then a quick set in about 4 min. It is usually bonded to the tray by a special adhesive.

The dimensional stability is excellent, being approximately equal to the polysulphides and better than the silicones. The recovery of polyether from permanent deformation is also good, being similar to the silicones, which are more satisfactory in this respect than the polysulphides. The shelf life is guaranteed by the manufacturers for two years. Allergic reactions to this material have been reported both with a patient (Nally and Storr, 1973) and nursing staff. This is associated with the catalyst which is a sulphonic acid ester named methyl paratoluene sulphonate; however, aromatic sulphonates are also used with Scutan, Lastic 55, Storra, Xantopren, Optosil and Verone.

The main disadvantage of the material is its hardness and high elastic modulus when set, which may give rise to difficulty when removing it from the mouth and from the working model. Moreover, its flow characteristics are not as good as those of a light-bodied polysulphide, particularly into small areas such as the gingival crevice. For all these reasons the use of polyether is not to be recommended for long span bridges.

* Espe, GmbH, Seefeld/Oberbay, W. Germany.
† L. D. Caulk Co., Div. of the Dentists' Supply Co. of NY, Milford, Del. Toronto, Ontario, Canada.

Technique

This material is used in a similar manner to the polysulphides, the method for which is described in detail in Chapter 16.

The mixing technique is straightforward, the catalyst being incorporated in the paste and stirred until an even colour is achieved. The viscosity of the material to be used in the syringe is usually reduced by adding a thinner.

As it is relatively rigid when set a greater thickness of material must be allowed for in the tray, otherwise removal will be difficult. This can be achieved either by using a stock tray or by constructing a special tray and allowing for more clearance than with a polysulphide, i.e. at least 6·0 mm.

To break the seal and remove the impression gradual pressure is advisable, in contradistinction to the 'snap' technique required for the alginates.

This material may be used in a copper ring if required, adhesive being painted on the inside. However, it is important that the ring be both rigid and a loose fit, so that it will not distort on removal.

Uses

The polyethers currently available are particularly valuable for taking an impression of one or two crown preparations or possibly a simple three-unit bridge. They have the advantage that they are quick and easy to use and are more pleasant for the patient than polysulphide. Their rigidity when set and relatively limited working time preclude their use for complex or long-span bridges and the results obtained when they are used for recording intracoronal preparations are not entirely satisfactory.

DIE MATERIALS

This subject will not be dealt with in any detail as it has already been covered in depth in the textbooks on dental materials and several articles have been written on the subject. However, it is desirable that the operator has some knowledge of the various materials which may be used for forming dies, the indications of each of these and their compatibility with the impression materials used.

The main properties required of a die are accuracy, surface hardness and smoothness and ease of production. There are two main ways in which a die may be formed, either by casting it in one of the improved dental stones or by electroplating the impression.

■ Stone Dies

The improved dental stones will produce a very accurate die which will be sufficiently hard for the fabrication of bridges by the experienced technician. However, where the dies have to be worked on to any degree, for instance if copings have to be employed which will be taken on and off several times, or where the stone would be thin or have a fine and fragile margin, then they are less satisfactory. Likewise, considerable care has to be taken if a platinum foil has to be burnished down to a stone model. In these instances an electroplated die is often preferable.

When a stone die is being made from a polysulphide or silicone impression then these must first be treated with a wetting agent to overcome their water-repellent nature and thus permit the close and ready adaptation of the stone to the impression. The reversible and irreversible hydrocolloids, because of their hydrophilic nature, do not require to be treated in this way. However, these materials tend to retard the set of the stone and may affect its surfaces because of the syneresis which occurs, matrix material being exuded from the hydrocolloid, and this has to be counteracted by using a fixing solution which also stabilizes the impression after its removal from the mouth by preventing water loss.

■ Electroplated Dies

There are two materials used for electroplating impressions to make dies copper and silver. The former is of particular value when producing individual dies from copper ring impressions. It gives both a hard and an accurate model.

Silver plating is indicated where it is desirable to coat a larger impression involving several teeth such as a complex bridge or one incorporating precision retainers (attachments) where copings may be required.

Because of the water-absorbent and relatively unstable nature of the hydrocolloids electroplated dies cannot be produced from these. However, the polysulphides are completely suitable for this purpose and respond better to silver than copper plating, possibly because copper is an acid-based bath whilst silver is deposited from a cyanide solution. The silicones can be electroplated; however, the results achieved are not nearly as satisfactory as with the polysulphides, possibly because the metal deposited fails to adhere very closely to the surface of the material and because of certain other chemical factors.

Similarly the polyether impression materials can be silverplated without difficulty, but it would seem likely that their hydrophilic properties might give rise to some distortion whilst they are in the plating bath.

DENTAL CEMENTS

Ideal properties required of a dental cement used for placing a bridge are:

1. *Good adhesion:* (*a*) to the underlying abutment preparations, the surface of which may comprise enamel, dentine, cementum or amalgam; (*b*) to the materials used for constructing the bridge retainers, which may be gold, porcelain, acrylic or a combination of these.

2. *Adequate strength* to resist the forces of mastication.

3. *Thin film thickness* to permit a casting to seat adequately. The less the film thickness the greater the retention. Any figure below 30–40 μm may be considered satisfactory, as in clinical practice few castings fit the tooth to within less than 100 μm (Jørgensen, 1960).

4. *Low solubility.*

5. *Low toxicity.*

6. *Satisfactory working properties* including good flow characteristics and a slow set giving adequate time for the seating of the castings.

There are three main groups of material which may be used for cementing a bridge; those based on zinc oxide and eugenol, the zinc phosphates and the polycarboxylates.

■ Zinc Oxide and Eugenol Cements

There are several types of zinc oxide and eugenol cement.

a. Simple Zinc Oxide and Eugenol

The very slow set, poor strength and high solubility of these means that they can only be used for temporary cementation or fillings.

b. Accelerated Zinc Oxide and Eugenol

These are usually reinforced with hydrogenated resin and incorporate an accelerator such as zinc acetate which reduces the setting time to 3–4 min. They are three to four times as strong as a simple mix of zinc oxide and eugenol. However, their compressive strength is still far too low to permit their use for the permanent cementation of bridges. Furthermore their solubility is too high.

c. EBA Cements

This group of cements was developed from the accelerated zinc oxide and eugenol materials, a large part of the eugenol being replaced by ethyl benzoic acid (hence EBA). Similarly some of the zinc oxide is replaced by finely ground quartz or aluminium oxide. The addition of this latter material would seem to provide the greater strength.

There is a considerable variation in the results obtained with the various EBA cements currently available; however, the best are almost as strong as a zinc phosphate cement.

They have a fairly long working time and then a rapid set in the mouth. This is because moisture is required for the setting process.

The average film thickness of the EBA cements when used for placing a casting has been found by some authorities to be considerably greater than that of zinc phosphate, which would seem to indicate that the flow characteristics are not so satisfactory. However, it is still probably within clinically acceptable limits. Their biggest advantage as compared with the phosphate and polycarboxylate cements is that they are not irritant to the pulp and one of their main disadvantages is their high solubility which usually contra-indicates their use for permanent cementation.

To summarize, this group of cements are very valuable as a lining material and are also occasionally of value for cementing full crowns where retention is excellent and it is essential to keep pulpal irritation to a minimum. They are positively contraindicated for post crowns, pinlays or any bridge in which the retention available on the abutment preparations is less than would ideally be desired.

■ Zinc Phosphate Cements

These cements have been used for luting bridges for longer than any of the other materials and as far as retention is concerned they still produce the best and most consistent results. However, they have a serious disadvantage in that at cementation they have a pH of the order of 2·5–3 and this relatively low figure may persist for a considerable time after the material is apparently set (*Table I*). Antonioli (1969) has shown that this may well produce a lowering of the pH in the pulp chamber itself by 1–2 units, which shows that appreciable leachable free acid is present in fresh cement.

It is extremely difficult to assess the clinical significance of the pulpal irritation caused by the phosphate cements. It would seem likely that this is quite often responsible for postoperative pain, but rarely causes death of the pulp.

Table I. The change of pH of zinc phosphate and polycarboxylate cements during the first 48 hours after insertion

Time	*Zinc oxyphosphate*	*Polycarboxylate*
15 min	4·9	4·8
30 min	5·4	5·4
24 hr	6·7	6·5
48 hr	6·9	6·6

Figures taken from Phillips R. W. et al. (1970) *J. Am. Dent. Assoc.* **81**, 1353.

The phosphate cements have reasonable flow characteristics, a minimal film thickness of 30–40 μm, and the relatively high compressive (crush) strength of up to 96 mN/m² (*Fig.* 4.13). They have an adequate working time which may be increased by using a cool slab and also by adding a little powder to the liquid before commencing the main mix. This latter technique will slow the reaction time by buffering the acid and thus also reduce the irritancy of the cement.

Once set the strength of phosphate cement builds up quite rapidly so that it is clinically usable in a relatively short time. Solubility in the oral fluids is fairly low and in clinical practice gives little trouble. It is essential that the correct proportioning and mixing of cements is carried out if their optimum strength and working time and minimal film thickness is to be achieved (Eames et al., 1977). This applies equally to the phosphate and polycarboxylate cement. Best results are obtained with phosphate cement if 0·5 g of powder is added, by increments, on a cool slab to 0·25 ml of liquid, over a period of 90 sec. Increasing the mixing time beyond 90 sec merely reduces the working time. The mix should be carried out on as large an area of the slab as possible to increase heat dissipation.

■ The Polycarboxylate Cements

The polycarboxylate cements are relatively new, having been developed by

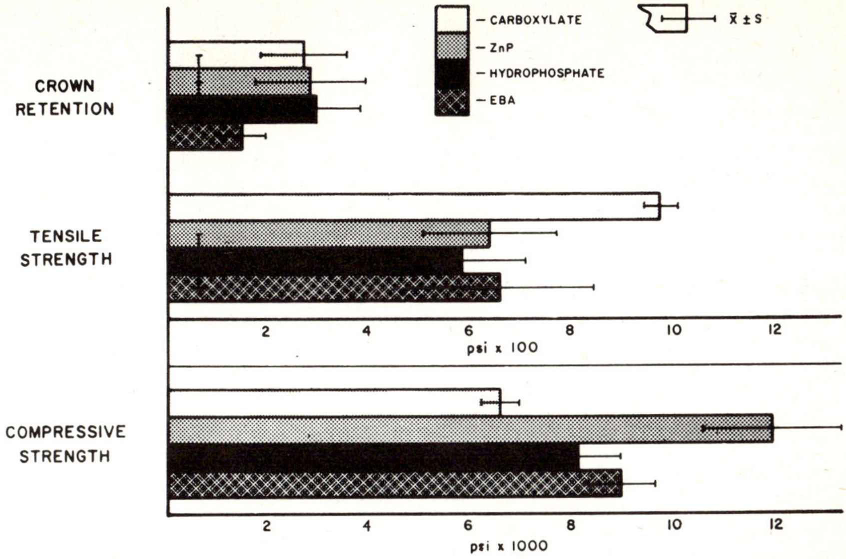

Fig. 4.13. *Comparison of crown retention to tensile and compressive strengths.* (Reproduced with permission from Richter W. A., Mitchem J. C. and Brown J. D. (1970) *J. Prosthet. Dent.* **24**, 301.)

D. C. Smith and first reported by him in 1967. They consist of zinc oxide powder to which magnesium oxide has been added and a liquid which is a solution of polyacrylic acid.

The primary aim is to produce a more positive bond with the tooth tissue than could be obtained with the other materials currently available. In this he has succeeded in that the bond to enamel is much stronger than with the phosphate cement and the retention available on dentine and cementum is also improved.

This is achieved by the residual acid groupings in the long-chain zinc polyacrylate produced by the setting reaction appearing to chelate (or bond to) the calcium in the enamel. Unfortunately, however, as far as crown and bridge work are concerned this is largely negated by their poor bond to porcelain and gold. Thus in clinical practice the retention obtained with these materials when cementing a casting, a crown, or a facing is actually inferior to that obtained with phosphate cement.

A further factor which may contribute to the relatively poor results obtained with the polycarboxylates, particularly when they are used for cementing post crowns and pinlays, is their fairly low crush (compressive) strength which compares unfavourably with the phosphates.

Under laboratory test conditions the solubility of the polycarboxylates is as low or lower than that of the zinc phosphates, although in clinical practice the results seem to be somewhat less favourable. However, they have a low cytotoxicity.

The viscosity of the polycarboxylate cements when first introduced was fairly high and thus the material did not flow readily; however, the latest materials have been improved appreciably in this respect. During setting it becomes rubbery and it is essential that the casting is fully seated before this stage is reached.

The working time of the material is somewhat limited and this makes it unsuitable for use with complex bridges, although this can be improved by using a refrigerated glass slab.

Correct proportioning and mixing of the material is essential if a satisfactory result is to be achieved. Because of the viscous nature of the liquid a fairly thick mix is necessary if the correct powder/liquid ratio is to be achieved. If this is not attained the strength will be appreciably reduced and the solubility increased. It is this characteristic which may well have resulted in some of the relatively disappointing clinical results achieved with this material.

A further factor to be borne in mind is that the cement should be mixed soon after the liquid is dispensed, otherwise it will lose water due to evaporation and this will appreciably alter the properties of the material.

To summarize, the polycarboxylate cements require precise handling if a satisfactory result is to be achieved. Their main advantages are their positive bond to enamel and their relatively low pulpal irritation when compared with phosphate cements. They are of value as a luting agent in all cases where the operator is certain that he has achieved adequate retention, but if he is in doubt then phosphate cement should still be employed. They are positively contra-indicated for the cementing of porcelain crowns and facings and should only be used with caution when placing pinlays and post crowns.

BIBLIOGRAPHY

Porcelain

McLean J. W. (1967) The alumina tube post crown. *Br. Dent. J.* **123**, 87.

McLean J. W. (1967) High alumina ceramics for bridge pontic construction. *Br. Dent. J.* **123**, 571.

McLean J. W. (1967) The alumina reinforced porcelain jacket crown. *J. Am. Dent. Assoc.* **75**, 621.

McLean J. W. (1974, 1976) *The Science and Art of Dental Ceramics*. A collection of monographs. Louisiana State University Medical Center, School of Dentistry, USA. Also published by Quintessence Publishing Co. Inc., Chicago, 1978.

McLean J. W., Kedge M. I. and Hubbard J. R. (1976) The bonded alumina crown. II. Construction using the twin foil technique. *Aust. Dent. J.* **21**, 262.

McLean J. W. and Sced I. R. (1976) The bonded alumina crown. I. The bonding of platinum to aluminous dental porcelain using tin oxide coatings. *Aust. Dent. J.* **21**, 119.

Mumford G. (1965) The porcelain fused to metal restoration. *Dent. Clin. North Am.* March, p. 241.

Mumford G. and Ridge A. (1971) Dental porcelain. *Dent. Clin. North Am.* **15**, 33.

Nally J. N. (1968) Chemico-physical analysis and mechanical tests of ceramo-metallic complex. *Int. Dent. J.* **18**, 309.

Schwartz M. (1969) Review of dental research. *J. Am. Dent. Assoc.* **79**, 901.

Southan D. E. (1969) *The Physical Properties of Modern Dental Porcelain*. Ph.D. Thesis, Sydney University.

Plastic

Crispin B. (1978) Acrylic resin copings. An adjunct to fixed restorative dentistry. *J. Prosthet. Dent.* **39**, 632.

Garver D. G. and Wisser R. C. (1978) A safe crown-removal technique. *J. Prosthet. Dent.* **39**, 56.

Henry P. J. and Mitchell D. F. (1966) Tissue changes beneath fixed partial dentures. *J. Prosthet. Dent.* **16**, 937.

Peyton F. A. (1963) Current evaluation of plastics in crown and bridge prosthesis. *J. Prosthet. Dent.* **13**, 743.

Gold and Non-precious Metals

Harcourt H. J., Riddihough M. and Osborne J. (1970) The properties of nickel-chromium casting alloys containing boron and silicon. *Br. Dent. J.* **129**, 419.

Kaires A. K. and Thompson J. C. (1959) The effect of heat treatment variables on the microstructure and hardness of a cast dental gold alloy. *J. Dent. Res.* **38**, 888.

McLean J. W. and Sced I. R. (1973) Bonding of dental porcelain to metal. (1) The gold alloy/porcelain bond. (II) The base-metal alloy/porcelain bond. *Trans. Ceramic Soc.* **72**, 229–235.

Nitkin D. A. and Asgar K. (1976) Evaluation of alternative alloys to type 111 gold for use in fixed prosthodontics. *J. Am. Dent. Assoc.* **93**, 622.

Sced I. R. and McLean J. W. (1972) The strength of metal/ceramic bonds with base metals containing chromium. *Br. Dent. J.* **132**, 232.

Trifunovic D. M., von Fraunhofer J. A. and Davies E. H. (1976) Transverse bond strength studies of base metal alloy-porcelain systems. *Surf. Technol.* **4**, 485.

Impression Materials

Asgar K. (1971) Elastic impression materials. *Dent. Clin. North Am.* **15**, 81.

Bell J. W., Davies E. H. and von Fraunhofer J. A. (1975) The dimensional changes of elastomeric impression materials under various conditions of humidity. *J. Dent.* **4**, 73.

Bell J. W. and von Fraunhofer J. A. (1975) The handling of elastomeric impression materials: a review. *J. Dent.* **3**, 229.

Causton B. and Braden M. (1970) *Polyether Impression Rubber*, IADR. British Division Report 8, 10 April 1970.

Chong M. P. and Docking A. R. (1969) Some setting characteristics of elastomeric impression materials. *Aust. Dent. J.* **14**, 295.
von Körber E. and Lehmann K. (1969) Vergleichende Untersuchungen bei Abdruckmaterialsen für Kronen und Bruken. *D. Zahnärztl. Z.* **24**, 791.
McLean J. W. (1961) Physical properties influencing the accuracy of thiokol and silicone impression materials. *Br. Dent. J.* **110**, 85.
McLean J. W. (1976) *The Science and Art of Dental Ceramics*. Monographs III and IV, Louisiana State University Medical Center, School of Dentistry, USA. Also published by Quintessence Publishing Co. Inc. Chicago, 1978.
Nally S. and Storr J. (1973) Hypersensitivity to a dental impression material—A case report. *Br. Dent. J.* **134**, 244.
Peyton F. A. and Craig R. G. (1971) *Restorative Dental Materials,* 4th ed. St Louis, Mosby.
Phillips R. W. (1973) *Skinner's Science of Dental Materials,* 7th ed. Philadelphia, Saunders.
Purrman R., ESPE. Personal communication.
Skinner E. W. (1958) Properties and manipulation of mercaptan base and silicone base impression materials. *Dent. Clin. North Am.* November, p. 685.
Talbot W. F., Kerr Manufacturing Co. Personal communication.
Wilson H. J. (1966) Elastomeric impression materials. 1. The setting material. *Br. Dent. J.* **121**, 277.
Wilson H. J. (1966) Elastomeric impression materials. II. The set materials. *Br. Dent. J.* **121**, 322.

Die Materials

Asgar K. (1971) Elastic impression materials. *Dent. Clin. North Am.* **15**, 94.
Markley M. R. and Krug K. S. (1969) Silver plating rubber base material for superior dies and casts. *J. Prosthet. Dent.* **22**, 103.
Myers G. E. (1958) Electroformed die technique for rubber impressions. *J. Prosthet. Dent.* **8**, 531.
Peyton F. A. (1965) Evaluation of materials used for indirect techniques. *Dent. Clin. North Am.* March, p. 213.
Peyton F. A. and Craig R. G. (1971) *Restorative Dental Materials,* 4th ed. St Louis, Mosby.
Peyton F. A., Leibold J. P. and Ridgley G. V. (1952) Surface hardness compressive strength and abrasion resistance of indirect die stones. *J. Prosthet. Dent.* **2**, 381.
Phillips R. W., Swartz M. L. and Norman R. D. (1969) *Materials for the Practising Dentist.* St Louis, Mosby, pp. 130–141.

Cements

Antonioli C. A. (1969) Etude sur le pénétration des ions H^+ de differents cements de scellenent a travers la dentine. *SSO* **79**, 533.
Eames W. B. et al. (1977) Proportioning and mixing of cements: A comparison of working times. *Op. Dent.* **2**, 97.
von Fraunhofer J. A. (ed.) (1975) *Scientific Aspects of Dental Materials.* London, Butterworths.
Grieve A. R. (1969) A study of dental cements. *Br. Dent. J.* **127**, 405.
Jϕrgensen K. D. (1960) Factors affecting the film thickness of zinc phosphate cements. *Acta Odontol. Scand.* **18**, 479.
Jϕrgensen K. D. and Holst K. (1967) The relationship between the retention of cemented veneer crowns and the crushing strength of the cements. *Acta Odontol. Scand.* **25**, 355.
McLean J. W. (1972) Polycarboxylate cements. Five years' experience in general practice. *Br. Dent. J.* **132**, 9.
McLean J. W. and von Fraunhofer J. A. (1971) The estimation of cement film thickness by an 'in vivo' technique. *Br. Dent. J.* **131**, 107.
Moffa J. P., Jenkins W. A. and Razzono, M. R. (1970) An evaluation of zinc-oxide and eugenol cements. IADR 48th General Meeting, New York, Paper No. 669.
Norman R. D., Swartz M. L. and Phillips R. W. (1966) Direct pH determinations of setting cements. I. A test method and the effects of storage time and media. *J. Dent. Res.* **45**, 136.
Paffenberger G. C. (1972) Dental cements, direct filling resins. Composite and adhesive restorative materials: A résumé. *J. Biomed. Mater. Res.* **6**, 363.
Peyton F. A. and Craig R. G. (1971) *Restorative Dental Materials,* 4th ed. St Louis, Mosby.
Phillips R. W. and others (1968) Zinc oxide and eugenol cements for permanent cementation. *J. Prosthet. Dent.* **19**, 144.
Phillips R. W., Swartz M. L. and Norman R. D. (1969) *Materials for the Practising Dentist.* St Louis, Mosby.
Phillips R. W., Swartz M. L. and Rhodes B. (1970) An evaluation of a carboxylate adhesive cement. *J. Am. Dent. Assoc.* **81**, 1353.
Plant C. G. (1970) The effect of polycarboxylate cement on tne dental pulp. *Br. Dent. J.* **129**, 424.
Richter W. A., Mitchem J. C. and Brown J. D. (1970) Predictability of retentive values of dental cements. *J. Prosthet. Dent.* **24**, 298.
Smith D. C. (1967) A new dental cement. *Br. Dent. J.* **123**, 540.
Smith D. C. (1971) Dental cements. *Dental Clin. North Am.* **15**, 3.

General References

Bergman B. (1977) The effects of prosthodontic materials on oral tissues. *Oral Sci. Rev.* **10**, 75.
Combe E. C. and Grant A. A. (1972) The selection and properties of materials for dental practice, Parts I to VIII. *Br. Dent. J.* **134**, 18, 95, 134, 197, 240, 287, 333.
Dickson G. and Cassel J. M. (ed.) *Dental Materials Research,* National Bureau of Standards Special Publication 354, Washington.
Hannah C. McD. and Smith D. C. (1972) Tensile strength of selected restorative materials. *J. Prosthet. Dent.* **26**, 314.
Phillips R. W. (1972) Report of the Committee on Scientific Investigation of the American Academy of Restorative Dentistry. *J. Prosthet. Dent.* **28**, 82.

5

PONTICS

Properties required of a Bridge Pontic
Pontic Design. Materials used
Types of Pontic
Choice of Pontic Type for Specific Cases

The main purposes of a bridge are the same as those already discussed in Chapter 2 when considering why missing teeth should be replaced. However, the two primary factors are usually aesthetics and function and if one or both of these cannot be materially improved then there is little point in proceeding.

PROPERTIES REQUIRED OF A BRIDGE PONTIC

The properties of the various materials used in the construction of a bridge pontic have already been discussed in Chapter 4 and the specific requirements of a pontic will now be considered.

■ Reliability

The most important property of a pontic and its associated facing is that it shall stay in place. This implies that it will outlast the life expectancy of the rest of the bridge. It is most disappointing when an otherwise satisfactory prosthesis has to be replaced after 2–3 years because of pontic failure, such as a facing repeatedly becoming detached (*Fig*. 5.1).

Should any distortion or flexing of the gold supporting an individual facing take place it will result in cementation failure, particularly if the facing is constructed of porcelain. Acrylic will tolerate some degree of flexion and thus it is rare for a facing made of this material to become detached. However, leakage may occur at the margins and give rise to staining and moreover the discoloration and wear of acrylic may shorten the life of the pontic. Undoubtedly the most reliable, hygienic and aesthetically pleasing pontics can now be produced by employing porcelain bonded to gold.

■ Good Aesthetics

The commonest reason for patients requesting a bridge is that the loss of a

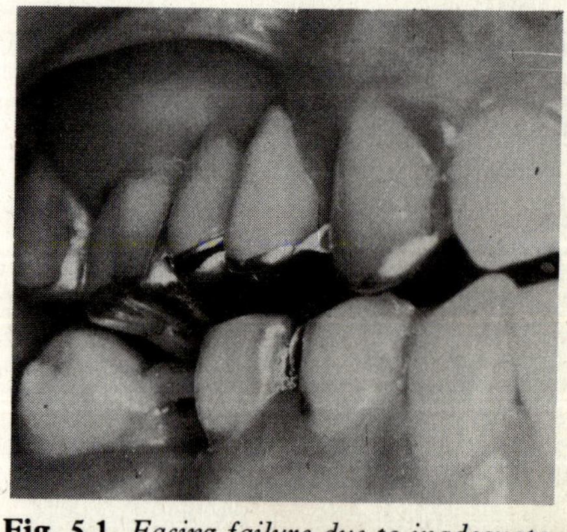

Fig. 5.1. *Facing failure due to inadequate occlusal gold and an incorrect occlusion.*

tooth is marring their appearance. Therefore, if at the end of treatment the pontic does little to remedy this situation then the bridge is obviously a failure. However, the degree of perfection required will vary with both the patient and the missing tooth. Thus if an upper second premolar is being replaced for an elderly man the aesthetic requirements are obviously far less than if an upper central is missing in a girl of 21.

■ Colour Stability

Not only must the pontic match the adjoining teeth immediately after cementation but it is desirable that it still does so 5, 10, or even 15 years later. In this respect acrylic is poor, often discolouring appreciably in a matter of 4–5 years and requiring replacement in the anterior region within 6–7 years. However, the expectation of life of an acrylic facing varies appreciably both with the acrylic used and with the patient. Porcelain does not discolour, which is generally an advantage; but it must be remembered that the natural dentition gradually darkens with age and thus after 15 years the porcelain pontic may well be considerably lighter than the other teeth.

■ Hygiene

All pontics should be designed so that they give rise to the minimum of food retention and plaque formation. They should also be constructed so that it is relatively simple for the patient to keep them clean by means of tape, dental floss, and interdental stimulators. Power-operated water cleaners may also be of use in this respect.

■ Non-irritant to the Soft Tissues

The pontic should not give rise to any soft-tissue irritation. Factors which effect this are its morphology and the material from which it is made. These will be considered under pontic design.

■ Will not Overload the Abutment Teeth

It is important that the pontic is designed in such a way that the periodontal tissues of the abutment teeth are not overloaded. This factor is, of course, interrelated with the choice of abutments.

LOAD APPLIED TO THEM.

PONTIC DESIGN

The following are the main factors to be considered when designing a pontic.

■ Interproximal Embrasures

The interdental spaces should generally be relatively large (*Fig.* 5.2) to assist natural self cleansing and also the use of

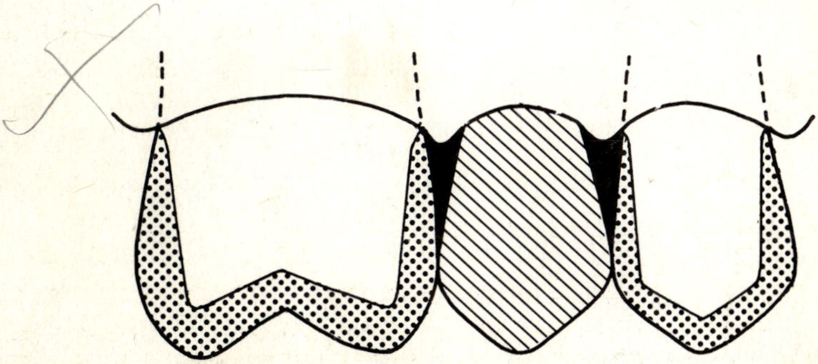

Fig. 5.2. *Wide interproximal embrasures are required to simplify cleansing by dental floss and other means to reduce plaque formation.*

dental floss and wood sticks, by the patient. This is mainly applicable to the posterior region. With the anterior pontic aesthetics demands as natural a contour as possible. However, in this region the provision of adequate interdental spaces is far less critical as they are much simpler to keep clean because of their small width buccolingually. A point to be guarded against, particularly with anterior bridges, is the creation of a large interproximal embrasure but a correspondingly weak solder joint (*Fig*. 5.3).

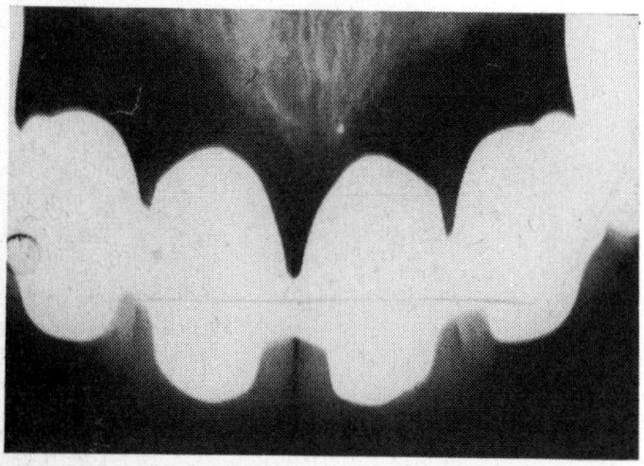

Fig. 5.3. *Relatively weak interproximal gold which may result in bridge failure. See also Fig*. 5.11.

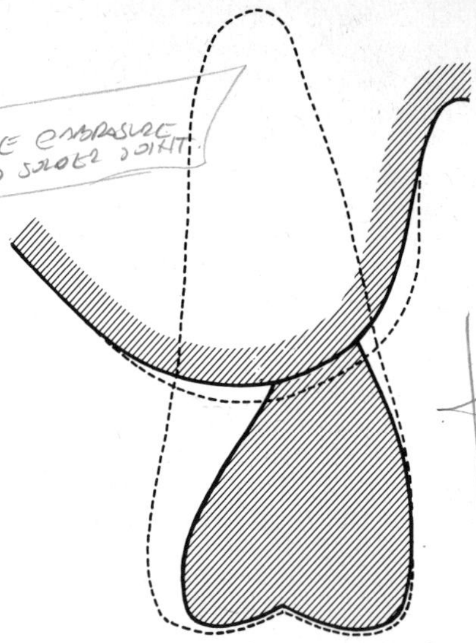

Fig. 5.4. *Soft-tissue contact of the pontic should be kept relatively small. This may be achieved by decreasing the occlusal width and curving the lingual aspect in considerably, and the buccal aspect a little, relative to the tooth it replaces (original tooth and ridge contour shown by dotted line).*

■ Tissue Covered

The tissue contact area of the pontic should be kept relatively small (*Fig*. 5.4). On the buccal or labial aspects its outline usually has to correspond fairly closely with that of the tooth it replaces, for aesthetic reasons, although it can be moved lingually or palatally a little as the case may be. This will vary to some extent with the smile line and the position of the tooth being replaced.

Aesthetics are not nearly so critical on the inner aspect of the pontic and thus this surface can be curved in so as to join the mucosa at a position approaching the crest of the ridge. This minimizes soft-tissue contact and ideally should be almost a straight line.

Some authorities consider that point contact is best for most pontics; however, this is only applicable where there is rather more than average vertical dimension in which to house the pontic and where aesthetics permit it. If the bite is close what should be an easily cleanable pontic becomes most unhygienic (*Fig*. 5.5).

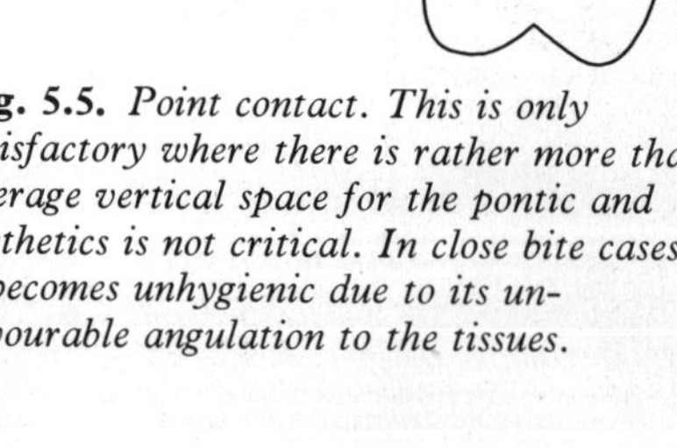

Fig. 5.5. *Point contact. This is only satisfactory where there is rather more than average vertical space for the pontic and aesthetics is not critical. In close bite cases, it becomes unhygienic due to its unfavourable angulation to the tissues.*

So far as the provision of an easily cleanable pontic is concerned the cantilever bridge is nearly ideal because it is bounded on the one side only by an abutment tooth and it is extremely easy for the patient to pass dental floss beneath it (*Fig*. 5.6).

■ Occlusal Surface

The occlusal form of the pontic should roughly correspond with that of the tooth it replaces. In the posterior region it is important that it be confined within the margins of the abutment teeth (*Fig*. 5.7). It is sometimes desirable to decrease the width by about 20 per cent to reduce any torque on the retainers and abutments and simplify the provision of an easily cleanable pontic with minimal soft-tissue contact. However, the width of pontic required will be governed by such factors as aesthetics, the length of span, the strength of the abutment teeth, the ridge form and last but not least the occlusion.

The angulation of the cusps depends on that of the neighbouring teeth and the articulation in general. If the tooth opposing the pontic has overerupted then it is important that it be either ground back to its correct occlusal contour or even crowned before proceeding with the bridge.

■ Tissue Contact

Ideally the tissue contact should be entirely of glazed porcelain as less plaque forms on this than any other dental material. If this cannot be employed then gold should be used; however, this does attract more plaque. The use of acrylic

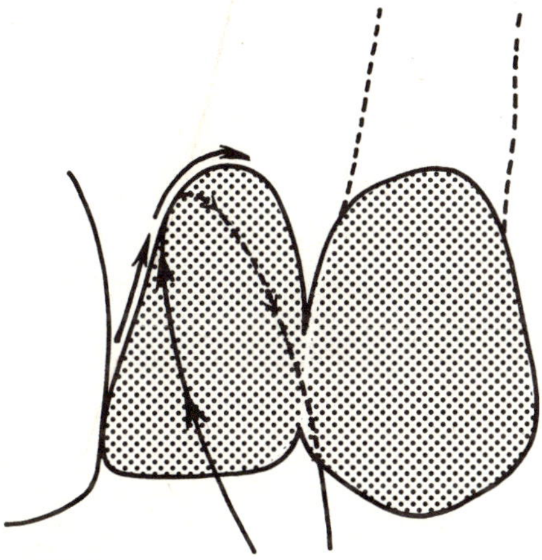

Fig. 5.6. *The passing of dental floss beneath a cantilever bridge.*

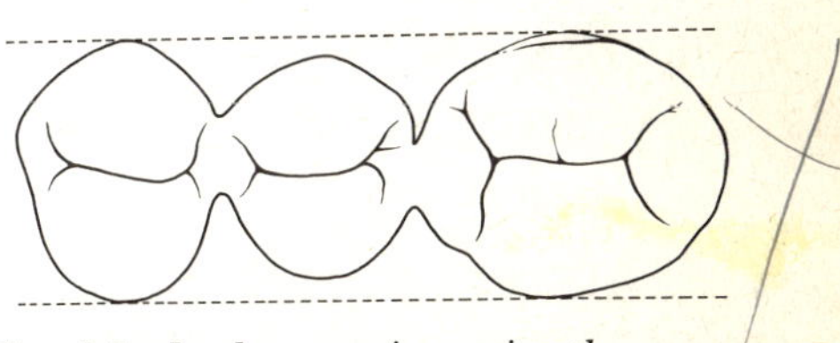

Fig. 5.7. *In the posterior region the occlusal surface of the pontic should be confined within the margins of the abutment teeth.*

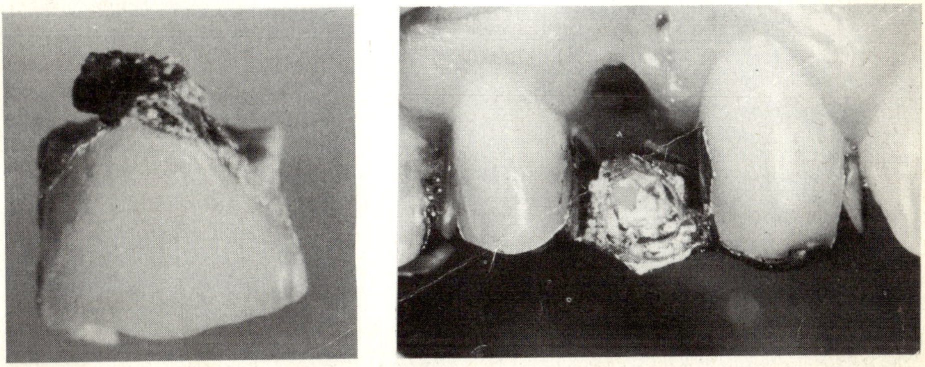

Fig. 5.8. *Calculus on the fit surface of a pontic and the resultant soft-tissue irritation.*

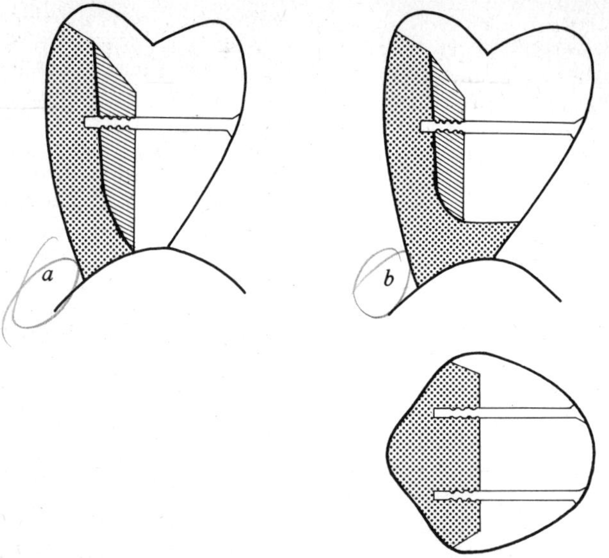

Fig. 5.9. *a, A long-pin pontic with an undesirable junction between the porcelain and the gold on the fit surface. b, An addition has been made to the facing to give all-porcelain to tissue contact.*

results in more gingival irritation than any other material, particularly after it has been in the mouth for a few years, has absorbed moisture, and possibly become foul. It also attracts calculus deposition (*Fig.* 5.8).

A junction between two different materials on the fit surface should be avoided so far as possible (*Fig.* 5.9) as, however perfect, it is bound to lead to increased plaque retention in this area. For the same reason all facings should be cemented to the gold work before the bridge is fitted so that the fit surface may be checked, thus avoiding any chance of residual cement impinging on the mucosa.

Similarly cold-curing acrylic should never be used to fix a bridge pontic in place, particularly in the mouth, and indeed should never be allowed to come into contact with the gingival tissues. The actual area of tissue contact should be kept to the minimum compatible with good hygiene and aesthetics.

When a bridge is placed the pontic should exert only *slight* pressure on the tissues. Should a space exist between pontic and mucosa this will usually close if it is 0·1 mm or less. If it is more than this, it may not close, particularly if the patient's oral hygiene is good. Should the pontic press too hard on the mucosa the tissues will tend to proliferate up around it (*Fig.* 5.10). Although initially it may give a very natural appearance it results in a pontic which is impossible for the patient to clean satisfactorily.

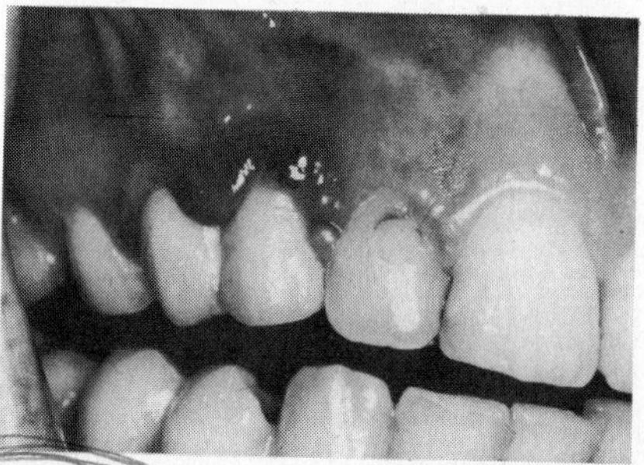

Fig. 5.10. *A bridge 1 year after placement in which the pontic has been let in too deeply and soft-tissue proliferation has resulted.*

■ Length of Span

It must be remembered that the longer the span of the pontic area the greater will be the stress imposed on both the pontics and the solder joints (*see Fig.* 3.9, p. 41) when a load is applied to them and thus the stronger they need to be. This is particularly true in the anterior region where the solder joint or interproximal metal tends to be weak (*Fig.* 5.11).

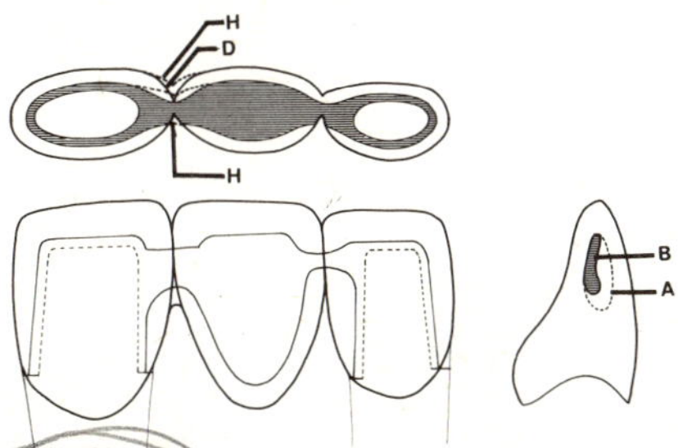

Fig. 5.11. *The interproximal area of an anterior bridge should not be excessively weakened* (B) *merely to improve aesthetics and give a good appearance of separation* (D). *The contact area should be enlarged* (A) *by increasing both the width of the junction* (H) *and also the depth.*

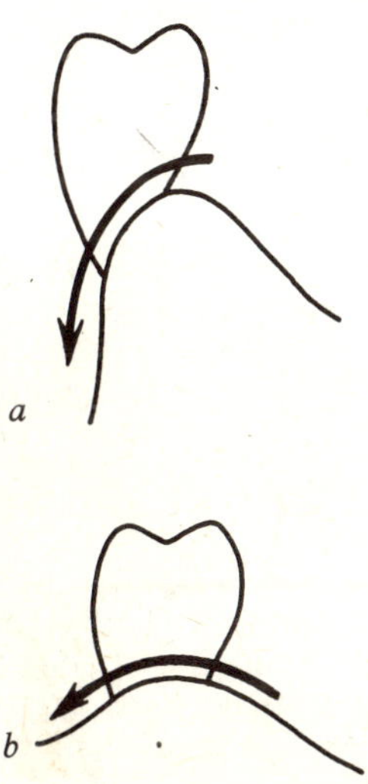

Fig. 5.12. *Favourable* (*a*) *and unfavourable* (*b*) *ridge forms for providing a pontic the fit surface of which is easy to keep clean.*

■ Relationship of Ridge Form to Pontic Design

Basically a fairly sharp ridge such as that shown in *Fig.* 5.12 *a* is favourable as it enables a self-cleansing pontic to be placed relatively easily, whereas a flat ridge makes the construction of a hygienic pontic difficult, particularly if the bite is close and there is a lack of vertical space with the teeth in occlusion. The food tends to accumulate beneath it as there is little natural shedding. Where there is adequate vertical clearance the problem may be overcome by placing a sanitary pontic.

MATERIALS USED

These have already been discussed in Chapter 4. Suffice to say here that a combination of porcelain and gold, preferably bonded, will produce the best pontic in the majority of cases. The tissue contact should usually be of porcelain and it is best if there is no junction between two different materials in this area as however well this is executed it will be bound to cause plaque formation.

TYPES OF PONTIC

The types of pontic employed in bridge work may be classified according to the means of retention employed for the facing. This may be by:

1. Rails.
2. Pins.
3. Cores and posts.
4. Bonding to the metal.
5. Mechanical locking.

As well as the foregoing the pontic may be constructed entirely of acrylic, porcelain, or gold.

■ 1. Retention by Rails

These may be divided into those having a vertical and those having a horizontal line

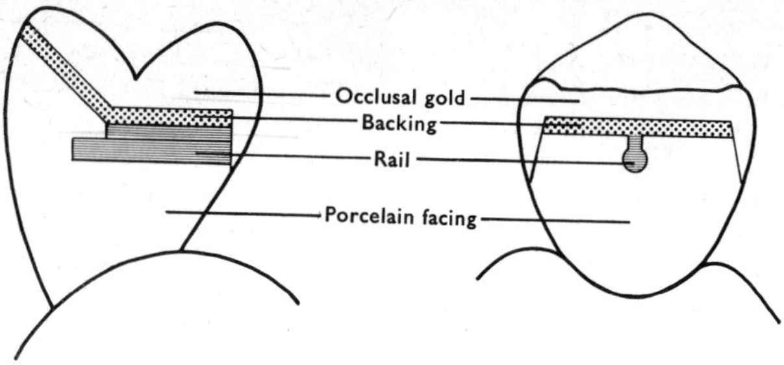

Fig. 5.13. *The Trupontic. The occlusal surface may be made either of a separate backing and occlusal gold or entirely of gold by incorporating a plastic backing in the wax-up. It is desirable to incorporate a lingual skirt of gold to seal the end of the rail and increase the rigidity of the casting.*

of insertion. An example of the former is the Steeles slotted facing and an example of the latter is the Trupontic.

a. Vertical Insertion

The basic design of this type is a rail on to which is slotted a porcelain facing. Gold is added to the backing on its lingual aspect so as to reinforce it and produce the correct contour.

It is a relatively fragile facing, partly because the porcelain is weakened by the slot cut in it to accommodate the rail and also because it is impossible to protect the incisal edge satisfactorily.

For these reasons the incisal withdrawal slotted facing is now seldom used.

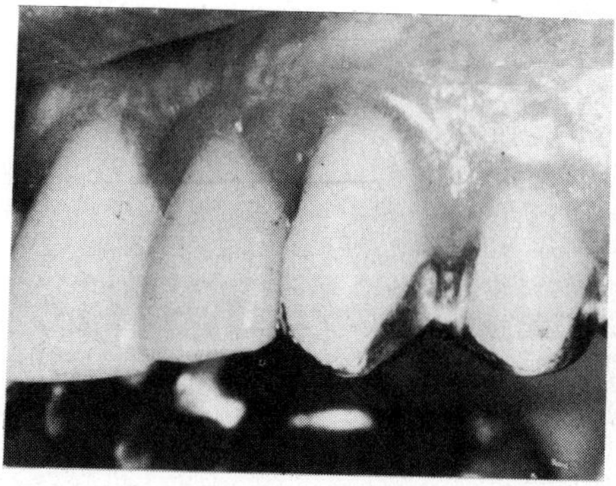

Fig. 5.14. *All-porcelain incisal pontics used to replace the upper incisors.* (*By courtesy of Mr T. R. Hill.*)

b. Horizontal Insertion

This type may be constructed in two ways, either to give a gold occlusal surface and a porcelain to tissue contact, or a porcelain occlusal and a gold fit surface. An example of the former is the Trupontic and of the latter the Steeles all-porcelain occlusal pontic. Neither has any advantage over the bonded porcelain pontic and they are far less reliable. However, they may sometimes be of use if no facilities are available for carrying out metal-ceramic work and the occlusion is favourable.

i. Trupontic

This may be employed in either the anterior or posterior regions, but is more commonly of use in the latter situation. It has the advantages that as it has a horizontal line of withdrawal its occlusal surface can be protected by gold and a porcelain to tissue contact may be achieved (*Fig.* 5.13).

Its main disadvantage is that it is unsuitable in cases where the vertical dimension is at all limited. This is because it is impossible to accommodate all the components, i.e. occlusal gold, backing, rail and porcelain, without a resultant weakness of one or more of these.

ii. Steeles All-porcelain Occlusal Pontic

This is the reverse of the Trupontic

which has already been described. Aesthetically it is very pleasing (*Fig*. 5.14) but it is fragile and should only be used in cases where the occlusion is very favourable. Its other disadvantages are that the tissue contact is mainly in gold and that there is a gold/porcelain junction on this surface.

2. Retention by Pins

This is probably the most versatile of manufactured facings. A popular form is the *long pin pontic* in which the pins are taken right through the gold and riveted on its lingual aspect (*see Fig*. 5.9), thus providing positive retention. However, the facing must still be carefully boxed in and occlusal protection provided if failure is to be avoided.

Advantages of this type of facing are that it permits a good thickness of gold to be used on the occlusal surface and that by baking on to its fit surface an all-porcelain to tissue contact may be achieved. It can be used satisfactorily in cases where the bite is close or the space is limited mesiodistally. Its failure rate is low and it can be accommodated in many cases where it would be impossible to house a Trupontic.

An alternative to the long pin is the *reverse pin facing* in which 4–5 parallel holes are drilled in a porcelain facing which has already been ground to size. A casting, complete with pins, is then made to fit the facing and complete the pontic.

3. Cores and Posts

a. Cores

An example of the use of cores, which are usually in the shape of a porcelain jacket crown preparation, is the gold subframe with porcelain jacket crowns placed over this (*Fig*. 5.15). They may also be used in the simple cantilever bridge. The advantage of this method is that an

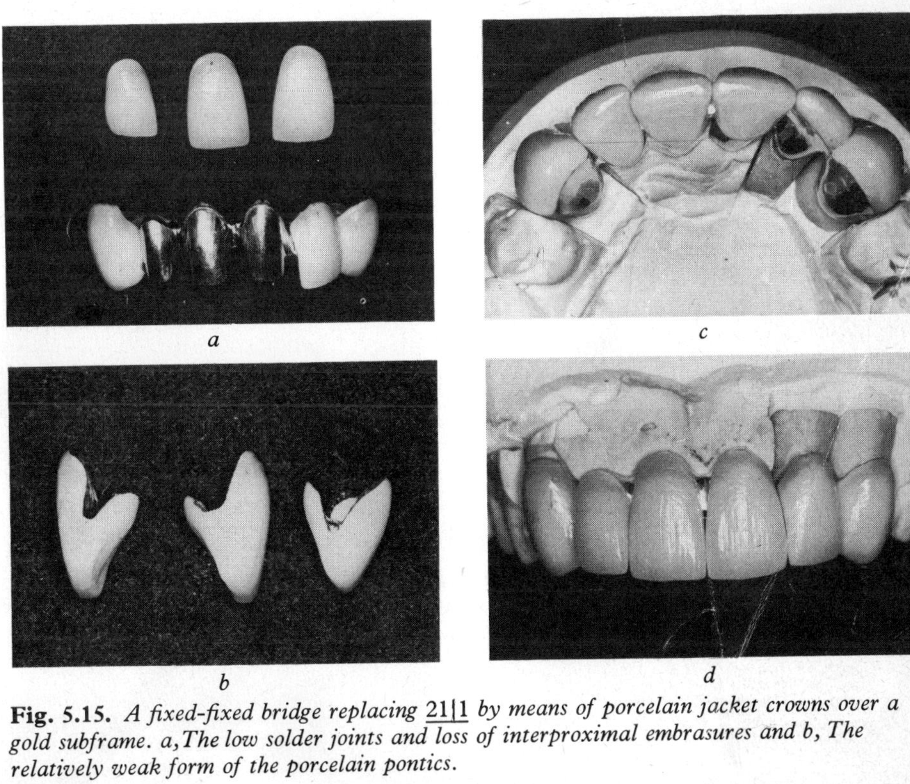

Fig. 5.15. *A fixed-fixed bridge replacing 21|1 by means of porcelain jacket crowns over a gold subframe. a, The low solder joints and loss of interproximal embrasures and b, The relatively weak form of the porcelain pontics.*

extremely good aesthetic result may be achieved even in the younger patient where the shades achieved with the bonded materials are sometimes unsatisfactory. Furthermore the facing can be adapted relatively easily to any given pontic space and individual facings may be replaced should they fail. The disadvantages are:

i. The gingivally placed solder joints (*Figs*. 5.16, 5.17) which make satisfactory oral hygiene difficult to carry out and so predispose to periodontal disease. This is of less importance with the anterior pontic, which is relatively thin linguobuccally, than in the posterior region.

ii. The junctions between the retainers and pontics of the bridge leads to a weakness in the porcelain jacket (*see Fig*. 5.15*b*) which can result in its failure. This is particularly likely to occur in the posterior region.

iii. There is gold rather than porcelain soft tissue contact.

A further use of the porcelain jacket type pontic is in the spring bridge (*Fig*. 5.18). Here it is nearly ideal. Excellent aesthetics may be achieved and because of the flexibility of the bar, which in effect provides a built-in shock absorber, it is rare for a pontic to fracture. Should it do so then it is relatively easily replaced without disturbing the bridge.

For aesthetic reasons and to minimize gingival irritation in this area a porcelain to tissue contact is used labially.

b. Post-retained Pontics

Examples of the post-retained pontic are the tube tooth, which has now largely gone out of favour, and the alumina tube pontic.

The basis of the latter is the use of an extremely strong oval alumina tube

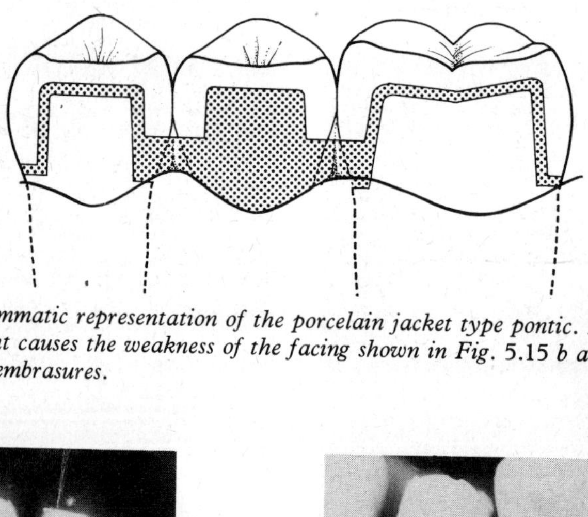

Fig. 5.16. *Diagrammatic representation of the porcelain jacket type pontic. It can be seen that the solder joint causes the weakness of the facing shown in Fig. 5.15 b and the loss of the interproximal embrasures.*

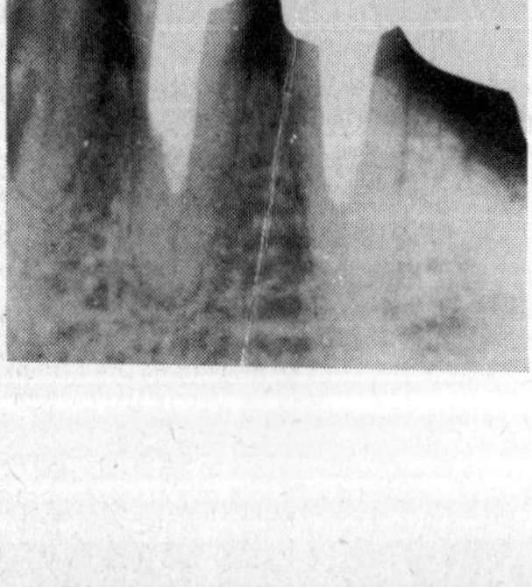

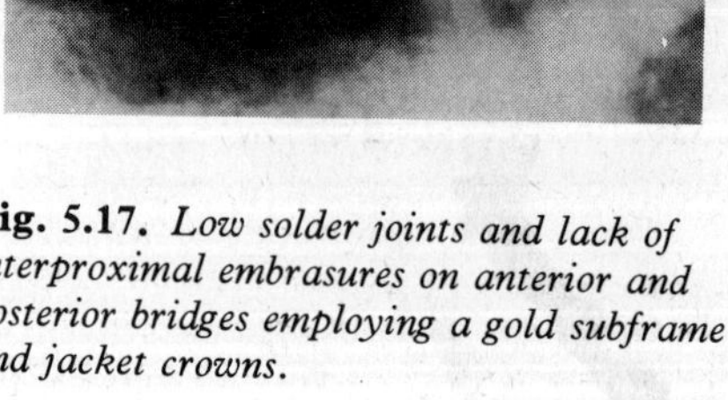

Fig. 5.17. *Low solder joints and lack of interproximal embrasures on anterior and posterior bridges employing a gold subframe and jacket crowns.*

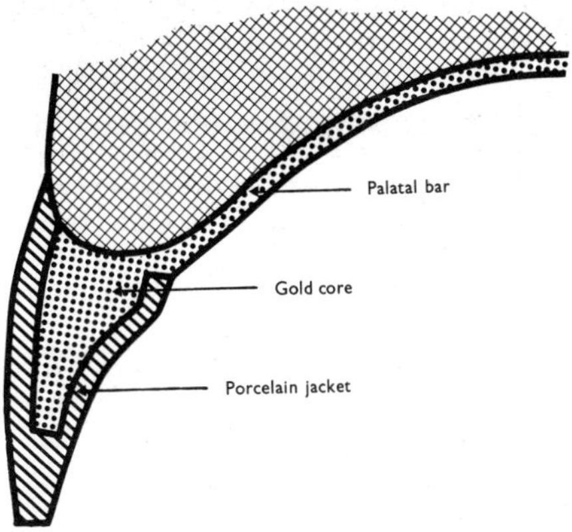

Fig. 5.18. *A porcelain jacket type pontic being used for a spring bridge.*

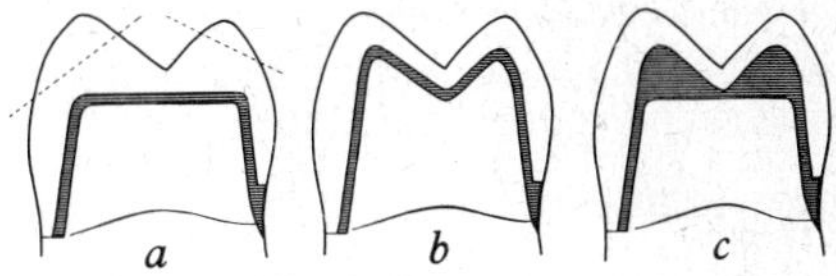

Fig. 5.19. *During preparation the orginal contour of the tooth should be followed as in (b) otherwise the porcelain will exceed its critical thickness (a) and be likely to fracture. The maleffects of a flat-topped preparation may be mitigated by making certain that the external surface of the goldwork follows the external surface of the tooth (c).*

positioned at an angle of approximately 30° to the occlusal plane. On to the tube is fired porcelain which is built up to tooth contour. This is then supported by a gold substructure incorporating the post which passes into the alumina tube. Unfortunately although the pontic has several theoretical advantages its use has now been largely discontinued because of its very high failure rate.

■ 4. Bonded Pontics

In many ways the ideal combination of pontic materials is porcelain bonded to gold, where it is probable that a chemical bond occurs between the two. Thus it is possible to obtain the strength of gold and at the same time have the excellent aesthetics and tissue tolerance of porcelain. The bond of the porcelain to the gold is such that the strength of the latter is thereby materially increased. It has the further advantage that there is little chance of the porcelain becoming detached from the framework as can happen, for instance, with the Trupontic. In the majority of instances both the fit and the occlusal surfaces may be made of porcelain, although in practice many operators prefer to have gold occlusally.

It is capable of producing pontics of widely varying shapes and sizes, even the most difficult of cases being possible. Its only disadvantage is in the lower anterior region (*see Fig*. 6.48, p. 108) where the limited space available to accommodate both the facing and its metal backing may result in an indifferent aesthetic result. Likewise it is a difficult material with which to achieve a satisfactory result when the lighter shades are required, for instance in a girl of 21. It is here that it may sometimes be better to use the porcelain jacket type pontic.

Probably the most important point to remember when building bonded porcelain pontics is that the porcelain should not exceed 1·5 mm in thickness particularly on the cusps, otherwise failure is likely to result (*Fig*. 5.19).

Base Metal Alloys

The bonding of porcelain to base metal alloys such as nickel-chrome has already been discussed in Chapter 4. The principal use of this technique would seem to be in the construction of long span bridges where the greater strength of the base metal when compared with gold may prove an advantage; however, in practice the less efficient bonding between the materials more than negates this.

■ 5. Mechanical Locking

An acrylic pontic may be prepared and then cured on to the gold work, mechanical retention being obtained either by means of surface irregularities of the gold casting which can be deliberately created, or by the boxing in of the acrylic. Thus it is scarcely surprising that it is extremely rare for this facing to become displaced. However, it does have most of the disadvantages of acrylic mentioned in Chapter 4.

When it is employed it is important that the whole of the fit surface is made of gold so as to keep any gingival irritation to a minimum. Moreover the occlusal surface should also be entirely in gold to provide a stable occlusion. It is best to use a manufactured acrylic facing as this will be harder and have better colour stability than one made in the laboratory.

■ The All-acrylic Pontic

On grounds of strength, wear, tissue tolerance and colour stability the all-acrylic pontic can be dismissed as being completely unsatisfactory as a permanent bridge pontic. However, it is an extremely useful material for the construction of a temporary bridge which may be required before fitting the permanent restoration. A further use is as an immediate replacement where it only has to last 4–6 months until healing is complete and the final bridge can be placed. This avoids the patient having to wear a denture.

■ The All-porcelain Pontic

This is only applicable to the all-porcelain bridge which is discussed in greater detail on pp. 45–46 and 132–135. However, it is worth noting here that the reliability of the all-porcelain cantilever bridge is good whereas with fixed-fixed designs the prognosis is poor. It produces an excellent aesthetic result and the pontic as such seldom fractures. It is the all-porcelain retainers on either side which are more likely to fail.

■ The All-gold Pontic

This may be of use in two instances:

a. Where there is very limited space and aesthetics is of little importance. Here the simplicity of just constructing the pontic in gold enables its morphology to be nearer the ideal than when a facing has to be accommodated. It is also relatively easy to provide satisfactory interproximal embrasures and a favourable ridge contact.

b. The sanitary pontic: Where aesthetics is of little importance, as in the lower posterior region, then the sanitary pontic may be employed (*Fig.* 5.20). This consists of a bar of gold connecting the two retainers which is kept well clear of the soft tissues (*Fig.* 5.21*a*). This latter is essential, otherwise food packing and gingival proliferation will occur beneath it (*Fig.* 5.21*b*). For the same reason this pontic can only be satisfactorily employed where there has been appreciable ridge resorption.

The undersurface should be curved in a buccolingual direction so as to make it as self cleansing and easily cleansable by the patient as possible. It should also be arched mesiodistally.

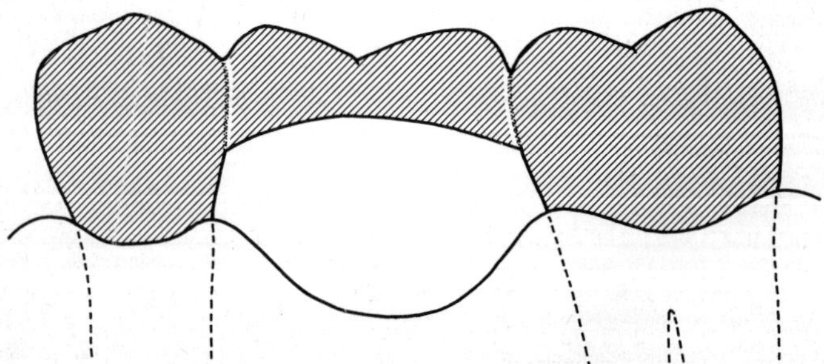

Fig. 5.20. *An all-gold sanitary pontic. Note the 'arching' of the undersurface to provide maximum clearance, thus simplifying cleaning and reducing food stagnation.*

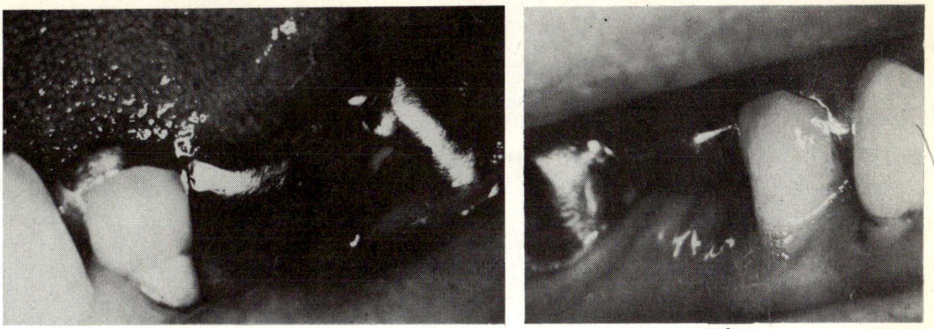

a b

Fig. 5.21. *a, A favourable case for a sanitary pontic where there is considerable soft-tissue loss. b, An unfavourable case for a sanitary pontic in which there is inadequate clearance and thus gingival proliferation occurred.*

CHOICE OF PONTIC TYPE FOR SPECIFIC CASES

The choice of pontic type for any particular case may vary with such factors as the materials being used for the retainers, the space and vertical dimension available, the angulation of the abutment teeth, the region involved, the aesthetic requirements and the ridge form.

Thus if the retainers being employed are bonded full crowns then the same materials will probably be used for the pontics. They are also the materials of choice for the majority of other anterior and posterior pontics.

In the posterior region if there is plenty of clearance and aesthetics is of little importance a sanitary pontic is best. However, if space is very limited the all-gold pontic touching the mucosa may be the answer.

In the average posterior bridge when full or three-quarter gold crowns are being employed the long-pin or reverse pin may be used instead of the bonded-porcelain pontic, providing that an occlusal display of gold is acceptable to the patient.

The porcelain jacket type pontic is ideal for all spring bridges and can also on occasions be valuable in the younger patient where aesthetics is at a premium and other bridge designs are being employed.

The use of gold and acrylic pontics is generally confined to bridges where the expectation of life of the prosthesis is only 5–7 years.

One further factor to be considered is that the golds used with bonded porcelain are softer than those generally employed for bridges and thus should be made somewhat thicker to allow for this. When used for the construction of the dovetail of a fixed-movable bridge they should be a little heavier than when a hard gold is used.

Bibliography

Cavazos E., jun. (1968) Tissue response to fixed partial denture pontics. *J. Prosthet. Dent.* **20,** 143.

Clayton J. A. and Green E. (1970) Roughness of pontic materials and dental plaque. *J. Prosthet. Dent.* **23,** 407.

Henry P. J., Johnson J. F. and Mitchell D. F. (1966) Tissue changes beneath fixed partial dentures. *J. Prosthet. Dent.* **16,** 937.

Perel M. L. (1972) A modified sanitary pontic. *J. Prosthet. Dent.* **38,** 589.

Peyton F. A. and Craig R. G. (1963) Current evaluation of plastics in crown and bridge prosthesis. *J. Prosthet. Dent.* **13,** 743.

Roche H. A. P. (1949) An assessment of the values of porcelain versus methyl-methacrylate in jacket crown and bridge work. *Br. Dent. J.* **87,** 25.

Sheets, C. E. (1966) A split cast procedure for the replacement of pontics. *J. Prosthet. Dent.* **16,** 948.

Skurow H. M. and Lyttle J. D. (1971) The interproximal embrasure. *Dent. Clin. North. Am.* **15,** 641.

See also references in Chapter 4.

6

ABUTMENTS AND RETAINERS

Abutments. Retainers. Specific Retainers

ABUTMENTS

Many factors affect the selection of the correct abutments. Amongst these are the following:

■ A. Type of Bridge

With a conventional fixed-fixed or fixed-movable bridge it is seldom possible to choose the abutment teeth to be employed. Those on either side of the missing tooth are the ones which must be incorporated in the design. However, one can vary the number used. Thus in a long-span bridge replacing the lower second premolar and first molar it may be desirable to use both the first premolar and the canine mesial to the gap.

If there is a weak or doubtful tooth on one side of the space it is sometimes better to extract this to allow the bridge to extend to a more suitable abutment.

The cantilever bridge has an advantage over previous bridges mentioned in that support is only required from one side. Thus the use of a weak tooth either mesial or distal to the gap may sometimes be avoided. An example of this is the replacement of the upper canine by a cantilever bridge, the first and second premolars being the abutments. If a fixed-fixed design had been employed the relatively weak upper lateral would have had to be used.

The fact that the spring bridge usually employs an abutment tooth remote from the one being replaced is often of value as it permits considerable flexibility when selecting the most suitable tooth. Thus when replacing the upper central, if the first premolar is unsuitable as an abutment then the second premolar or possibly the canine may be employed.

■ B. Effective Root Surface Area

The effective root surface area or bony support available will determine whether or not a tooth will be able to bear the additional load imposed on it by a pontic. Generally speaking, in fixed-fixed and fixed-movable bridges a periodontally sound tooth can support at least a pontic of equal size and in many instances this load may be safely exceeded. However, in the case of the cantilever bridge the load imposed must be reduced. This is particularly true in the posterior region where only limited cantilevering may be carried out if a single abutment is used. Where the cantilevering is part of a complex fixed prothesis then far more extensive cantilevering may often be possible and indeed even desirable if it is part of the overall periodontal and occlusal treatment of the patient.

The approximate order of strength of

the teeth as bridge abutments, i.e. their ability to bear an additional load, is:

Maximal ⟶ Minimal
Upper 6 3 7 4 5 1 2
Lower 6 3 7 5 4 2 1

However, each tooth requires individual assessment, when such factors as the shape and size of its roots, the degree of eruption and its angulation all need to be taken into account.

■ C. Periodontal Condition

The periodontal condition must always be considered when assessing how suitable a tooth will be as an abutment. The greater the recession and bone loss the less the load that tooth will be able to bear. Whereas with periodontally sound teeth the use of just one abutment on either side of a single tooth replacement may be adequate, if the periodontal condition is unsatisfactory then two or more may have to be utilized.

If the periodontal condition is poor the benefits of splinting imparted by a fixed-fixed bridge may be indicated.

■ D. Crown of Tooth

The condition, degree of eruption, shape and surface area of the crown of the tooth are of paramount importance in assessing its suitability as an abutment.

1. Condition. If the crown is carious and heavily filled it is always desirable to remove the caries and all existing fillings and then restore the tooth with amalgam (*see Fig.* 15.12, p. 197), incorporating pins as necessary, before proceeding with the bridge. Where excessive restoration is required the crown may be too weak to be suitable for bridge work.

2. Degree of Eruption. The degree of eruption of a tooth is the most important factor in determining the amount of retention available. The more fully the tooth is erupted the greater the surface area covered by the retainer, the thicker and more rigid the casting will be, and the more nearly the preparation can be made to approach the ideal of having nearly parallel sides (*see Figs*. 3.4, 3.5, pp. 35, 36). Jørgensen's work with regard to this has already been mentioned in Chapter 3. Other aspects relating to the degree of eruption are dealt with in greater detail in the section on retainers.

3. Shape and Surface Area of Crown. The greater the surface of a crown the more retention can be achieved. Similarly the shape of the crown of a tooth materially affects the degree of retention available (*Fig*. 6.1). This is because retention depends to a large extent on the degree of parallelism between the various aspects of the preparation. It can be seen that on a patient with fairly conical crowns the retention is reduced because the sides of the preparation are relatively divergent. It is usually possible to gain far more retention on a posterior than an anterior

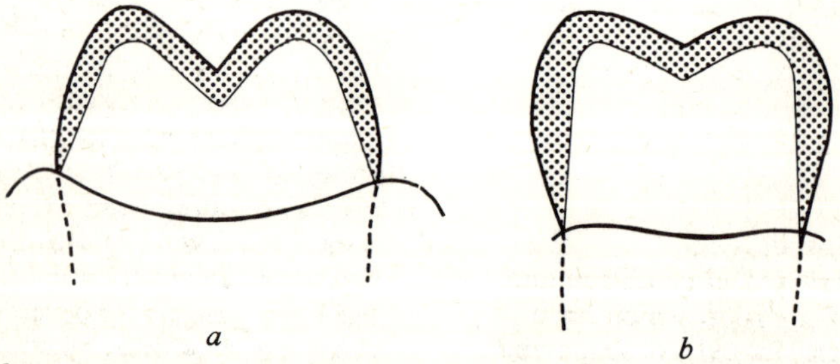

Fig. 6.1. *The degree of retention available on a tooth is materially affected by the shape of the crown. a, Unfavourable, giving widely divergent sides and a thin casting. b, Favourable. Retention would be improved in (a) by using a chamfer finish.*

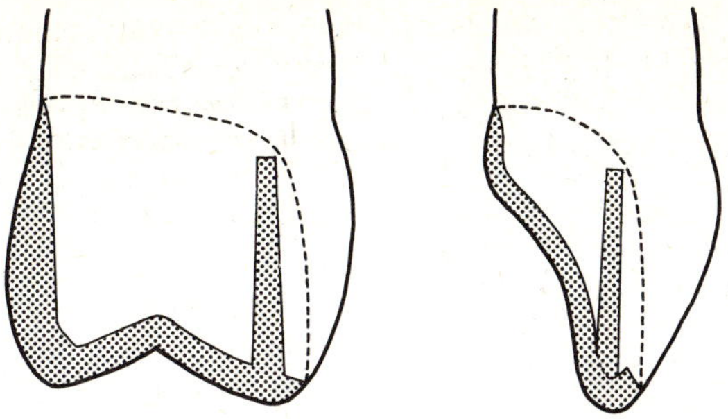

Fig. 6.2. *A comparison of three-quarter crowns on anterior and posterior teeth. It will be seen that only a very short lingual skirt can be obtained on the former and thus retention is correspondingly decreased.*

tooth especially when a three-quarter crown is employed. This is because the area of the surfaces of the preparation opposing each other determine, with other factors, the total retention available. Obviously if any aspect of the preparation, in particular the lingual, is small, as in most anterior teeth, then the resistance to displacement is minimal.

This may be illustrated by comparing a three-quarter crown on the canine with that on a premolar (*Fig.* 6.2). The degree of retention of the former is probably only one-half of the latter, because of the short lingual skirt on the canine preparation. It must also be remembered that it is only the lingual aspect of the slot which aids retention and in the case of the canine this is shorter than the buccal aspect.

The approximate degree of retention available from the different teeth is:

Excellent	⟶						Poor
Upper	6	7	4	5	3	1	2
Lower	6	7	5	4	3	2	1

■ E. Condition of Root

Besides the periodontal condition and surface area of the root, which have already been considered, its shape and apical condition must also be taken into account. If it is non-vital the form of the root canal may be important.

The shape of the root has an appreciable effect on the load which a tooth is able to withstand. Thus the upper first premolar, which is normally two-rooted, is a better abutment tooth than the single-rooted second premolar.

Apical Condition

If a tooth is non-vital then its apical condition must be ascertained and any necessary endodontic therapy carried out.

When a root filling is placed it is desirable to fill only the apical third or less of the root canal so as to leave the rest free for the post which may subsequently be required. After root-canal therapy it is usually desirable to wait at least 6 months so as to be reasonably certain of the tooth's prognosis before using it as a bridge abutment. However, one's approach will vary with the urgency of the bridge and the complexity and prognosis of the root-canal therapy. Thus if an anterior tooth is involved as an abutment the prognosis of any endodontic therapy is usually excellent and should a conventional root filling fail then an apicectomy can be resorted to without disturbing the bridge, so there is little necessity for delay. With a posterior bridge, and particularly where the gap has been present for several years and complex endodontic treatment is involved, then it may well be best to delay construction of the bridge for up to 2 years.

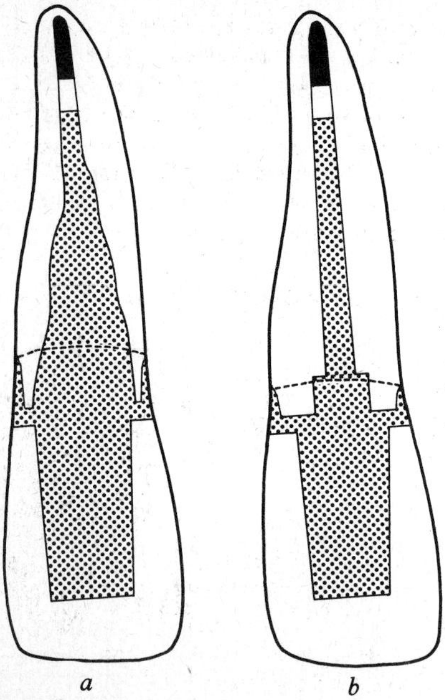

Fig. 6.3. *a, Caries in the root canal appreciably decreases retention and renders the root more liable to fracture. This may to some extent be compensated for by providing a deep cervical collar. b, This technique is also desirable when incorporating the majority of post crowns in bridge work.*

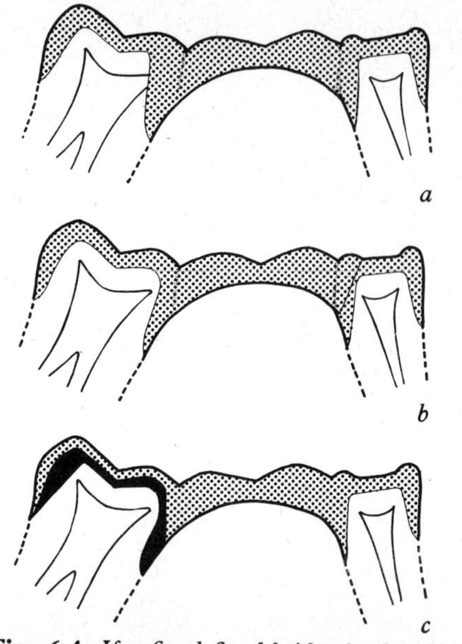

Fig. 6.4. *If a fixed-fixed bridge is placed (a) when teeth are badly tilted then it will result in unretentive preparations and a possible exposure. A fixed-movable bridge (b) will overcome this difficulty. Alternatively, if a fixed-fixed design is essential, then a telescopic (double) full crown technique may be employed (c). Here an initial crown (shown in black) is placed on the molar and the external surface of this milled so that it has the same line of withdrawal as the second retainer.*

■ F. Shape and Number of Root Canals

The shape and number of the root canals will have a material effect on the adequacy of any post crown which may be placed. Thus an extremely satisfactory post can usually be placed in the long straight root canal of an upper canine, whereas the divergent roots of an upper first premolar make adequate retention by a conventional post difficult. Indeed, in this case it is often best to rebuild the tooth with a pinned amalgam with screw posts going down the root canals, and after this carrying out a full crown preparation.

Caries in a root canal may appreciably weaken the root (*Fig.* 6.3) and make it liable to fracture if a post is placed. Similarly, caries in the upper part of the root canal may seriously shorten its effective length.

■ G. Rotated and Tilted Teeth

When the abutment teeth are tilted or rotated it may prove impossible to align the preparations on them for a fixed-fixed bridge without risking either an exposure of the pulp or an unretentive preparation (*Fig.* 6.4*a*). In these instances a fixed-movable bridge is usually indicated (*Fig.* 6.4*b*). However, if a fixed-fixed bridge is required, for instance because the span is long or the periodontal condition poor, it may be possible to achieve this either by using a telescopic full crown technique (*Fig.* 6.4*c*) or by the incorporation of precision retainers in the prosthesis.

When badly tilted or rotated teeth have to be prepared it is wise to have a study model available to refer to, so that the operator always knows exactly how much tooth tissue has been removed and can thus avoid the risk of an exposure.

■ H. Multiple Retainers

When a relatively large number of retainers are employed in a fixed-fixed bridge it may prove impossible to prepare these to give a common path of insertion. This can be overcome by locking the various retainers together with precision attachments.

■ I. Curvature of Arch

In the posterior region the pontics can usually be kept within the width of the abutment teeth. However, in the anterior region the curvature of the arch often precludes this (*Fig*. 6.5) and thus greater care is required if overloading is to be avoided.

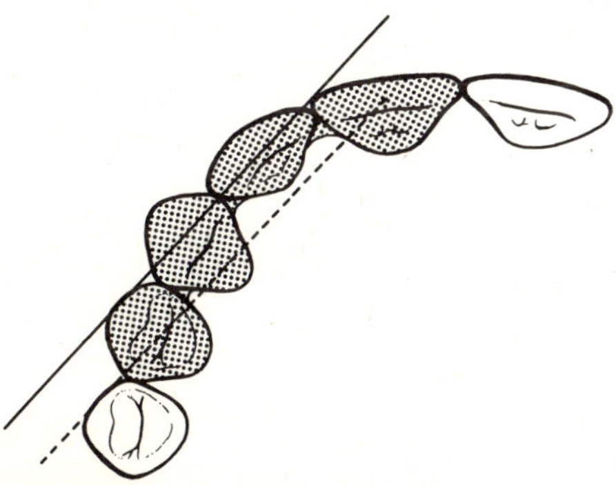

Fig. 6.5. *In the anterior region it is generally impossible to keep the pontics within the width of the abutment teeth because of the curvature of the arch and thus greater stresses are likely to be imposed on them.*

RETAINERS

A retainer may be defined as a casting cemented to an abutment tooth which retains, or helps to retain, a pontic. Its primary function must always be to keep the bridge in place and this consideration should override all others. Cementation failure of a retainer is probably the most serious disaster that can befall a bridge. All too often, particularly in the case of a fixed-fixed design, it leads to rapid caries (*Fig*. 6.6) and the possible loss of the abutment tooth.

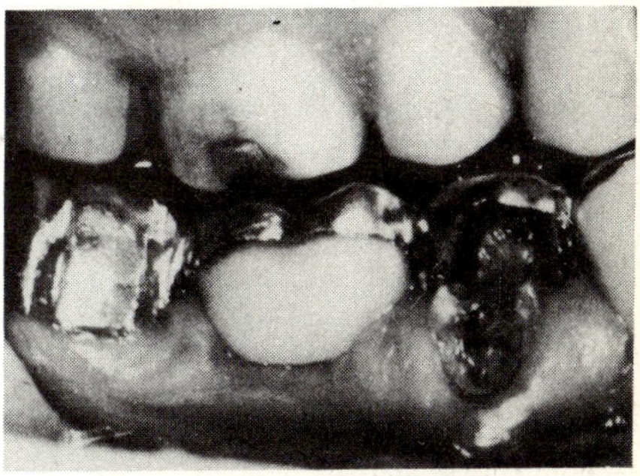

Fig. 6.6. *Rampant caries below an uncemented bridge retainer.*

■ Factors affecting Retention required

The main factors which determine the degree of retention required in any specific instance are:

1. Length of span.
2. Type of bridge.
3. Occlusion.
4. Tooth or teeth to be replaced.
5. Habits of patient.
6. Periodontal condition.

1. Length of Span. The longer the span the greater the stress on the retainers and the more the likelihood of their becoming uncemented. Similarly the castings will be more liable to flex, and therefore great care must be taken to make certain that they are sufficiently rigid. Indeed, the longer the span the stronger must be all the components of a bridge, not only the retainers but also the pontics, solder joints and any connectors.

2. Type of Bridge. Certain types of bridge impose greater stresses on the cementing media of a casting than others. Thus far stronger retainers are required for a fixed-fixed than a fixed-movable bridge. Indeed, comparatively little retention is needed for the minor retainer of a fixed-movable design. This is illustrated by the fact that the failure rate of the three-quarter crown when used as a minor retainer is only one-tenth of that experienced when it is used as a major retainer (*see Fig.* 6.15, p. 91). Similarly the Class II although relatively unretentive is perfectly satisfactory as a minor retainer. Thus where it is desirable to preserve tooth tissue the fixed-movable bridge is normally indicated as far lighter retainers can be used. An example of this is the replacement of the upper first premolar by a fixed-movable bridge using a three-quarter crown on the second premolar as the major retainer and a Selburg modified three-quarter crown on the canine as the minor retainer. In this way any labial display of gold on the canine is avoided and only the minimum of tooth tissue is destroyed. A further advantage is that the incisal edge of the tooth is not involved, which is of particular value when it is subject to a heavy bite in lateral excursions, as in occlusions which possess a canine rise.

3. Occlusion. The occlusal stresses applied to a bridge obviously determine the degree of retention required to resist these. It will vary with the age, sex and muscular development of the patient concerned. The heavier the occlusion the stronger and thicker the gold needed to prevent failure of the retainers or pontics.

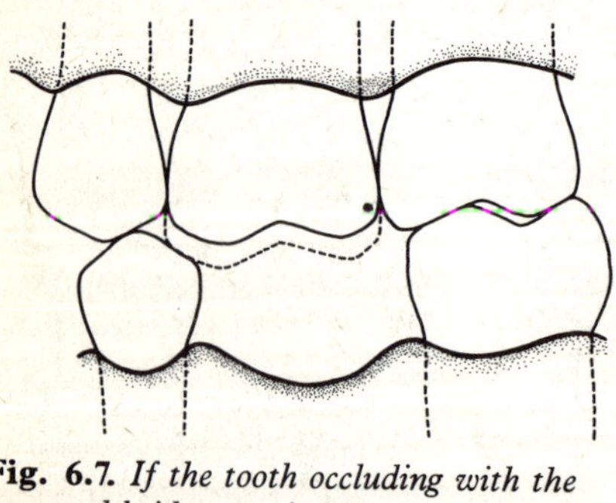

Fig. 6.7. *If the tooth occluding with the proposed bridge pontic has over-erupted it should either be ground or crowned to re-establish the correct occlusal contour.*

The articulation will always influence the selection and design of a retainer, an example being the avoidance of heavy wear facets. However, irregularities in the occlusion should usually be dealt with before commencing the construction of a bridge. Quite frequently the tooth opposing the pontic area has over-erupted and will need equilibrating or even crowning to restore it to the correct occlusal level (*Fig.* 6.7).

4. Tooth or Teeth to be replaced. The size and position of the pontic will have a direct bearing on the type of retainer required. Thus the replacement of a molar will obviously impart a greater stress to the abutments than a lower central. Similarly the occlusal forces applied to a canine are likely to be more than those acting on a central.

5. Habits of Patient. Various habits of the patient may affect a bridge, the most important of these being grinding, which may or may not be amenable to treatment. If a large number of the patient's natural teeth are severely attrited then any gold occluding surface will be similarly worn unless the habit can be corrected. Therefore the castings will have to be thicker and stronger than normal.

Another habit which may lead to difficulties is that of pipe smoking, where the clenching of the teeth on the stem of the pipe will greatly increase the load. The playing of wind instruments may also pose problems.

6. Periodontal Condition. The more rigidly the teeth are retained in their sockets, i.e. the better the periodontal condition, the more they will resist any displacing force. Thus if one abutment of a simple fixed-fixed bridge is moved in a periodontally sound mouth then considerable stress will be created when the second abutment, to which it is rigidly joined, is forced to move also. This may result in failure either in the structure of the bridge or in the cement bond; however, if the periodontal condition is poor and the teeth mobile then little stress will be created when either tooth is displaced as the other one will move readily also. Thus the chances of structural or cementation failure occurring are greatly reduced in these patients. The most unfavourable situation is created when one abutment tooth is firm and all the others are highly mobile, thus imposing a great strain on the retainer on the periodontally sound tooth.

■ Factors affecting Retention Available

The degree of retention which may be obtained from any casting varies with:

1. The tooth involved.
2. The surface area of the retainer.
3. The degree of parallelism that can be obtained as between the various aspects of the preparation.
4. The rigidity of the casting.
5. The cementing media used.
6. The material employed in the construction of the retainer.

The foregoing do not take into account the various methods of achieving additional retention, which will be discussed later.

1. Tooth involved. A guide to the degree of retention available from the various teeth has already been given (p. 83). Another factor to be considered is the size and shape of the teeth of the person being treated. Thus a tooth with a short conical crown will provide far less retention than one with a relatively long crown with near-parallel sides.

2. Surface Area of Casting. The greater the surface area of the casting the more retentive it will be. Thus in the younger patient the relatively short crown of the tooth results in a casting with a low surface area and this must often be compensated by taking the preparation to the maximum depth permitted by the gingival crevice. If necessary a gingivectomy may have to be performed.

In the older patient with well-erupted teeth, particularly if these have become elongated by gingival recession due to periodontal disease, adequate retention may be achieved with supragingival preparations which will result in the minimum of gingival irritation.

3. The Degree of Parallelism between the Various Aspects of the Preparation. Although the relationship between the convergence angle of the two sides of a preparation and the retention available has already been discussed in Chapter 3 it is worth reiterating here that this is probably the most important single factor in retainer design. It is extremely significant that by paying the greatest attention to a preparation and reducing the degree of convergence between its two sides from 10° to 5°, retention, according to Jϕrgensen, is doubled.

The ways of increasing the retention of a preparation with relatively divergent sides is discussed at a later stage in the chapter.

4. Rigidity of the Casting. Lack of rigidity is probably a contributory factor in most retainer failures. Only a very small degree of flexion is needed for the cement seal to be broken and the casting to become loose.

The direct relationship between rigidity and retention can be illustrated by the observation that it is extremely rare for a porcelain jacket crown, which is completely rigid, to become uncemented, whereas the comparatively flexible acrylic jacket frequently fails to stay in place.

The relative lack of rigidity of the three-quarter crown, especially when compared with a full crown, is easily appreciated if it is likened to a cardboard box which, when one side is removed, is reduced to only a fraction of its original strength. The simile may be taken a little further by comparing the conventional MOD slice preparation to a box with two sides missing.

Due to the normal independent vertical movement of the teeth during mastication the leverage on the slice portion of a retainer such as the three-quarter or full crown, particularly in the case of a fixed-fixed bridge, is great. This is because the slice is rigidly joined, via the pontic, to the other retainer.

Thus in the example shown in *Fig.* 6.8, when the molar is depressed the slice attached to the pontic, if weak, is levered away from the tooth at the cervical margin and the cement seal broken. When the masticatory force is released the retainer returns to its original position and looks a perfect fit, but rapid caries will usually ensue.

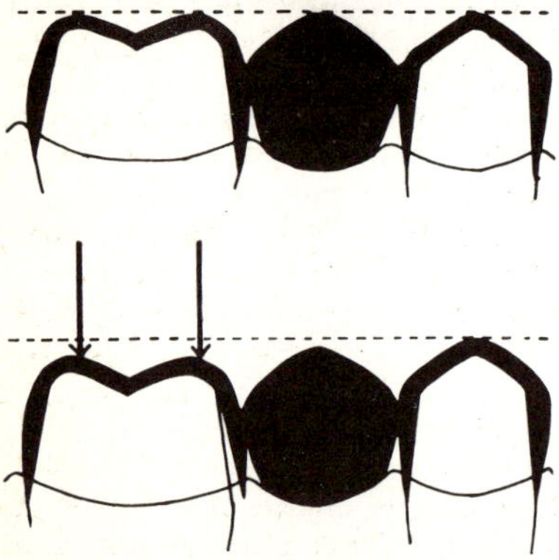

Fig. 6.8. *If a casting lacks rigidity then cementation failure will occur. In this example, depression of the molar will cause flexion of the mesial slice and the breaking of the cement seal.*

The failure is not generally obvious on a radiograph as the lingual gold of the three-quarter crown or full crown masks

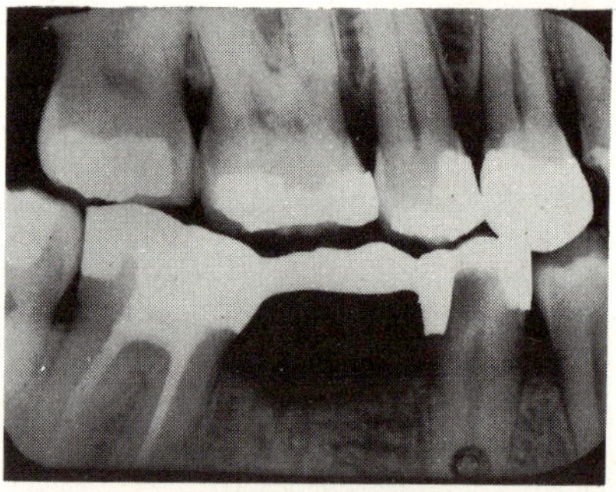

Fig. 6.9. *A fixed-fixed bridge in which flexion of the MOD inlay in 5| has resulted in cementation failure of the distal box.*

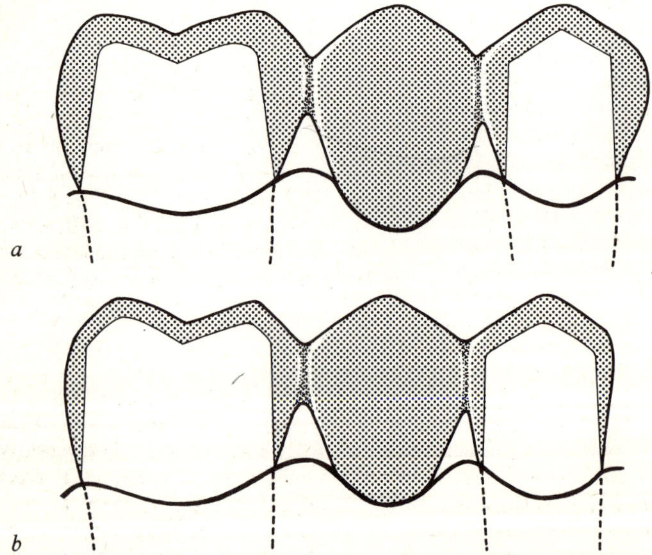

Fig. 6.10. *The thickness of the slices obtainable with a three-quarter crown depends to some extent on the morphology of the teeth. a, Favourable; b, Unfavourable tooth form. Were a chamfer finish to be employed then the thickness of the castings would be increased and retention improved correspondingly, particularly in b (see Fig.* 6.58, p. 113).

nearly all the tooth substance. However, it can normally be seen clearly in the case of an MOD inlay and the radiograph (*Fig.* 6.9) illustrates this. It should be noted that this inlay was still firmly held in place by the mesial box, although the distal box was completely uncemented.

The thickness of the slices in a three-quarter crown depends on the morphology of the teeth involved (*Fig.* 6.10), the amount of tooth tissue which can be removed, and the shape of the finishing margin. This will obviously be directly related to the rigidity of the casting.

5. Cementing Media. The strength of the cement bond obviously directly affects the degree of retention of a casting. With the phosphates and those cements based on zinc oxide and eugenol such as the EBAs, it is probable that no actual chemical bond exists between the cement and the tooth tissue or the gold. Thus the degree of retention they provide is directly related to their compressive and tensile strengths and their film thickness. The thinner the layer of cement the stronger the bond between the materials being joined.

The minimum film thickness is theoretically limited by the size of the cement particles. However, in clinical practice this is of little significance as the thickness of the cement between the casting and the tooth is seldom less than 100 μm, whereas the cement particle size does not usually exceed 30–40 μm.

The polycarboxylates, unlike the other cements currently employed, appear to bond chemically to enamel and possibly to a lesser extent to dentine. However, the results obtained when they are used to join porcelain to gold are poor and even when cementing gold castings in place, particularly post crowns, the bond achieved is inferior to that experienced with the phosphates, as the polycarboxylate fails to adhere to the gold. This may be because of the cement's lower crush strength.

The relative merits of the various types of cement have already been discussed in Chapter 4 and their use will be described in Chapter 18.

6. Material used in the Construction of the Retainer. The material used in the construction of a retainer may vary the degree of retention available for several reasons. If it lacks rigidity, as does acrylic, then it will flex under the stresses of mastication and cause cementation failure. Similarly, if its rate of thermal expansion differs markedly from that of the tooth tissue, as does acrylic, this will lead to a breakdown of the cement bond.

To prevent flexion it is important that only hard golds be used in bridge prostheses. For the same reason all castings should be heat-treated before cementing them in place so as to obtain their optimum strength.

The golds used in porcelain bonded to gold techniques are softer and wear more rapidly than the hard dental golds and this must be taken into account when designing the retainer.

THE RELATIVE RETENTION OF VARIOUS RETAINERS

The correct choice of retainer is of critical importance in any bridge design and emphasis must always be laid on providing too much rather than too little retention. Retainers may be divided into two groups: (A) major retainers which are all those used in fixed-fixed, spring, and cantilever bridges, and (B) minor retainers, implying the lesser retainer of a fixed movable bridge into which the connector from a pontic fits.

A. Major Retainers

Research was carried out at the Institute of Dental Surgery (Roberts, 1970) using similar criteria to those regarding the relationship between the age of the patient and the failure rate of bridges (Roberts, 1970) and expressing the results in the same way. From this it becomes apparent (*Fig.* 6.11) that as a major retainer the posterior full crown with a failure rate of only 0·5 per cent per year is by far the most reliable, and where there is any doubt regarding retention it is the restoration of choice.

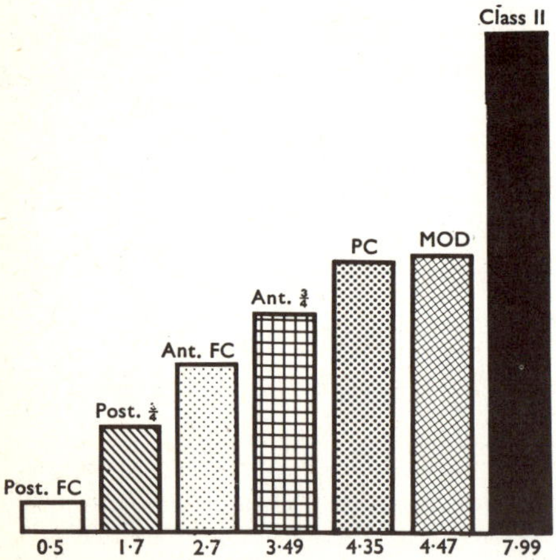

Fig. 6.11. *Relative failure rates per cent per year of major bridge retainers.*

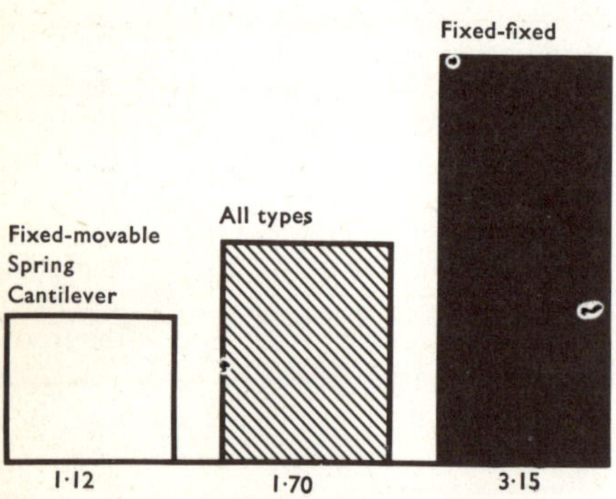

Fig. 6.12. *Relative failure rates per cent per year of the posterior three-quarter crown when used as a major retainer in (a) fixed-fixed and (b) other types of bridge.*

1. Posterior Three-quarter Crown. The failure rate of only 1·7 per cent per year for the posterior three-quarter crown is an acceptable figure which would indicate that a well prepared three-quarter crown is a completely satisfactory retainer for the majority of bridges. However, it is interesting to see (*Fig.* 6.12) that when the use of the posterior three-quarter crown is confined to fixed-fixed bridges its failure rate almost doubles. Thus it would seem that, unless a considerably longer than average clinical crown is available and greater retention is possible than will generally be the case, the conventional posterior three-quarter crown should not be used in fixed-fixed bridges.

When the use of the posterior three-quarter crown is confined to fixed-movable, spring, and cantilever bridges then the failure rate falls to only 1·12 per cent per year.

2. Anterior Three-quarter Crown. The failure rate of the anterior three-quarter crown when used as a major bridge retainer is relatively high, being double that of the posterior three-quarter crown which emphasizes the care which must be taken if this preparation is used as a major bridge retainer.

It is interesting to note that its failure rate is far less when it is used for fixed-movable and cantilever than fixed-fixed and spring bridges. *Fig.* 6.13 shows the far greater demands made on retention by the latter group.

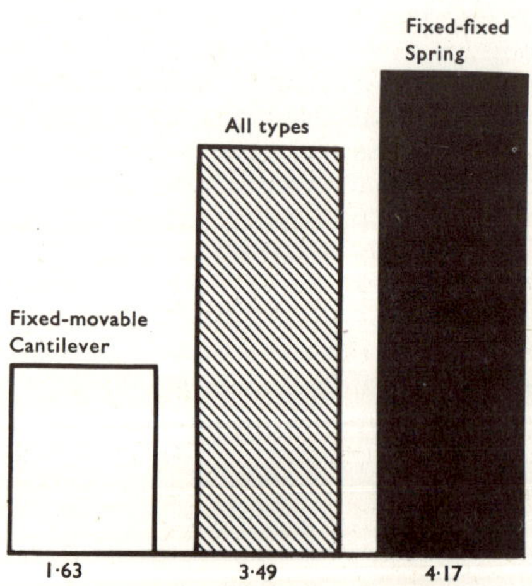

Fig. 6.13. *Relative failure rates per cent per year of the anterior three-quarter crown when used in (a) fixed-fixed and spring bridges and (b) fixed-movable and cantilever designs.*

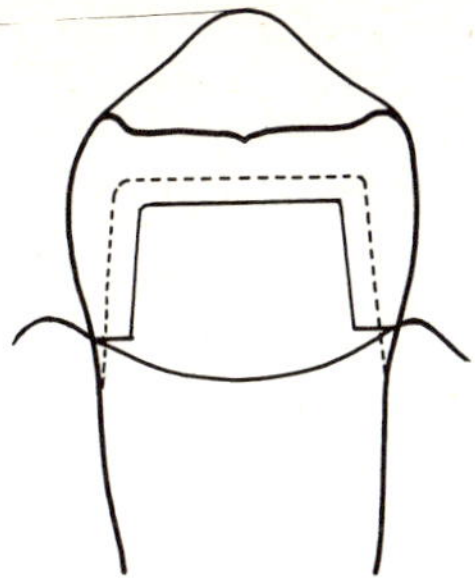

Fig. 6.14. *This cross-sectional diagram shows three-quarter and MOD preparations. It can be seen that the three-quarter crown preparation penetrates less deeply into tooth tissue, but gives better protection cervically. Its fit is also less critical in this region.*

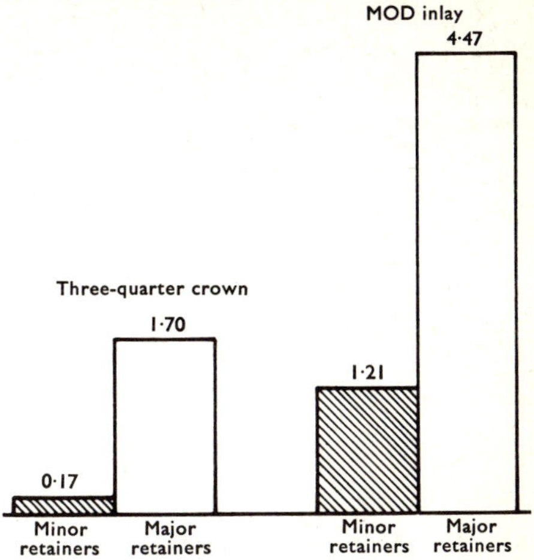

Fig. 6.15. *The failure rates of the three-quarter crown and MOD inlay when used as minor and major retainers.*

3. The MOD Inlay. The high failure rate of this restoration would indicate that it should not normally be employed as a major bridge retainer unless there is a definite indication for its choice. The poor performance of the MOD is not only due to its greater liability to either partial or complete cementation failure but also to its increased susceptibility to recurrent caries when compared with the three-quarter crown (*Fig.* 6.14). There are several reasons for this, possibly the most important being that when an extracoronal preparatión is used the tooth can first be restored in amalgam. Because of the foregoing the posterior three-quarter or full crown is nearly always to be preferred.

4. The Post Crown. The post crown, like the MOD inlay, has a relatively high failure rate. Although its use as a major bridge retainer cannot sometimes be avoided, great care must always be taken to secure the maximum of retention when preparing the tooth. A partial or full gold collar is desirable in all instances (*Fig.* 6.65, p. 117).

B. Minor Retainers

The fact that a minor retainer is not directly joined to the major retainer of a fixed-movable bridge reduces the stress which may be applied to it and means that the chances of cementation failure are greatly reduced. This is borne out by the failure rates shown in *Fig.* 6.15, where it can be seen that the failure rate of the posterior three-quarter crown when used as a minor retainer is only one-tenth of that when it is employed as a major retainer. Similar results were obtained with the MOD inlay.

It is because of the lesser demands made on minor retainers that such relatively unretentive preparations as the Class III inlay, albeit prepared with care, may occasionally be used with success for this purpose.

■ Methods of Increasing Retention

One of the most commonly employed methods of improving the retention of a casting is by the incorporation of pins. Other techniques are mainly directed towards increasing the degree of parallelism in the retainer or improving its rigidity.

The Retention of Castings by Pins

Pins may be incorporated in retainers

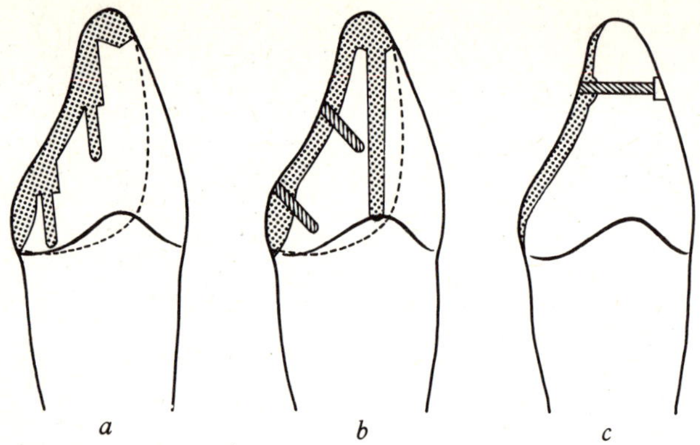

Fig. 6.16. *Alternative methods of pin fixation: a, Vertical, when the pins are incorporated in the casting; b, Non-parallel; c, Horizontal. In these latter cases the pins are placed after the main casting is cemented in situ.*

merely to increase retention a little or they may be used to provide the majority of the retention necessary.

There are two ways in which pins may be employed:

a. By making them part of the castings, in which case they must have the same line of insertion as the rest of the retainer.

b. By placing the pins after cementation of the casting, when they can have a different line of insertion and will thus positively lock the restoration in place (*Fig*. 6.16). This would seem the more logical approach.

The advantage of method (*a*) is that the pins may be cast with the gold work or, in the case or iridioplatinum pins, the metal is cast directly on to them. The advantage of the method (*b*) is that the retention available is far greater and indeed is limited only by the sheer strength of the pins or screws used. This may well prove a disadvantage when the time comes to remove the bridge for renewal or repair.

The value of inserting pins at an angle to the line of withdrawal of the inlay is illustrated by a case in which a Class IV inlay was placed in a girl of 15. Because of the large pulp and the loss of tooth tissue the preparation was shallow and retention proved inadequate, the casting becoming uncemented three times in as many months. After the third failure the inlay was recemented and retention reinforced with two iridioplatinum pins inserted at right-angles to the line of withdrawal of the inlay. This casting is still in situ some 12 years later. The method used in this case was a very simple one and since then more efficient techniques have been evolved.

Parallel or Vertical Pin Fixation

There are two main types of pin which may be used with this technique, wrought and cast. The advantage of the former is strength and of the latter adaptability. They can literally be made to any size or shape required. Thus, generally speaking, if a pin hole is irregular in outline, or short and thick, then cast pins are the more desirable. However, if the pin hole is long, wrought iridioplatinum is the best material. A cast pin usually has to taper whereas a wrought one is generally parallel sided, which gives greater retention.

The wrought pins are available in two forms, either smooth or roughened. The latter are usually to be preferred because of the increased retention available.

Technique

A. Wrought Pins

i. When a direct wax technique is being employed the pin hole is drilled with a bur corresponding in size to that of the iridioplatinum wire used. After this the wire is seated in the hole and the end bent over into the lock so that it will not protrude beyond the external surface of the wax-up, which is now completed in the usual way.

ii. When an indirect technique is used the pin holes are made with the correct drill, the pins, usually of iridioplatinum or stainless steel, are placed in the pin holes and the protruding ends bent to ensure that they are withdrawn with the impression material. Before casting the impression each pin is sleeved so that it may be easily removed from the model. If stainless-steel pins have been used for the impression these are replaced by iridioplatinum ones prior to waxing up.

iii. An alternative is to use a standardized technique such as than described by Karlström (1968) or Goransson (1967) in which the drills, impression pins and retention pins are all matched.

Starting points for the pin holes are made with a half-round bur. This is then followed up with a spiral twist drill of a suitable thickness and length such as the Spirco drills marketed by the Svenska Dental Instrument Co. of Stockholm (*see Fig.* 6.70 *f*, p. 122). These may be either 0·6, 0·7, or 0·8 mm in diameter and either 21, 23, 28, or 31 mm long. They incorporate a 'stop' so that the pin hole will always be of an exact known depth. If multiple pin holes are being used then it is advisable to use a paralleling device such as the Prec-in-Dent, which is described later.

After all the pin holes have been prepared, matching plastic pins are inserted in them which are 0·01 mm narrower. These are colour-coded for length and diameter to avoid any confusion. With those designed by Karlström a very fine point at the tip of the plastic pin maintains a small space at the bottom of the pin hole, so as to create some clearance for the pin at cementation. A small amount of oil will help the seating and removal of the pins and to centre them in the pin holes.

An overall impression is now taken in a suitable material, such as polysulphide. Care is needed to see that the tray will not impinge on the plastic pins when inserted and that all the pins are fully seated at the time. After removal of the impression the pin holes may be protected by plastic pins which are specially made for this purpose. An alternative is to use paper points which have previously been soaked in cavity varnish. If used alone they will take up water, swell and stick in the canal.

A stone die is now made from the impression and the plastic pins removed from it. This is relatively straightforward as they elongate and become thinner as they are pulled out.

The correct knurled iridioplatinum pins, which will have a similar colour-coding to the plastic ones, but are 0·04 mm less in diameter, are now inserted in the model and the pinlay waxed up and cast.

To summarize, if the Spirco drill used is 0·8 mm diameter the plastic pin will be 0·79 mm and the iridioplatinum pin 0·75 mm in diameter.

B. Cast Pins

Where cast pins are employed then it is necessary to record the shape of the pin holes accurately. This may be achieved by using plastic pins which match the size of the holes drilled. They are incorporated in the wax-up and burnt out of the investment with the wax. Alternatively an accurate impression of the pin holes may be recorded with an impression material such as polysulphide. This is either injected down the pin holes with a syringe fitted with a very fine nozzle, or introduced by means of a spiral root-canal filler. After this a piece of fine stainless-steel wire coated with adhesive is inserted to reinforce it. The rest of the cavity is then injected with impression material and the overall impression taken. Where the pin holes are relatively wide and short then the stainless-steel wire may be dispensed with.

Vertical Non-parallel Pin Fixation

Where it is desirable to increase or

indeed provide the majority of the retention for an intracoronal inlay such as the MO, DO, or MOD, non-parallel pin fixation may be employed (*Fig*. 6.17). This may also be used with extracoronal restorations.

The most important criterion is that the casting through which the pin passes is of sufficient thickness to provide adequate retention for the pins. This is often more of a problem with extra- than intracoronal restorations. The retainer must also be of sufficient rigidity to exclude all chance of it flexing during use. The pins should be in dentine.

There are three main methods of providing non-parallel pin fixation:

a. By cementing the bridge in place and then drilling the required number of holes with a twist drill through the gold at approximately 45° to the line of withdrawal of the castings and continuing these into the dentine for approximately 1 mm.

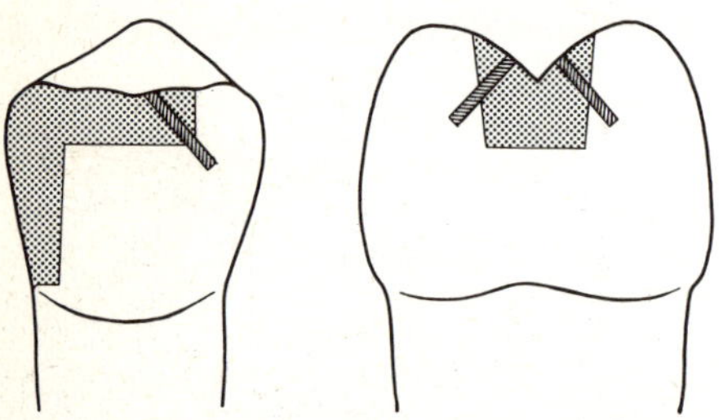

Fig. 6.17. *Non-parallel pin fixation on a Class II inlay.*

Matching self-tapping pins such as those marketed by Whaledent under the trade name of TMS are then inserted, using a hand wrench. If an engine is used the pins are liable to sheer.

b. By drilling the holes in the retainers and tapping threads in these with a special tool prior to cementing the bridge. After cementation the excess cement is removed with a twist drill which is driven approximately 1 mm into the dentine. The pins are then inserted.

Both the foregoing methods (*a* and *b*) should only be used if additional retention is required for either a bridge which has repeatedly become uncemented, but in all other respects is sound, or one which at try-in is felt to possibly have inadequate retention but otherwise is suitable for cementation.

Where it has been determined from the outset that pins are going to be used to provide additional retention then only (*c*) should be employed. This has the advantage that the pin screws only into the dentine and not the gold and thus 'pulls' the casting onto the tooth. With (*a*) and (*b*) the thread is in both the gold and dentine. Moreover if the pin is inserted too far (i.e. to the bottom of the hole), it will act like a car jack and elevate the casting from the tooth, a principle used by one form of full crown remover.

c. The third and best method is to incorporate pins (*Fig*. 6.23) in the wax-up at different angles of insertion both to the casting and to each other.

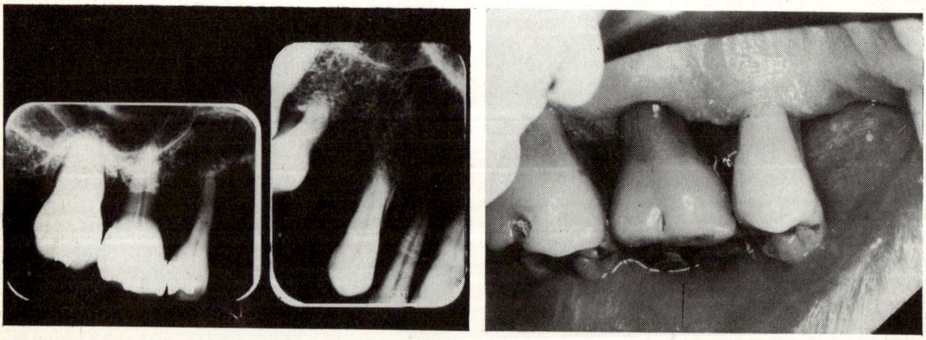

Fig. 6.18. *A patient who has had periodontal therapy including the removal of the buccal roots of* 6| *and now requires splinting and bridgework.*

The teeth are prepared and the position and angulation of the various non-parallel pins decided on. Channels are started with a half-round bur, which act as a guide for the 0·6 mm drill which is then used. This is limited in depth of insertion to 3 mm. A stone is now employed to bevel the aperture of the channels, and it is important at this stage that no enamel is left overlying the pinhole. An additional parallel channel is drilled in each tooth to a depth of 1–1·5 mm to provide guide pins which simplify insertion of the bridge.

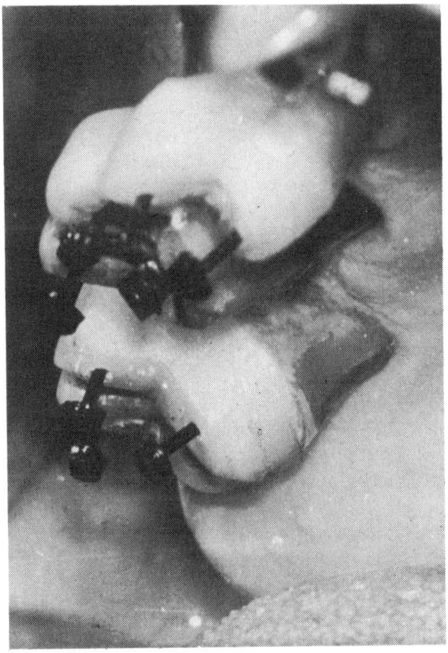

Fig. 6.19. *The completed preparations with plastic pins inserted in the pinholes immediately before the impression.*

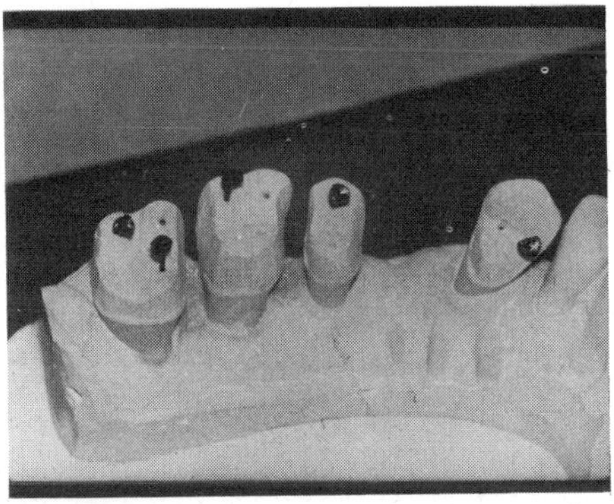

Fig. 6.20. *The stone model with some of the plastic pins removed.*

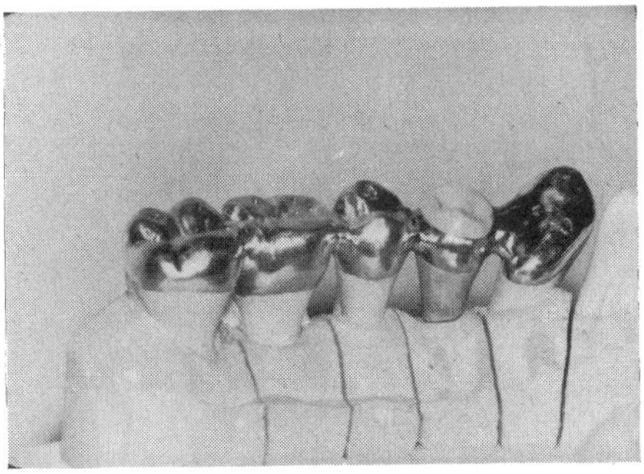

Fig. 6.21. *The completed bridge.*

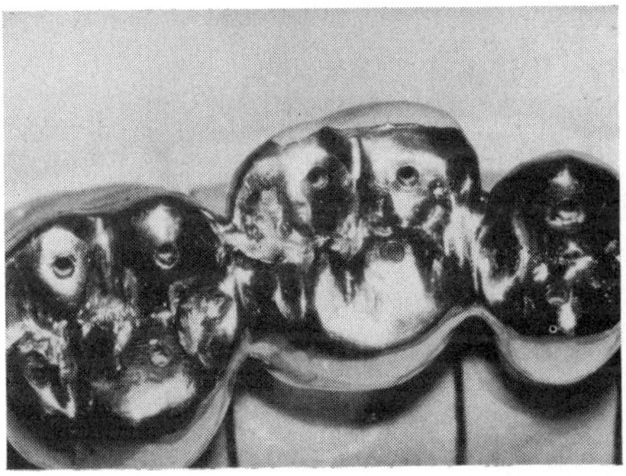

Fig. 6.22. *A close up of the castings showing the tapped holes in their occlusal surfaces.*

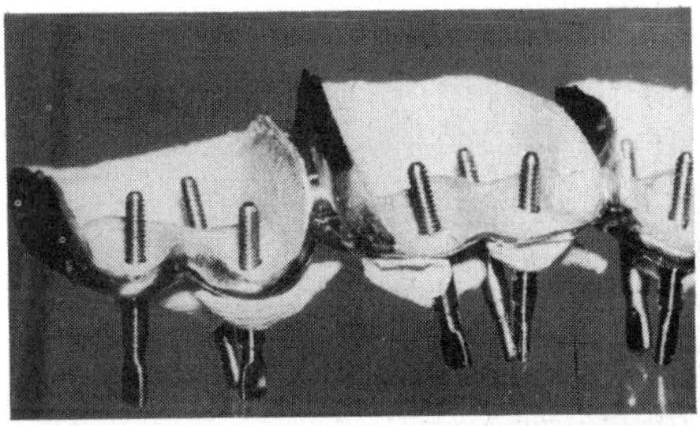

Fig. 6.23. *The casting with pins inserted to show their divergent angles.*

Matched plastic pins (*Fig*. 6.19) are now inserted into the pinholes and an overall impression taken which is cast in the usual manner, after which the plastic pins are removed. Into the parallel pinholes are now inserted serrated pins which are adjusted to clear the occlusion.

Into the non-parallel pinholes the special nickel-silver technique pins are placed, making certain that they seat to the full depth of their shoulders. The pattern is now roughly waxed; the nickel-silver pins are removed to clear the occlusion and the wax-up completed. The patterns are removed from the die and the pins reinserted and sealed into place, after which it can be cast.

The nickel-silver pins may now be removed from the casting by dissolving them out in nitric acid and the pinholes in the casting are then refined with a 0·8 mm drill. The VSMS self-threading screws are tried in the channels to check their seating prior to returning the castings to the model for finishing. The castings may now be tried in the mouth and any necessary adjustments to the occlusion and fit carried out. The non-parallel channels are enlarged from 0·6 to 0·7 mm prior to cementing the prosthesis. The final threaded pins used are 0·03 mm shorter than the depth limited drills so that they cannot 'bottom' in the pinhole. To further facilitate the insertion of the final pins the technique pins have 1° less taper.

The slowest possible setting mix of cement should always be used to give maximum working time to be able to remove the cement from the holes and insert all the threaded pins. This may be done either with the auto-clutch in a handpiece or with a hand wrench. Should the holes have been over-enlarged then oversize pins are available 0·05 mm greater in diameter. When the cement has set the pins are cut off flush with the gold and final polishing is carried out.

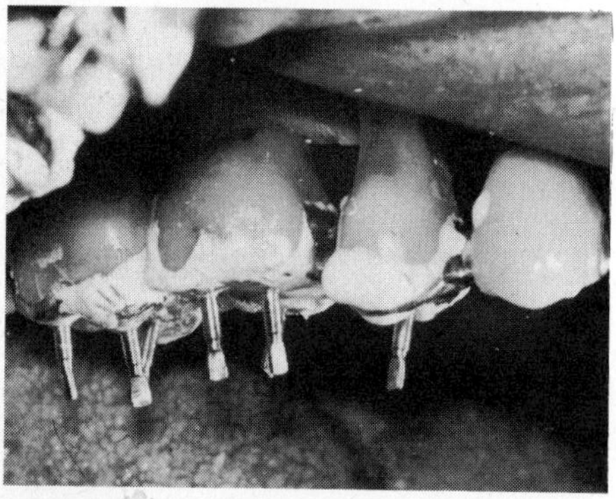

Fig. 6.24. *The bridge cemented and screwed into place.*

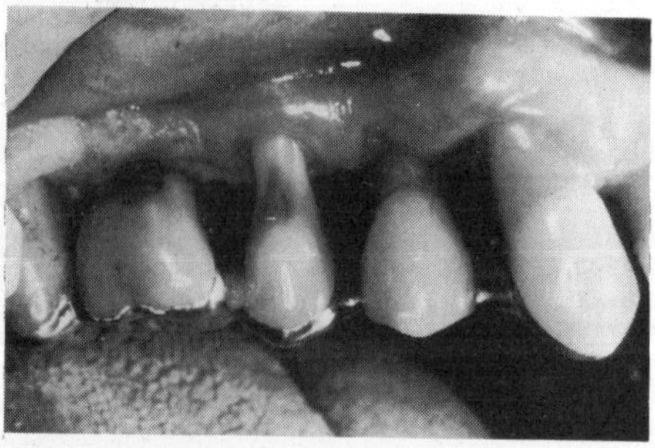

Fig. 6.25. *The completed prosthesis.* (*Figs*. 6.18–6.25 by courtesy of Mr P. Russell.)

Horizontal Pin Fixation

This technique is particularly useful in the lower anterior region and is especially valuable when fixed periodontal splinting is required (*Fig*. 6.26). It was first described by Weissman in 1965 and subsequently modifications have been suggested by Gerard L. Courtade. A complete kit for carrying out the procedure is marketed by Whaledent (*Fig*. 6.27).

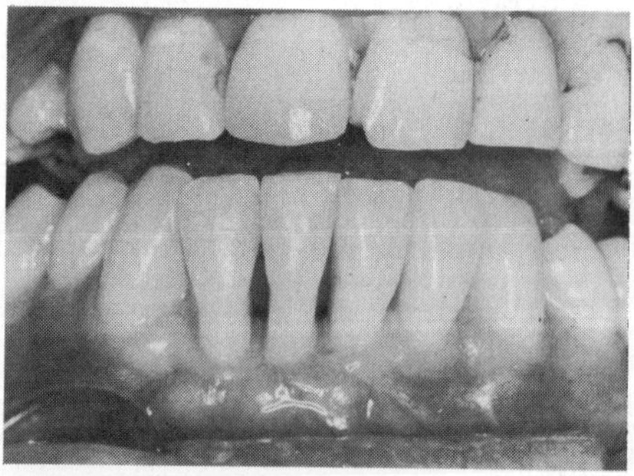

Fig. 6.26. *Teeth which have undergone periodontal therapy and require splinting.*

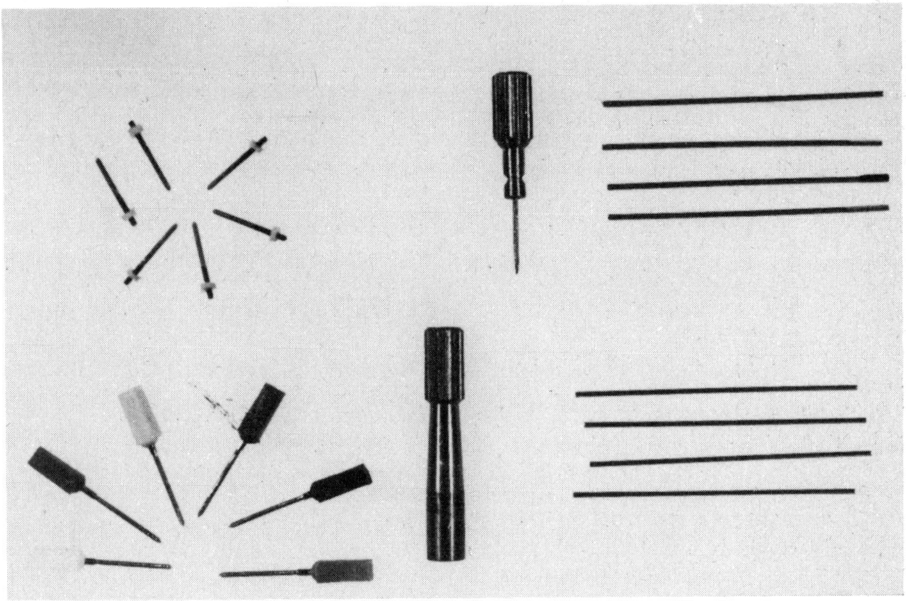

Fig. 6.27. *Whaledent kit for horizontal pin fixation:* Top left, *Nickel-silver threaded positioning pins.* Bottom left, *Acrylic-headed screws for splint fixation.* Top centre, *Tap for refining threads in lingual plate.* Top and bottom right, *Positioning pins for use in impression and model.*

The technique consists of the use of a lingual plate with a supragingival finishing margin which is fixed to the teeth by bolts passing through them (*Fig.* 6.28). The plate may have either a horizontal or vertical line of insertion. However, the advantage of the latter is that undercuts are less likely to be encountered and that vertical pins can be incorporated in the casting in the region of the cingulum which appreciably increases retention by counteracting any rotational forces.

The case should first be assessed on study models, when it can be seen whether it will be necessary to remove any tooth tissue to allow of one line of insertion for the splint. At the same time X-rays are referred to and the highest position of the pulps of the teeth is estimated and marked on the model. A line is then drawn on each tooth between this point and the incisal edge. This will indicate the correct level for drilling the horizontal channel (*Fig.* 6.29).

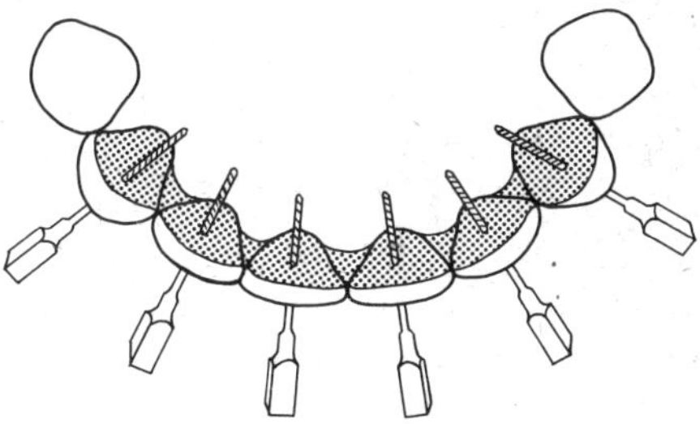

Fig. 6.28. *Horizontal pin fixation using threaded pins and a lingual plate.*

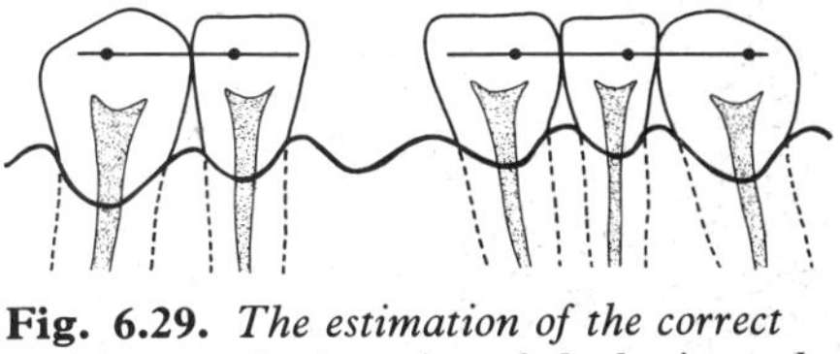

Fig. 6.29. *The estimation of the correct position for the insertion of the horizontal pins. This is midway between the incisal edges of the teeth and the highest points of the pulps.*

Should any lingual tooth tissue have to be removed because of undercuts then this is carried out first. The horizontal pin holes are then drilled. Initial penetration is obtained with a half-round tungsten carbide bur in a high speed handpiece. This is followed up by a special long-shank bur (Whaledent SMSR-3) to complete the hole (*Fig.* 6.30). After this a matching end-cutting bur (Whaledent SMSE-4) (*Fig.* 6.30) is used to enlarge and refine the channel so that the impression pin will pass through it easily.

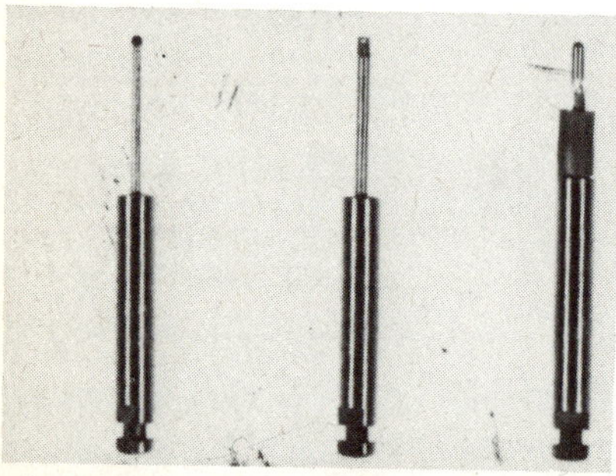

Fig. 6.30. Left, *Whaledent SMSR-3 long-shank bur for drilling horizontal channel through the tooth.* Centre, *SMSE-4 bur used for enlarging and refining channel.* Right, *SMSG-5 bur used for creating labial countersink.*

The next stage is to provide for a greater thickness of gold on the lingual aspect of the tooth where the threaded pin emerges. This may be achieved by creating a half-round countersink with a number 5 round bur or a diamond of similar size. However, this must not be too deep or an undercut will be created relative to the vertical cingulum pins.

The final stage in the preparations is to drill the vertical pin holes. A step is cut on the cingulum of each tooth and on this starting points are made with a half-round bur. This is followed by a spiral twist drill of appropriate size which is inserted to approximately 2 mm, care being taken to make certain that all the vertical pin holes are parallel.

The preparation of the teeth is now complete and the impression may be taken. Should they be mobile it is desirable to stabilize them either at this stage or prior to preparation, by such means as circumferential wiring.

A special tray is constructed with stops in the posterior region to provide positive location. It is cut away completely on the labial or buccal aspects in the region of the horizontal pin holes so as to avoid the impression pins (*Fig.* 6.31).

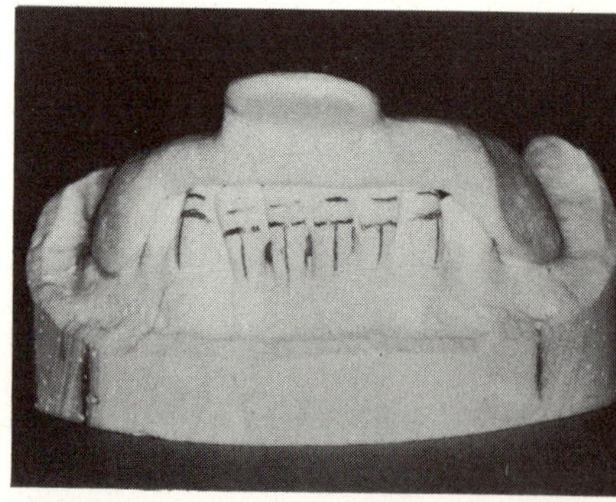

Fig. 6.31. *A line is drawn on the model midway between the incisal edge and the top of the pulp which indicates the position for insertion of the pins. The tray is designed to avoid this area.*

As this technique is often used when periodontal splinting is required it is likely that there has been appreciable gingival recession and thus large interproximal embrasures will be present. These will require blocking out with wax before taking the impression.

Plastic pins matching the drill size used are now inserted into the vertical pin holes and the horizontal (Whaledent SMS A) pins are passed through the teeth. An impression is then taken in the usual manner, making certain that the material is injected over the whole of the fit surface and around the pins. There must be sufficient impression material on the labial aspect of the teeth to provide positive location for the horizontal pins.

After the impression has set, the horizontal pins are removed and the impression is then taken out of the mouth, when the pins can be relocated.

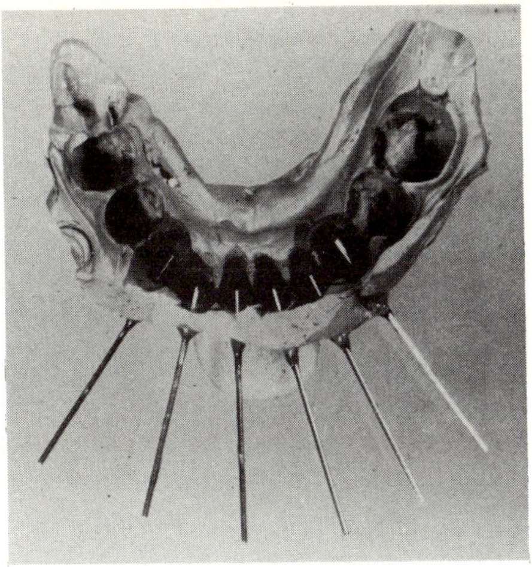

Fig. 6.32. *Prior to pouring up of the refractory model the pins are reinserted into the impression and waxed in place.*

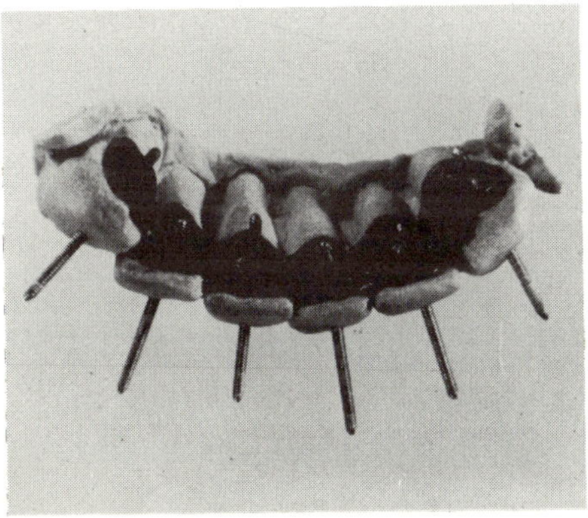

Fig. 6.33. *The nickel-silver threaded pins are inserted into the refractory model and the wax-up completed.*

In the laboratory the pins are removed from the impression again, lubricated and then reinserted into their correct position and fixed firmly with wax (*Fig.* 6.32). Any gross undercuts in the impression should be blanked out, as it is essential that it can be removed from the first cast without damage. A refractory model is now poured and when this is set the pins are carefully eased out of this before

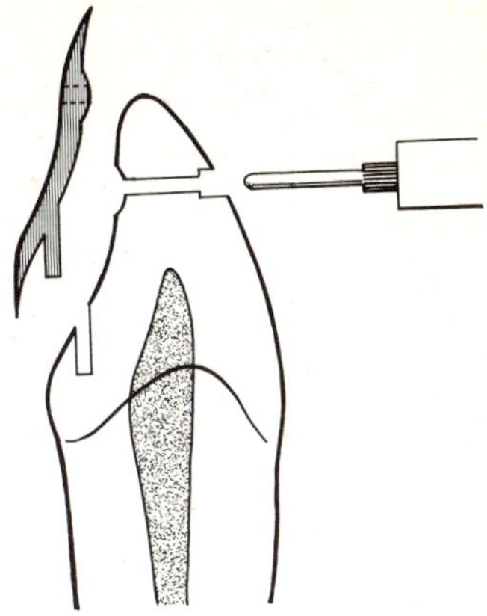

Fig. 6.34. *a, SMSC-5 bur used to create labial countersink in the tooth.*

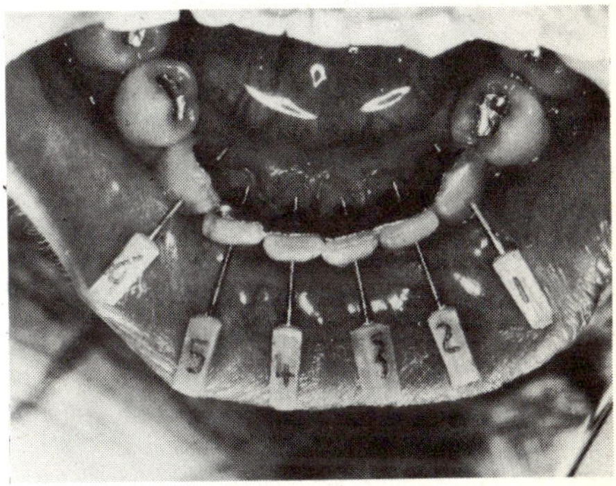

Fig. 6.34. *b, The splint is tried in the mouth with the horizontal threaded pins.*

removing the impression. This is now cleaned and slightly larger pins than the SMS A ones are inserted into the same holes in it. These can be identified by their flattened end and should be treated with a lubricant and fixed in place before the stone model is cast.

The outline for the bridge is now drawn on both models. It can usually be made well clear of both the gingival margins and incisal edge. The nickel-silver pins, complete with their plastic sleeves which give an indication of the thickness of gold required on the lingual aspect, are now inserted into the refractory model from its lingual surface

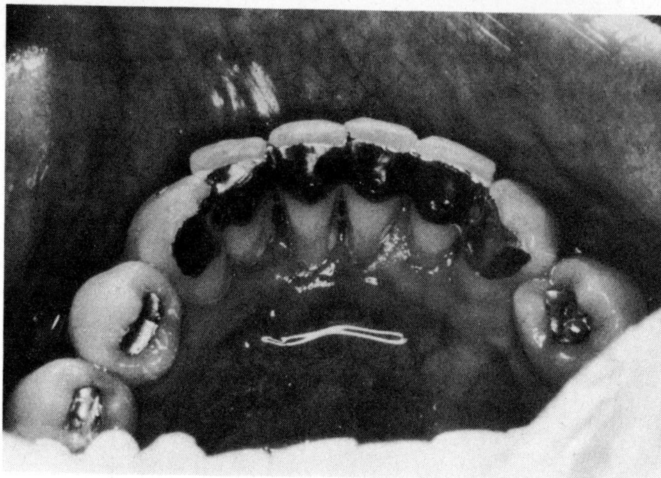

Fig. 6.35. *The completed splint with the pins ground smooth on the lingual aspect.*

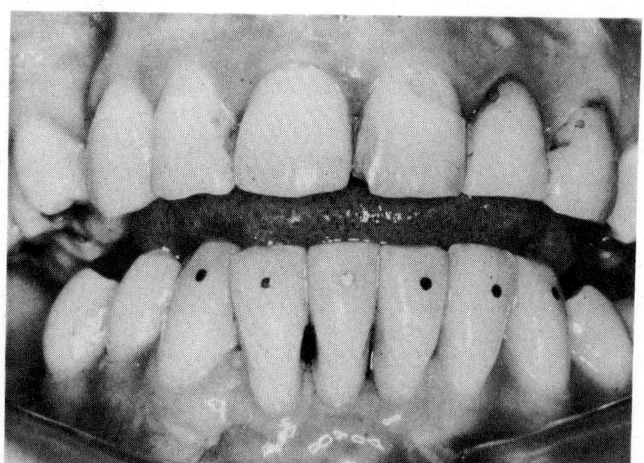

Fig. 6.36. *The heads of the pins are ground smooth on the labial aspect and polished. Where necessary they can be reduced and covered with composite.* (*Figs.* 6.26–6.36 by courtesy of Mr T. R. Hill.)

and waxed securely into place (*Fig.* 6.33). Iridioplatinum pins of the correct diameter are inserted into the vertical pin holes and shortened if necessary before the wax-up of the bridge is commenced.

This is now completed and the prosthesis cast in the conventional manner, using a hard gold such as Chicago 4 to ensure adequate rigidity. After this the nickel-silver pins can be removed with nitric acid.

The prosthesis is transferred to the master model on which it is finished. The threads are refined as necessary with a special tool and finally the acrylic-headed screws which will be used in the mouth to retain the prothesis are tried into place. If all is satisfactory the bridge is ready to be checked in the mouth.

However, before doing this a counter-sink is created on the labial aspect of all horizontal pin holes in the teeth to house the heads of the threaded pins (*Fig.* 6.34*a*). This is done with a Whaledent SMSC-5 drill, which will penetrate to a depth of 1·5 mm. The prosthesis may now be tried in, initially without and then with the horizontal pins (*Fig*. 6.28, p. 97) before finishing.

It is important that the pins are kept in their correct order, which, as they are colour-coded, is relatively simple.

Zinc phosphate is the cement of choice, all the usual methods being used to retard the set as far as possible. The vertical pin holes are filled with an endodontic spinner, the retainers coated with cement and forced firmly into place, when the excess should run out through the horizontal pinholes. The horizontal pins are now all loosely inserted and gradually tightened in rotation until they are fully seated. It is important not to overtighten them, otherwise it is possible to chip or craze the enamel or even break off the corner of a tooth.

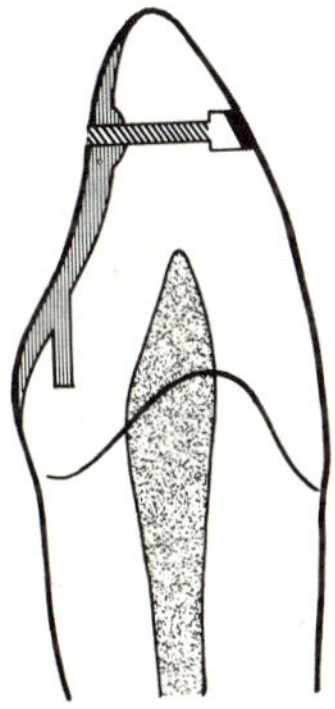

Fig. 6.37. *The completed splint. Note lingual countersink around bolt hole to increase the thickness of gold in this region. The head of the screw has been reduced labially to allow a silicate to be placed, thus masking it.*

After the cement has set the pins are cut off flush with the labial and lingual aspects, ground smooth, and polished (*Figs*. 6.35, 6.36). Should the patient object to their metal heads showing on the labial aspects of the teeth they can be reduced to 0·5 mm below the surface and a suitable filling material placed over them as a mask (*Fig*. 6.37). Alternatively, self-shearing pins may be used which will fracture off 1 mm below the tooth surface when tightened (*Fig*. 6.38).

Although it is unlikely that a bridge retained in this way will ever become

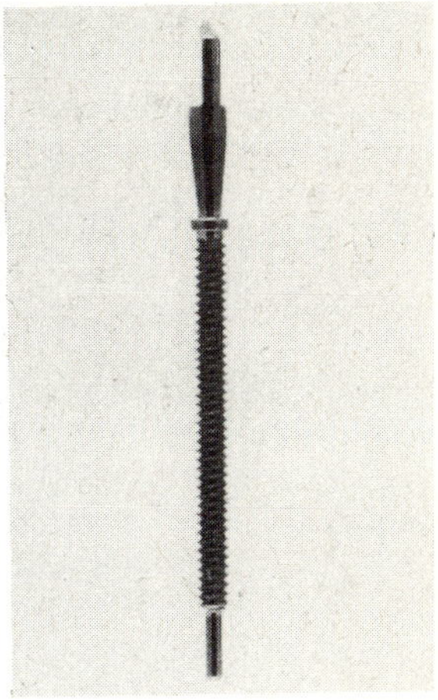

Fig. 6.38. *Syncron pins which will shear off approximately 0·5 mm below the surface of enamel and then leave space for a composite filling to mask them.*

detached it is important to check it regularly and in particular to make certain that no flexing of the gold has taken place which will result in a break of the cement seal and possible caries.

■ Further Methods of Increasing Retention

1. Use of Double Slots in the Three-quarter Crown Preparation. The retention of the three-quarter crown can be increased very considerably by providing two slots both mesially and distally (*Fig*. 6.39). However, although this is usually possible in the premolar and molar it cannot always be achieved in the canine because of the lack of length and width of the slice.

The provision of two slots increases retention by:

i. Increasing the degree of parallelism in the preparation. This is especially true in the canine where, without the extra slots, little parallelism is achieved in a buccolingual aspect. This is aggravated by the fact that the surface area of the slice on the average canine is relatively small, especially when compared with a premolar or molar.

ii. Making the retainer more rigid.

iii. Increasing the total surface area of the casting.

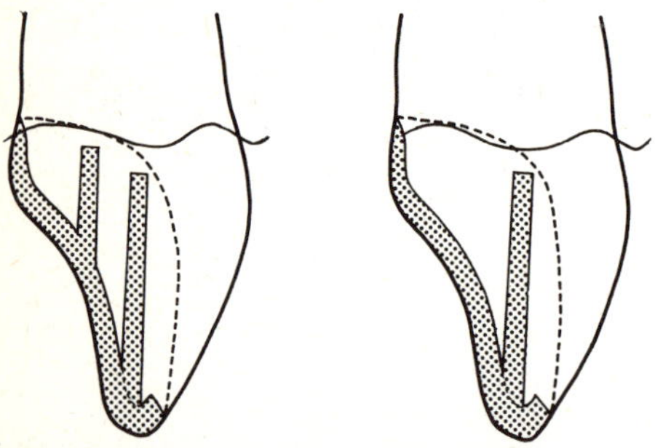

Fig. 6.39. *The use of double slots mesially and distally to improve retention by increasing the rigidity and the degree of parallelism present in the casting.*

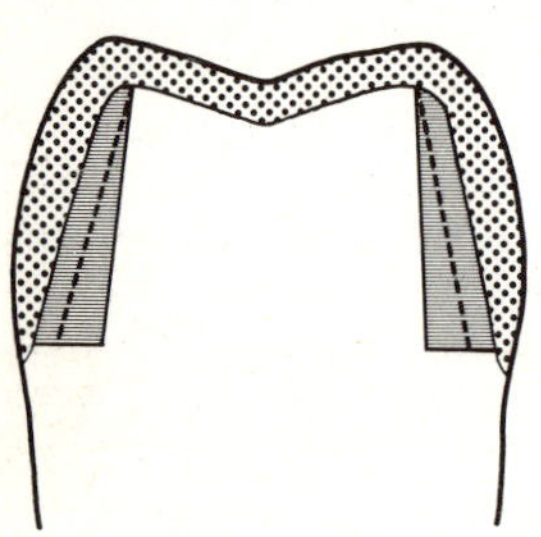

Fig. 6.40. *Where the mesial and distal slices are markedly divergent the slots should be cut in cervically so that they, at least, are within 5° of parallel to each other.*

2. Modification of the Angulation of Slots. When a three-quarter crown preparation is carried out on a poorly erupted tooth it may prove impossible to make the mesial and distal slices parallel to each other. However, in these cases it is still possible to make the rails nearly parallel by cutting them in at the cervical margin (*Fig.* 6.40).

3. The Addition of Rails to a Full Crown. When a full crown lacks retention this may be remedied by the incorporation of slots in the mesial and distal aspects of the preparation and on occasions the buccal and lingual surfaces also. This latter has the advantage that the slots can usually be made somewhat longer.

Additional methods of increasing retention will be covered when describing the specific types of bridge retainer.

■ Other Factors in Retainer Design

Although the provision of adequate retention is of paramount importance, the following points must also be considered.

Aesthetics

The aesthetics of the retainer must be acceptable to the patient. If this cannot be achieved without prejudicing the retention it is best not to proceed with the bridge.

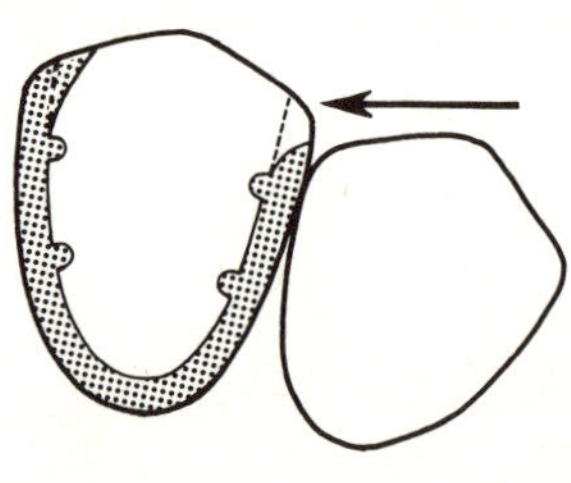

Fig. 6.41. *The mesial slice of a three-quarter crown should be curved so as to minimize the display of gold. Straight slices are shown in dotted outline. The distal slice, which is not normally visible, is curved mesially to increase retention.*

Aesthetics, so far as retainers are concerned, is generally related to the amount of gold displayed. If a faced full crown is employed then the quality of that facing will also be a factor. An intracoronal restoration will normally display less gold than an extracoronal one. However, these restorations, in conventional form at least, are only

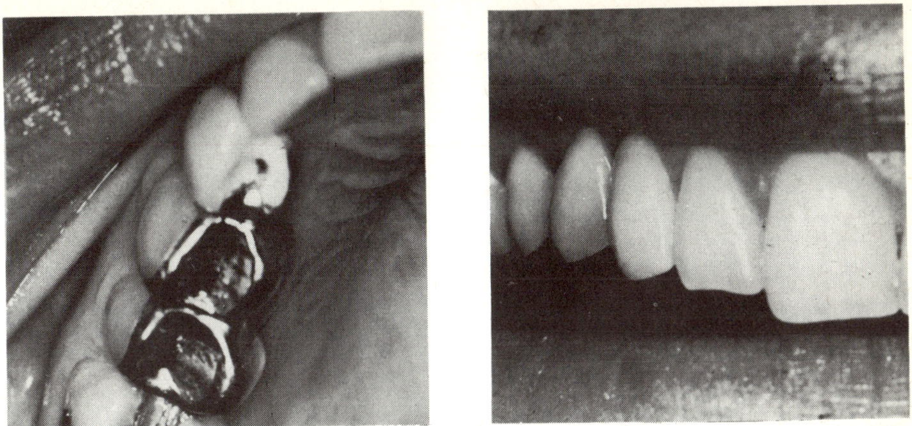

Fig. 6.42. *A cantilever bridge replacing* 3| *and supported by three-quarter crowns on* 54|. *Note how little gold is displayed.*

satisfactory as the minor retainers of fixed-movable bridges. Thus if an upper first premolar is missing and a fixed-movable design is employed, a three-quarter crown may be used as the major retainer on the second premolar and a Selberg modified three-quarter crown as the minor retainer in the canine. In this way no gold will be displayed on the latter tooth.

The gold that is shown on the mesial slice of a three-quarter crown can be reduced by curving it as shown in *Fig.* 6.41.

The gold of a retainer which is noticeable on the buccal or labial aspects can be further reduced by adjusting its angulation so that it does not reflect any light.

This is best carried out at the chair-side, prior to cementation of the bridge, by observing the gold work from the varying positions normally assumed during conversation, i.e. with the patient sitting upright or even standing in front of the operator, and gradually altering the angles of the gold. In many instances it can be made almost to disappear (*Fig.* 6.42).

Some patients are worried about any gold being displayed on the occlusal surfaces of the posterior teeth. This is difficult to prevent, but can be ameliorated by sand blasting the gold. The only alternative is the bonded full crown. However, quite drastic occlusal reduction, which is not always possible or desirable, will be necessary if a reasonable aesthetic result is to be achieved.

Occlusal Coverage

There are several reasons why full occlusal coverage is nearly always indicated for bridge retainers. It gives the abutment tooth complete protection during mastication and there is no fear of a cusp fracturing. This is especially likely to occur when an MOD inlay is placed in a premolar, particularly if the isthmus is cut too deeply.

Because of the increased fragility of non-vital abutment teeth, full occlusal coverage is essential in all instances. Indeed, in these cases it is also desirable to cement a post into the root canal to reinforce the crown and root of the tooth and thus reduce the risk of their fracturing.

Full occlusal coverage is always indicated in fixed-fixed bridges to decrease the chance of cementation failure caused by the tooth being literally bitten out of (down from) its gold inlay, which is being held rigidly in position via the solder joint and pontic to the other retainer (*Figs.* 6.43, 6.44).

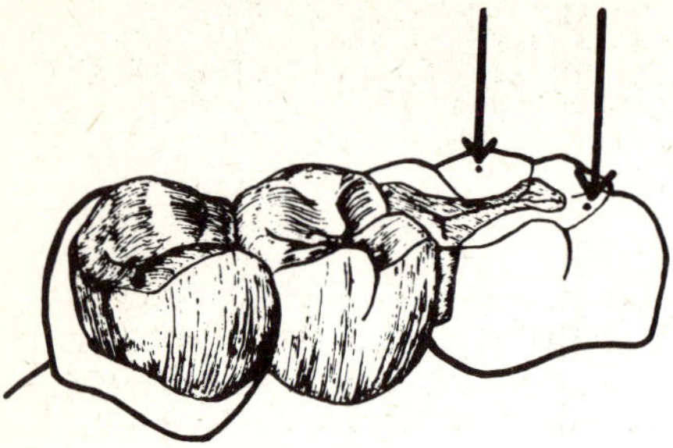

Fig. 6.43. *If full occlusal coverage is not provided for a fixed-fixed bridge then when an occlusal force is applied to an uncovered cusp it will depress the tooth and literally bite it away from the inlay.*

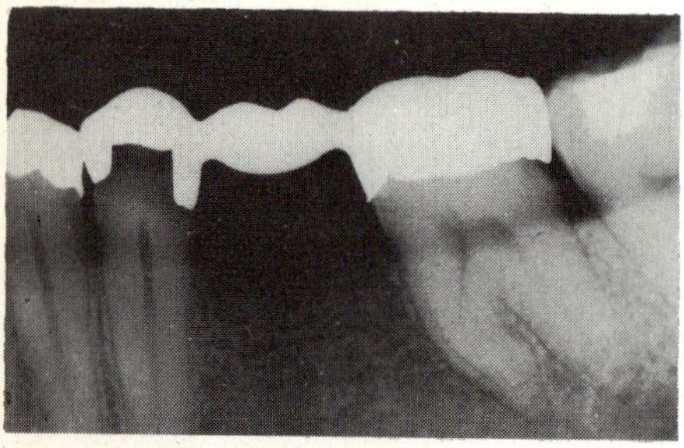

Fig. 6.44. *A fixed-fixed bridge in which the MOD in |5 has become uncemented because of the lack of full occlusal coverage.*

The occlusal gold should always be thick enough to provide sufficient rigidity for the casting. Approximately 1 mm of gold is usually adequate for this purpose, but if there is any doubt about the amount required an occlusal slot can be provided to help stiffen the casting and if an occlusal cavity is present this should always be carried out. However, care must be exercised as in the premolars, especially if cut too deeply, the slot is likely to weaken the tooth structure, resulting in possible fracture of a cusp, even in spite of occlusal coverage.

When preparing the tooth it is very important to make certain that sufficient clearance has been allowed for an adequate thickness of gold in both centric occlusion and lateral excursions of the bite. All too often the latter is neglected, either accidentally or for aesthetic reasons. In these cases the gold is worn away surprisingly quickly and eventually the margin fails or the casting becomes uncemented.

Destruction of Tooth Tissue

It is desirable to keep the destruction of tooth substance to a minimum and also to avoid any undue depth of preparation because:

a. The trauma inflicted on the pulp during cavity preparation is directly proportional to the depth and extent of the preparation. However, the correct use of watersprays should keep any adverse effect on the pulp to a minimum.

b. The irritant effect of the cement on the pulp obviously increases with the depth and surface area of the preparation.

c. The more extensive the preparation the more the abutment tooth will be weakened.

In the three-quarter crown the amount of tooth substance removed is relatively small because of the shallowness of the preparation, and at no point does this usually approach anywhere near the pulp. This is illustrated in *Fig.* 6.14 (p. 91) where in cross-section a three-quarter crown is shown superimposed on an MOD gold inlay preparation.

Prevention of Recurrent Caries

The design of any retainer should always be such that the liability to recurrent caries is minimal. To achieve this, particular attention must be paid to finishing the margins of the preparation in an easily cleansable area. This includes the provision of wide interproximal embrasures. In the young patient in particular it is important that the edge of the preparation is taken beyond any carious or decalcified area, or the margin of any existing amalgam. Mesially and distally this is easier to accomplish with a three-quarter crown than with the conventional MOD, since to finish a box to anything like the same depth as a slice would involve excessive depth of preparation and destruction of tooth tissue (*see Fig.* 6.14 p. 91).

■ Choice of Retainer

The choice of retainer for any particular bridge depends on many factors, such as:

Degree of Retention Required

This is the most important consideration and must override all others. Factors which affect this are whether the retainer is going to be a major or a minor one, the type of bridge for which it is required, the length of span, weight of bite, and the articulation.

Condition of Abutment Tooth

If a specific retainer is required to restore a tooth satisfactorily then provided this will give adequate retention for the bridge it will obviously be the restoration of choice. Thus if, for instance, a post crown is the only possible restoration that can be used for a particular tooth this will have to be employed. However, the design of the retainer will need modification to increase its retention and make it more suitable for bridge work. In the posterior region it is often better to restore a non-vital tooth with amalgam retained by pins and screws and then to place a full crown over it. Alternatively, a split post technique (*Fig*. 15.16, p. 198) may be employed.

Aesthetics

The aesthetic requirements of the patient will affect the choice of retainer. Thus in a fixed-movable bridge extending from the upper second premolar (the major abutment) to the canine (the minor abutment) a Selberg modified three-quarter crown will generally be used in the latter tooth in preference to a three-quarter crown to avoid any display of gold (*Fig*. 6.45). Likewise a bonded full crown may often be preferred to a three-quarter crown in an anterior bridge.

Material used for Pontic

The materials used for the pontic and the retainer are obviously interrelated. Thus

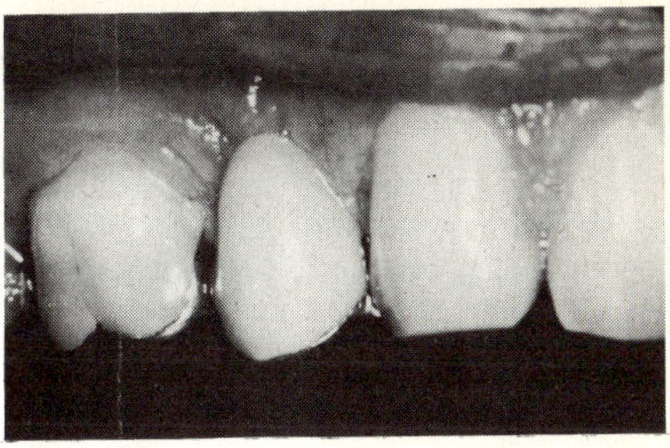

Fig. 6.45. *A fixed-movable bridge replacing 4|. By using this design only a Class III inlay is required as a minor retainer in the 3|, thus producing a more aesthetic result and avoiding the heavy bite incisally.*

if it has been decided that bonded pontics are required then in the majority of cases bonded porcelain will be indicated, for aesthetic reasons, for the retainers also. The converse also applies. However, bonded porcelain pontics may also be used in conjunction with full or three-quarter gold crowns.

Periodontal Condition

The periodontal condition may affect the choice of retainer in several ways. The more advanced the bone loss the greater the amount of gingival recession which is likely to have taken place and the more important it is to avoid any further plaque formation and thus gingival irritation. Fortunately the lengthening of the clinical crown in these instances enables the margin to be finished well supragingivally whilst still obtaining adequate retention.

Furthermore the three-quarter crown may often be safely employed in preference to the full crown because of the greater surface area, rigidity and parallelism which can be achieved in the casting.

SPECIFIC RETAINERS

In this chapter it is assumed that the reader has some knowledge of the standard intra- and extracoronal preparations. It is largely the modifications of these for bridge work which will be described.

The retainers used in fixed bridge prostheses may be divided into two groups, major and minor; the latter, which require considerably less retention, are the lesser retainers of fixed-movable bridges into which a dovetail usually slots.

The retainers which will be considered in this chapter are:

A. Major Retainers:
The full gold crown.
The faced full crown.
Posterior three-quarter crown.
Anterior three-quarter crown.
MOD inlay.
Post crown.
Three-quarter pinlay and pinledge.

B. Minor Retainers:
Three-quarter and full crowns.
Selberg modification of the three-quarter crown.
Class III incisal withdrawal inlay.
Class II inlay including the MOD.

All restorations used as major retainers can also be used with modification as minor retainers but the converse does not apply.

■ Major Retainers

The Full Gold Crown

The posterior full crown is the strongest of all restorations and should always be used where maximum retention is required, for instance in long-span fixed-fixed and compound bridges. It is also nearly always desirable in castings incorporating precision retainers.

The tooth should be prepared so as to allow approximately 1 mm of gold over the whole of the occlusal surface. To make certain that this can be achieved the occlusion should be checked, not only in centric but also in the lateral and protrusive excursions. So far as possible the natural contours of the occlusal surface of the tooth should be followed, but sometimes diagnostic wax-ups may be a better guide.

If the gold is likely to be thin in the region of the solder joint the preparation should be modified, for example by cutting a box, so as to increase the thickness of metal at this point (*Fig.* 6.46).

If any one aspect of the preparation is likely to lack retention this must be compensated. Thus when it is difficult to achieve any depth to a preparation on the

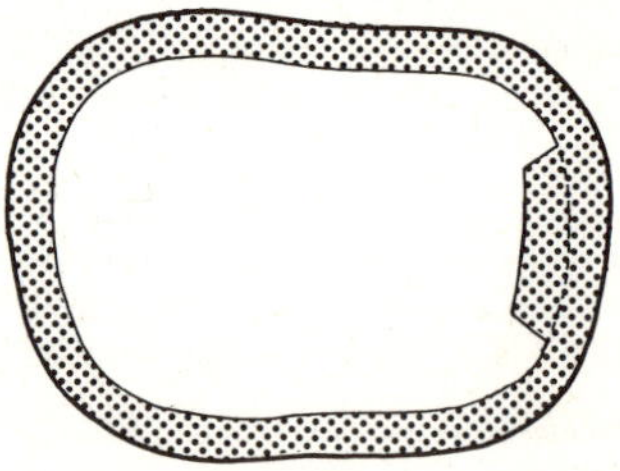

Fig. 6.46. *Full crown preparation modified to provide an increased thickness of gold in the region of the solder joint.*

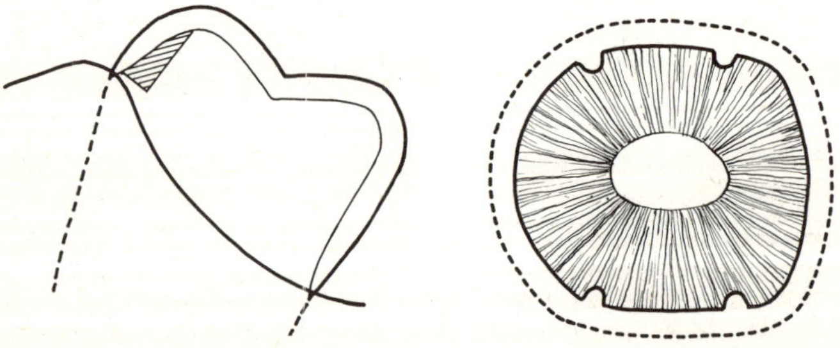

Fig. 6.47. *Increasing retention of a full crown by providing slots (a), distally or (b), buccally and lingually.*

distal aspect of the lower second or third molars, either one or two rails or a box may be incorporated at this point to compensate for this (*Fig*. 6.47). An alternative is to cut grooves in the buccal and lingual aspects of the tooth. Pins can also be used. The finishing margins of three-quarter and full crowns will be discussed at the end of the chapter.

The Faced Full Crown

The faced full crown gives excellent retention and providing it is sufficiently rigid, seldom becomes uncemented. However, its design is complicated by the necessity to supply a facing which may be fabricated either in acrylic or porcelain.

Gold and Acrylic

The simplest faced full crown is that made of gold and acrylic. This has some of the disadvantages of the latter material but these can to some extent be minimized by correct design. Thus the whole of the fit and articulating surfaces of the crown should be of gold so as to provide accuracy of fit and minimize wear. If acrylic is used on the occluding surfaces wear will be rapid and not only will this shorten the life of the retainer but it will allow the opposing tooth to overerupt until it comes into contact with the prepared surfaces, thus making any subsequent replacement far more difficult. Usually the incisal edge should be protected by gold, but occasionally if the bite is favourable this may be omitted.

The preparation is normally shoulderless on the inner aspect where only gold will be required, with a chamfer finish. On the labial, either a shoulder 1·2–1·5 mm wide will be required to accommodate the gold and the acrylic or a fairly deep chamfer may be provided with a gold finishing margin 1–1·5 mm deep. If necessary the gold may be omitted on the upper part of the labial surface to improve aesthetics, by preventing it shadowing through the acrylic.

Because of the large amount of time and expense involved in the construction of a bridge the comparatively small saving in cost achieved by using acrylic as opposed to porcelain facings would scarcely seem to be justified when their relatively short life, possibly 5–7 years, is considered. Thus it is only where the prognosis for the bridge as a whole or indeed all the standing teeth is less than 7 years that this restoration should be employed.

Bonded Porcelain

A porcelain facing may be fitted to a full crown in two ways, either by cementing it in place or bonding it to the metal. However, as the aesthetics and strength of the full crown with a cemented facing is inferior to the bonded variety their use has now been largely discontinued and they will not be considered further in this book.

The bonded full crown is the most commonly employed bridge retainer and thus its design will be considered in some detail.

1. *Strength*. The most important advantage of metal ceramic crown and bridgework is its strength and durability. This stems from the bonding of the two materials and greatly exceeds that of either when used on its own. Thus the modulus of rigidity of 'Degudent' metal used alone is 60 000 mN/mm whereas when porcelain is bonded to it the figure increases to 500 000 mN/mm. It is because of their great strength that failure of metal-ceramic restorations is rare.

2. *Wear*. The gold alloys used in metal-ceramic crowns and bridges are relatively soft and thus liable to wear more rapidly than conventional hard golds. To overcome this they should be protected by porcelain in situations such as the area of contact of the canine rise where attrition may be appreciable and in this way any wear can be reduced to a minimum. There is remarkably little risk of the porcelain fracturing, provided it is adequately supported by the gold substructure and its thickness does not exceed 1–1·5 mm. In the early days of metal-ceramic crowns several restorations were placed by the author in which the thickness of the porcelain in high stress

areas was reduced to only about 0·2 mm and even then the porcelain did not fail.

3. Aesthetics. Because bonded porcelain is able to withstand greater stresses than porcelain alone it can safely be used on unprotected incisal edges, thus avoiding any display of gold. A particular advantage, which patients are increasingly aware of, is the ability to be able to provide tooth-coloured occlusal surfaces in the posterior region, something we are unable to achieve reliably with any other material.

However, although aesthetics is usually better with bonded crown and bridgework than with gold-backed porcelain facings the difficulty of providing adequate space for the gold core, the opaque layer and the surface porcelains is often great and thus, especially where the lighter shades are being employed, may not be entirely satisfactory. This is likely to be a particular problem in young patients where it is difficult to carry out sufficient tooth tissue reduction to allow for adequate thickness of both metal and porcelain; this difficulty being further aggravated by the light shades required. In the older patient it is far easier to obtain a reasonable aesthetic result.

The greatest problem arises in the young patient with a Class II, division 2 malocclusion who requires a lower incisor crowned. In these instances the space between the palatal surface of the upper incisors and the pulp of the tooth to be crowned is often insufficient to permit the provision of adequate space for the porcelain and gold of the crown (*Fig.* 6.48).

However, the problem of providing satisfactory aesthetics is the price we must pay for the provision of adequate strength. Indeed it is very little easier to obtain a good aesthetic result with a crown with an alumina than with a metal core although somewhat less space is required with the former.

The two things which will assist in the production of a reasonable aesthetic result are:

a. An adequate and even reduction of tooth tissue so as to allow a thickness of at least 1·5 mm labially and 2 mm

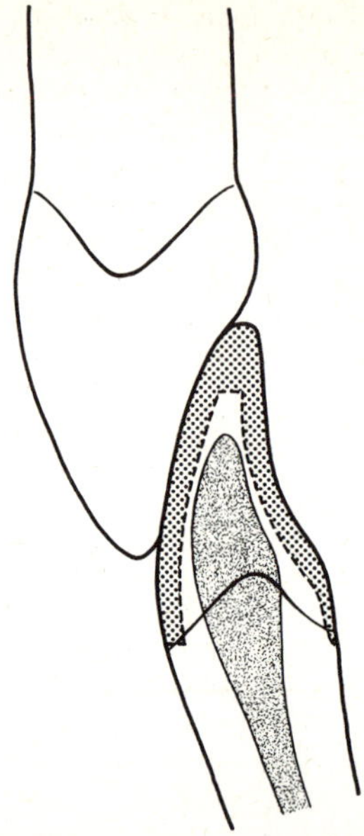

Fig. 6.48. *The space available between the occluding surface of the upper tooth and the pulp of the lower incisor which is being prepared often determines the maximum thickness of the crown and thus the aesthetic result which can be obtained.*

occlusally, for the layer of metal, the opaque mass and the porcelain.

b. Stopping the metal short of the buccal or labial aspect of the cervical margin of the crown on anterior teeth and upper premolars.

i. Prevent any metal being visible at the cervical margin.

ii. Avoid an additional junction of the materials in this region.

iii. Reduce the degree to which the gold will reflect through the porcelain in the cervical region, thus making it appear grey.

iv. Prevent distortion of the gold casting in this region (*Fig.* 4.8, p. 49).

When building a crown, once an adequate fit is obtained with the core porcelains at the cervical margin it will be maintained during the subsequent firing cycles when adding the surface porcelains, as these have an appreciably lower fusing point. To make certain that the correct crown contour is achieved it is usually best to wax-up the crown in full and then cut back the wax to allow for an even thickness of porcelain. To prevent the porcelain powders sticking to the stone die a separating medium such as Biodent varnish may be used.

4. Cost. The main disadvantage of metal-ceramic prostheses is their relatively high cost because of the considerable laboratory time required for their fabrication and the high price of gold alloys to which porcelain can be bonded. The latter cost could be reduced somewhat if the gold alloys were replaced by non-precious metals. However, the reliability of the porcelain-metal bond is not as good as with those consisting mainly of gold and the fit of the castings is not entirely satisfactory. This has already been discussed in greater detail in Chapter 4.

Tooth Preparation

Preservation of tooth tissue. The temptation when preparing a tooth for a bonded full crown is to over-reduce it to make certain of adequate space for both the metal and the porcelain so as to achieve a satisfactory aesthetic result; however, all too often this weakens the remaining tooth tissue so much that it is liable to break.

To reduce the chance of tooth fracture:

a. Have a shoulder on one surface only, usually the labial or buccal. On the other aspects of the tooth a chamfer or even occasionally a feather edge may be employed which should permit a thickness of gold of at least 0·75 mm.

b. Remove any existing restorations and where necessary pin the replacement restoration firmly into place so that it will give support to the remaining tooth tissue rather than rely on it for retention (*Fig.* 6.49).

c. Modify the preparations so as to save as much as possible of the existing tooth tissue. This is particularly important where posterior teeth, especially premolars, have been restored with MOD amalgams. In these instances it is often best to overcontour the bonded crown a little and have a gold finishing margin and collar so as to preserve the strength of a weak buccal or palatal cusp (*Fig.* 6.49). The shoulder for the porcelain is

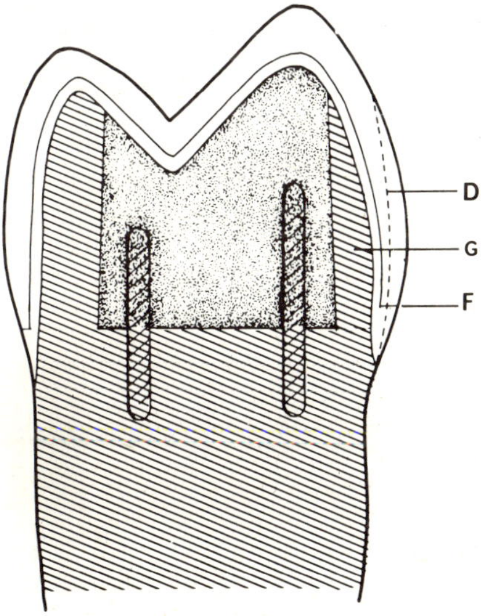

Fig. 6.49. (1) *Always pin extensive restorations to underlying tooth tissue;* (2) *A weak buccal cusp* (G) *may sometimes be retained by increasing the original contour of the tooth* (D) *having a gold finishing margin and establishing a shoulder* (F) *for the porcelain in the gold at a higher level.*

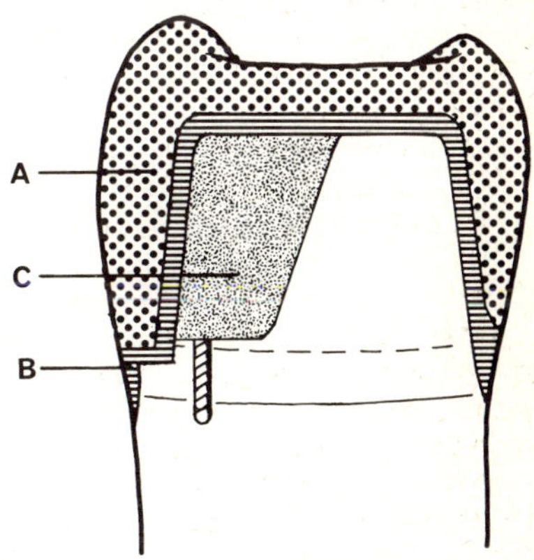

Fig. 6.50. *The extension of a gold chamfer beyond any restoration and onto sound tissue will reduce any risk of recurrent caries and help to transfer any stress onto the tooth tissue rather than the restoration.* A, *Porcelain;* B, *Gold;* C, *Amalgam.*

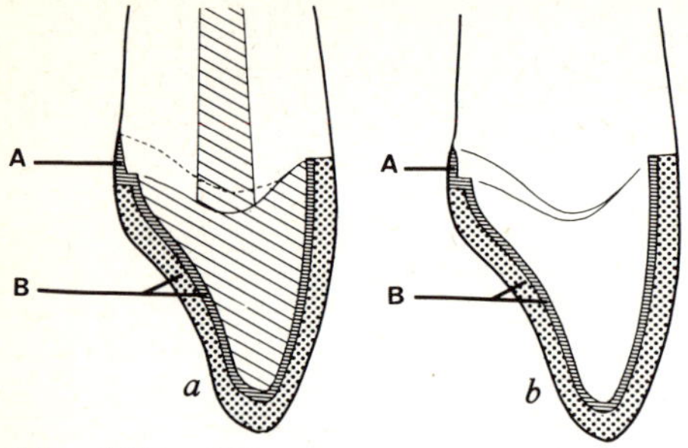

Fig. 6.51. *a Where a bonded full crown* (B) *is placed over the top of a post/core unit the provision of a palatal collar* (A) *transfers an appreciable proportion of the loading from the post to tooth tissue. Note that there is porcelain to tooth tissue contact on the labial aspect, to improve aesthetics. b The provision of a palatal collar* (A) *increases retention and transfers at least part of the occlusal load from a relatively weak to a much stronger part of the tooth.*

prepared in the gold at a higher level. Although over contouring, even if slight may be undesirable from a periodontal viewpoint it is on occasions the lesser of two evils.

d. Extend a chamfer in gold beyond any existing restoration so that the finishing margin of the gold is on tooth tissue, thus minimizing any risk of recurrent caries and helping to throw any occlusal load onto tooth tissue rather than the restoration (*Fig.* 6.50).

ii. Extend a chamfer beyond any shoulder preparation that may prove to be necessary, particularly on the palatal aspects of the upper incisors (*Fig.* 6.51*a*). This increases retention and transfers the occlusal load from a relatively weak to a much stronger part of the tooth. Where the restoration is being used as a bridge retainer a full collar is often indicated to increase retention. A collar is particularly useful where bonded crowns are being placed over a post/core unit as an appreciable proportion of the occlusal loading will be transferred from the post to the gold collar of the bolded crown, which in effect is a shallow full crown (*Fig.* 6.51*a*).

Anterior Teeth. When preparing teeth consideration must always be given to the requirements, strengths and weaknesses of the materials to be used. Thus the golds employed for metal-ceramic work are relatively soft and for this reason the point of occlusion is normally best taken on porcelain (*Fig.* 6.52). This is desirable in all instances in the anterior region and essential when restoring a canine. In the posterior region the relatively high surface area of the occlusal contacts usually reduces the wear to acceptable levels and gold is best employed.

a. Canine preparation. Where there is a canine rise all the forces of mastication are directed onto this point of contact and if this is provided by the relatively weak bonded gold it may wear quite rapidly. In severe cases particularly where bruxing is present or the occlusion faulty a bridge may well fail after 5–6 years because 1–1·5 mm of bonded gold have literally been worn away until eventually the lower teeth are occluding with the prepared palatal surfaces of the canine. At this stage cementation failure occurs and the remake because of the loss of vertical dimension is invariably difficult.

If the occlusion is taken on the porcelain then wear is minimal and moreover failure of the porcelain is rare.

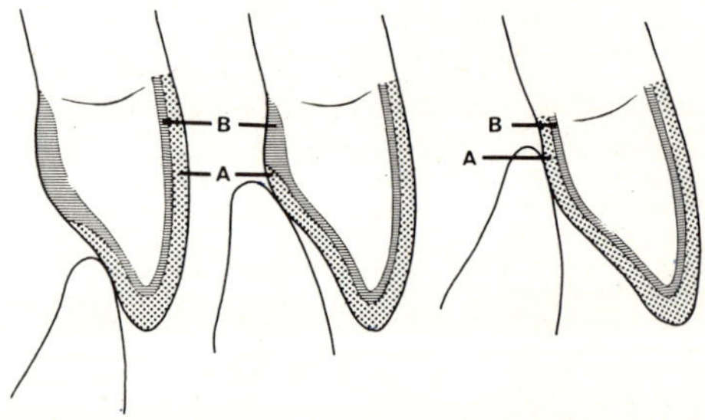

Fig. 6.52. *To make certain that the point of occlusion on an anterior tooth, particularly a canine, is always on porcelain, the further gingival the contact the further must the porcelain be extended. In severe examples* (right) *a full shoulder preparation is necessary.* A, *Porcelain;* B, *Gold.*

Thus the further gingival the point of occlusion the further must the porcelain be extended until in relatively severe examples a full shoulder should be provided so that the porcelain may be continued to the cervical margin (*Fig.* 6.52).

b. Upper Incisor Preparation. When preparing incisors it is not always possible, particularly in Class II, division 2 malocclusions, to reduce the tooth tissue sufficiently to provide sufficient space for the extension of a layer of porcelain over the gold at the point of occlusion; however, the lack of porcelain to protect the gold is not so critical in these instances as with the incisors group function is usually present and this means that the relatively soft gold is protected by the enamel of the teeth on either side during protrusive and lateral excursions. When all the incisors are crowned this argument does not apply so forcibly; however even here the load factor on any one incisor is normally far less than for a canine. Wear will be particularly severe if the gold palatal surfaces of the upper anterior teeth are opposed by porcelain lower incisors, which have lost their glaze.

A further cause of failure is the extension of the metal up to the incisal edge. In these instances the relatively

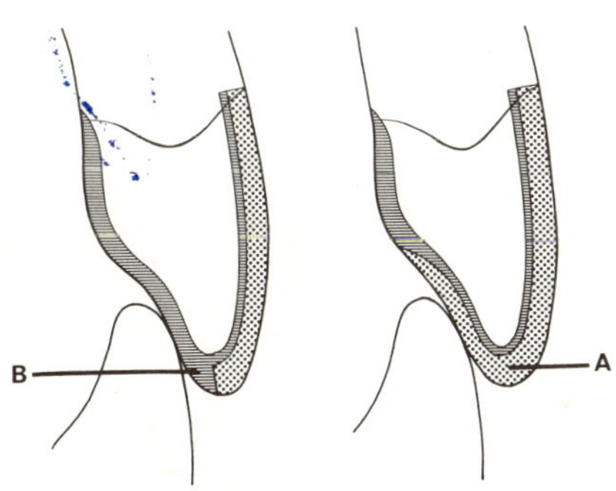

Fig. 6.53. *The incisal edge should always be in porcelain* (A) *which will be stronger than gold and aesthetically more pleasing. If the relatively weak metal used in bonded crowns is extended up to the incisal edge* (B) *it will bend or flow and cause fracture of the labial porcelain.*

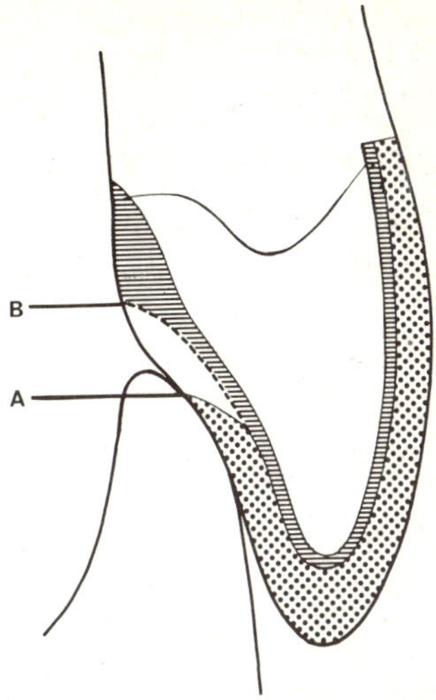

Fig. 6.54. *The porcelain/gold junction should always be kept well clear* (B) *of the point of occlusion. If it is not* (A) *then any metal flow which occurs will induce crack propagation in the porcelain.*

weak metal is prone to bend or flow and cause fracture of the labial porcelain (*Fig.* 6.53). Similarly, if the point of occlusion is at the porcelain/gold junction the metal will flow, induce stresses in the porcelain and cause crack propagation (*Fig.* 6.54).

Finishing Margins

Where possible it is always desirable to finish margins supragingivally and this it is possible to achieve with the majority of preparations. Even on the labial aspect of anterior teeth it may be practical to stop the preparations 'just' supragingival and still achieve a reasonable aesthetic result particularly if the smile is favourable, the gingivae are healthy and the patient is in the older age group. On the lingual or palatal aspects of all teeth and the buccal aspect of most posterior teeth margins can usually be finished supragingival unless such considerations as retention, the extension of the gold beyond an existing amalgam restoration or some such similar factor dictate otherwise.

The actual way in which the margin is prepared will vary with the tooth involved, which aspect of that tooth is being prepared, the materials being used

for restoring it and to some extent the individual operator's personal preference.
Labial Aspect. On the labial aspect of all incisors, canines and the first, and sometimes second, upper premolars a shoulder preparation with a slightly rounded internal line angle is to be preferred. When a bonded porcelain crown is placed on these teeth then a porcelain to tooth contact should be achieved on the labial aspect (*Fig*. 6.55).

If with a bonded full crown, the gold is extended to the margin of a shoulder preparation and it is finished to a knife edge to minimize its display then a poor fit will result because of:

a. Metal creep due to the close approximation of the melt temperatures of gold and porcelain.

b. The difference in thermal expansion and contraction of the two materials.

c. The sintering shrinkage of porcelain which, because it is bonded to the gold, will literally distort it and pull it away from the shoulder when it contracts (*Fig*. 6.56). This is the reason why a casting may fit perfectly at try-in but fails to do so after the porcelain has been fired onto it.

The only way in which distortion of the gold margin can be avoided is by increasing the thickness of the metal to at least 0·5 mm (*Fig*. 6.56*c*) which is generally only acceptable clinically in the posterior region.
Buccal Aspect. On the buccal aspect of all posterior teeth with the possible exception of the first and second upper premolars a gold finishing margin is to be preferred to porcelain because of its accuracy of fit and the reduced destruction of tooth tissue. Two techniques may be employed, either a strong chamfer or a combination of chamfer and shoulder

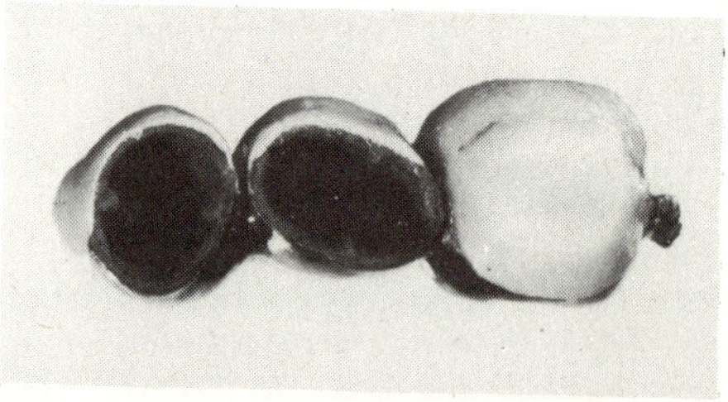

Fig. 6.55. *Porcelain finishing margins on the buccal aspects of bonded full crowns on* |45.
(By courtesy of Mr. B. J. Parkins.)

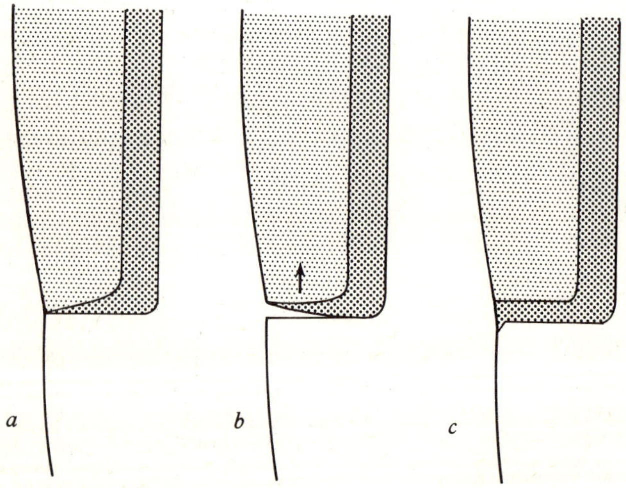

Fig. 6.56. *Although the casting may fit accurately* (*a*) *the sintering shrinkage of the porcelain when it is added and adheres to it may result in distortion of the margin* (*b*) *and a poor fit. To avoid this either a porcelain finishing margin should be employed* (*Fig*. 6.57) *or a thickness of gold of at least 0·5 mm provided* (*c*) *which will be sufficiently strong to resist distortion by the porcelain.*

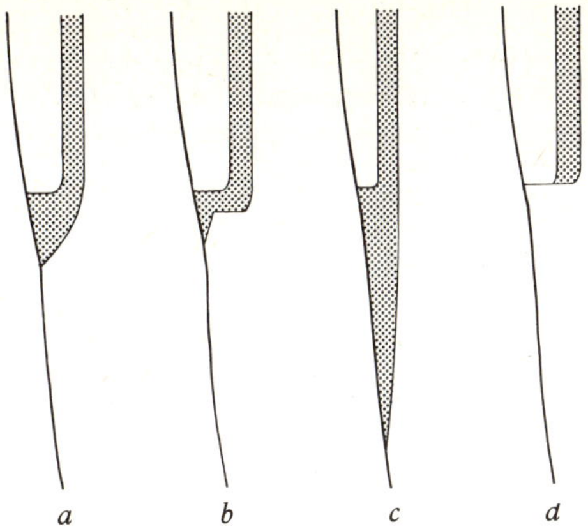

Fig. 6.57. *Alternative finishing margins for posterior bonded full crowns. Adequate space must always be provided for the porcelain cervically if a satisfactory aesthetic result and adequate strength are to be obtained. This may be achieved by: a, A strong chamfer; b, A combination of shoulder and chamfer; c, A long chamfer is of value when the preparation has to be extended well beyond the amelodentinal junction, possibly because of caries. This avoids the excessive destruction of tooth tissue which would occur with other techniques, particularly the full shoulder preparation; d, With a porcelain finishing margin a good aesthetic result is achieved but a shoulder has to be provided and the fit will not be as good as with a gold chamfer.*

(*Fig.* 6.57*a, b*). The advantage of the latter is that less gold is displayed and of the former that a shoulder does not have to be provided and that there is somewhat less destruction of tooth tissue.

A long chamfer (*Fig.* 6.57*c*) is of value where the preparation has to be extended beyond the amelodentinal junction, for instance because of caries or existing restorations. This again minimizes tooth tissue reduction, which will be excessive if a shoulder preparation is taken too far.

The Lingual, Palatal, Mesial and Distal Aspects of all Teeth. On these surfaces a chamfer finish can nearly always be employed and in the majority of instances this can be kept supragingival. Moreover because space does not usually have to be created for porcelain the chamfer only has to be sufficiently deep to provide for a layer of gold which will be thick enough to provide complete rigidity for the casting. The advantage of the chamfer over the feather or straight bevel finish is that it provides a more positive finishing margin for the technician to work to in the laboratory and that it increases the rigidity of the casting where it is most needed (*Fig.* 6.58). It is only where the crown of a tooth tapers markedly, as for instance on some lower incisors and occasionally premolars that a straight bevel should be employed to avoid any undue destruction of tooth tissue.

Crown Contour. If plaque retention is to be reduced to a minimum and the

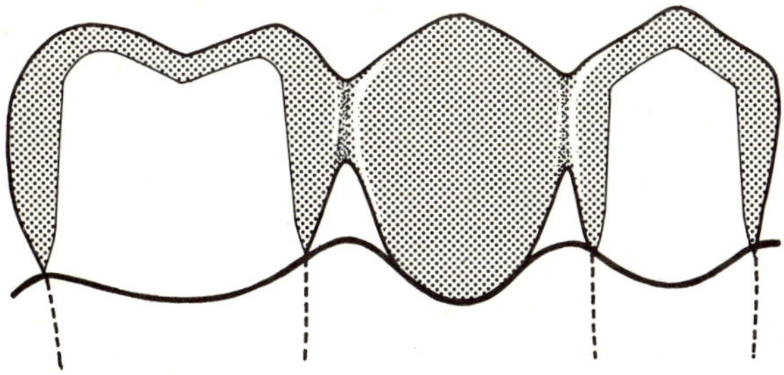

Fig. 6.58. *Where the casting will be thick, a straight bevel may be employed, as in Fig. 6.10a; but if it is likely to be thin and thus weak, the margin should be curved to increase the strength of the gold.*

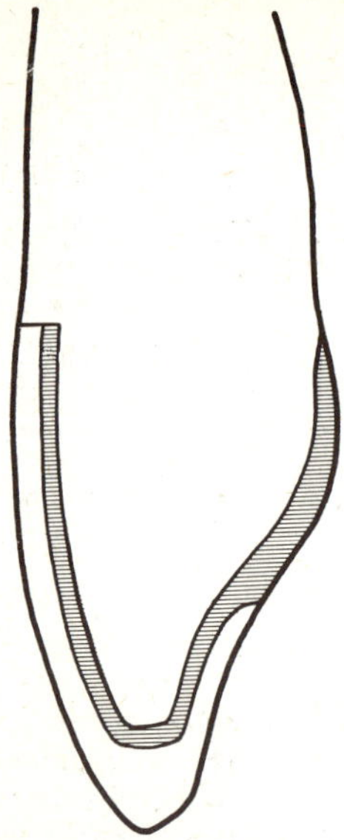

Fig. 6.59. *A porcelain bonded to gold full crown. Note that the porcelain is carried down a considerable distance on the palatal aspect.*

periodontal health of the patient maintained it is essential that the crown is not over contoured. This is probably the commonest error seen on bonded crown and bridgework and usually occurs because the operator has provided insufficient space for both the porcelain and the gold, particularly near the cervical margin. Unless a full shoulder has been prepared it is better to have a gold finishing margin and commence the porcelain 1–2 mm above this.

Summary

To prevent failure of metal-ceramic crowns it is necessary to:

a. Always provide a minimum space of 1·5 mm in which to accommodate the porcelain and gold.

b. Make certain that the subframe is of adequate thickness to prevent its flexion, particularly interproximally in bridges where movement will cause fracture of the porcelain.

c. Avoid the porcelain exceeding a thickness of 1·5 mm in any region but particularly on the cusps of posterior teeth. This can be achieved by correct tooth preparation and where necessary modification of the gold substructure (*Fig.* 5.19, p. 77).

d. Use one-piece castings when practical and in instances where this is contraindicated any soldering techniques should be carried out in the furnace. The area of the solder joint should always be relatively high.

e. Preserve as much of the tooth tissue as is compatible with providing an adequate thickness for the porcelain and gold. Avoid full-shoulder preparations where possible except on the labial aspect of anterior teeth and pin any underlying restorations firmly to tooth tissue.

f. On anterior teeth, especially canines, the point of occlusion should be on porcelain. This is essential in canines where there is a canine rise. On posterior teeth this requirement is far less critical because of the relatively large occlusal surface area and indeed in this region gold is to be preferred.

On occasions, for instance where there has been attrition, the amount of tooth tissue left may be small. This can be compensated to some degree by sinking a pin on the palatal and occasionally the mesial and distal aspects of the preparation. These are usually incorporated in the full crown but may on occasions be used in a separate subframe (*Fig.* 6.60) to build a tooth up to the shape normally required for a full crown preparation, prior to placing the final crown.

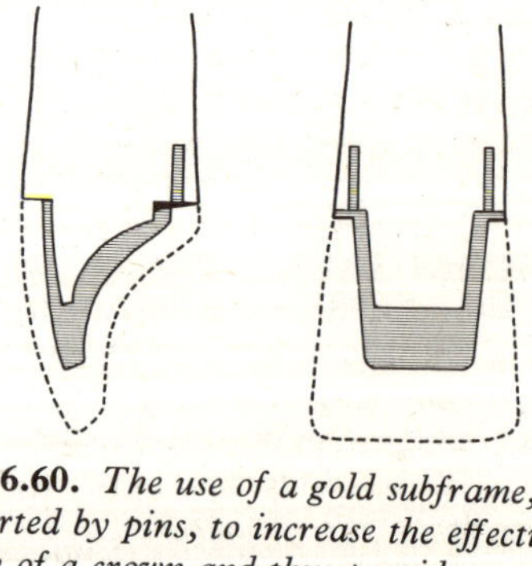

Fig. 6.60. *The use of a gold subframe, supported by pins, to increase the effective length of a crown and thus provide additional retention.*

The Posterior Three-quarter Crown

This retainer is of particular use in fixed-movable bridges and may also be of value in fixed-fixed prostheses if more than average retention is available. However, it is worth pointing out that its failure rate when used for this latter group is nearly three times as high as for fixed-movable bridges, so caution must always be employed.

It has two advantages over the full gold crown:

i. It is aesthetically more pleasing because the buccal aspect of the tooth is not covered by gold.

ii. It only extends around a little more than half of the cervical margin, thus appreciably decreasing any liability to plaque retention.

It is debatable whether a well executed three-quarter crown or the bonded full crown is the more pleasing aesthetically. Although the latter avoids any display of gold the colour match of the facing can never be as perfect as a natural tooth and will only deteriorate with time.

When preparing a tooth for a three-quarter crown it is important that the mesial slice be curved so as to avoid any undue display of gold anteriorly (*see Fig.* 6.41, p. 102). To compensate for any slight loss of retention this may cause, the distal slice may be extended and wrapped round the tooth further on the distobuccal aspect, thus in effect creating something akin to a seven-eighths crown.

If possible the slots should be placed on sound dentine, but if this is impractical they may safely be cut in amalgam provided that this is strong and preferably pin-retained. They should be positioned as far to the buccal aspect as practical taking into account that adequate length is required, and they should not extend to the margin of the preparation (*Fig.* 6.61). Where retention is suspect two rails may be provided in each slice instead of one (*see Fig.* 6.39, p. 102). An alternative to slots, when an existing amalgam or an interproximal carious lesion is present and this is not too extensive, is to use a box.

It is important to get the mesial and distal slices as near to 5–6° of parallel to each other as possible. Where this cannot be achieved the rails should be cut deeper into tooth tissue cervically to make them more nearly parallel to each other (*see Fig.* 6.40, p. 102).

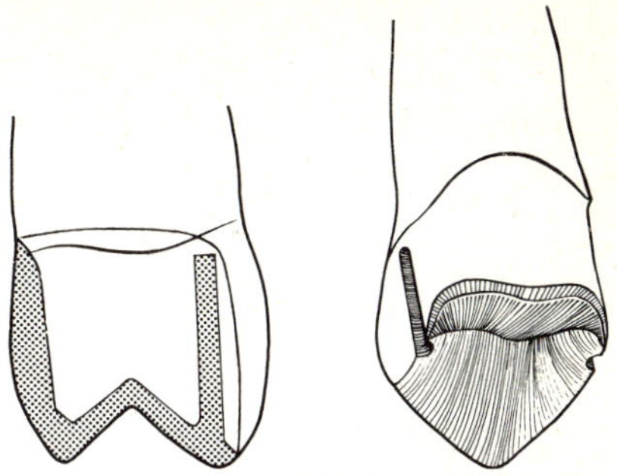

Fig. 6.61. *A standard three-quarter crown preparation suitable for use with bridge work.*

The casting should be rigid, and where there are any doubts it can be strengthened by, as mentioned previously, increasing the number of rails mesially and distally and also by providing an occlusal groove. This latter is of particular use when an occlusal amalgam is present in the tooth. It is nearly always satisfactory in the molar region but with the premolar care must be exercised otherwise the tooth will be weakened, particularly if the slot is taken too deeply, and this may result in its fracture, with the possible loss of a cusp.

Where the slices or palatal aspect of the retainer are likely to be thin a curved finishing margin is indicated (*see Fig.* 6.58, p. 113) to increase the overall thickness of the casting and thus provide it with greater rigidity at its most vulnerable point. Indeed the chamfer finish is the one of choice in the vast majority of cases.

In the lower arch the three-quarter crown preparation, particularly on the first and second premolars, may need modification, otherwise the finishing line will occur where the buccal cusp of the upper tooth impinges. This will cause breakdown of the enamel prisms in this region and caries at the margin of the

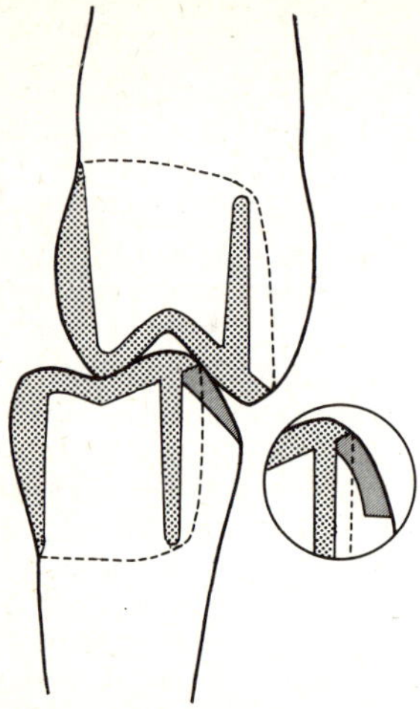

Fig. 6.62. *The three-quarter crown preparation will frequently need modification and extension in the lower arch to clear the bite and protect the margin of the preparation. Two alternatives are shown in the diagram.*

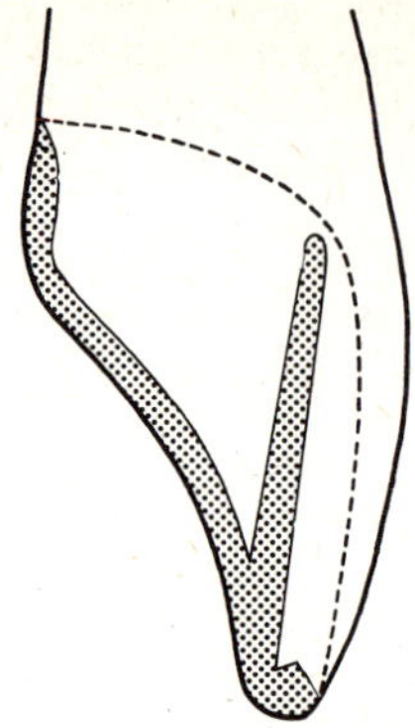

Fig. 6.63. *The anterior three-quarter crown preparation. The grooves should be kept as far labially as is compatible with good aesthetics and the lingual aspect kept as long as possible so as to provide maximum retention.*

retainer. The preparation should therefore be modified to that shown in *Fig.* 6.62.

Anterior Three-quarter Crown

This retainer has far less retention than the posterior three-quarter crown and for this reason is not usually suitable for use as a major retainer in fixed-fixed bridges. It is only where very long clinical crowns are present that its use may be contemplated for this purpose. However, it can be used to advantage on the canine for a simple cantilever design replacing the lateral incisor and is also satisfactory for the fixed-movable bridge, either as the major or minor retainer.

Because of the dictates of aesthetics the preparations should only be taken just through the contact points. It is important that the rails be placed as far labially as possible so as to achieve the maximum of retention (*Fig.* 6.63). At least 1 mm of gold should be provided incisally. This can be bevelled so as to minimize any display of gold.

When the clinical crown is short the preparation should be taken well down into the gingival crevice on the palatal surface to obtain the maximum of retention or, better still, gingival recontouring carried out prior to tooth preparation. It is important that the palatal aspect of the preparation be kept as long and as near parallel to the rails as possible. When the incisal edge is reasonably thick, as for instance on the majority of maxillary canines then it should be grooved; however on a thin incisor grooving of the incisal edge may merely weaken it. Retention can be increased, when necessary, by providing a cingulum pin.

MOD Onlay

On rare occasions an MOD gold inlay may be indicated as a major bridge retainer. However, it should never be used without full occlusal coverage. Its disadvantages are that it is more susceptible to recurrent caries and penetrates more deeply into tooth tissue than the three-quarter crown. It also weakens the tooth and makes it more susceptible to cuspal fracture, particularly if this is a premolar. One of its main advantages is that the length of the finishing margin next to the gingivae is less than with a three-quarter or full crown and thus plaque retention in a susceptible area is reduced.

Post Crown

More care is probably required in the preparation of a tooth for a post crown which will be used as a bridge retainer than any other. This is particularly true when the root is short. The possible cause of the high failure rate of the post crown when used in bridges is the relatively low surface area of the post and the high loading (per sq mm) placed on the cementing medium because of this.

When constructing a post crown the most satisfactory approach is generally to consider how best to restore the tooth to a classical full crown preparation over which the bridge retainer may then be placed.

To achieve this, all sound tooth tissue, as far as possible, is preserved and that missing is then made good with gold (*Fig*. 6.64). This has the advantage that not only is the surface area of the preparation on which the retainer is placed increased but the effective length and surface area of the post is also greater.

Where it is impossible to save any of the crown of the tooth every effort must be made to achieve maximum retention. Thus the post should always be made as long and as rigid as possible. When root filling the tooth only the apical 2–3 mm of the root canal should be occluded and the rest left free for the post. Should the entire root canal be filled for endodontic reasons then the canal must be prepared so that a post will go within 2–3 mm of the apex. To make certain of this a diagnostic x-ray should be taken with a piece of wire or the actual post in place.

A diaphragm is usually required and also a gold collar which extends either half or the whole of the way around the circumference of the tooth (*Fig*. 6.65). This is particularly important on the palatal aspect as the cuff will take a lot of the direct load off the post. This will also greatly reduce the likelihood of the root fracturing.

In favourable circumstances the collar can be omitted on the labial aspect, but where there are any doubts it should always be employed, even though it may mean showing approximately 1 mm of

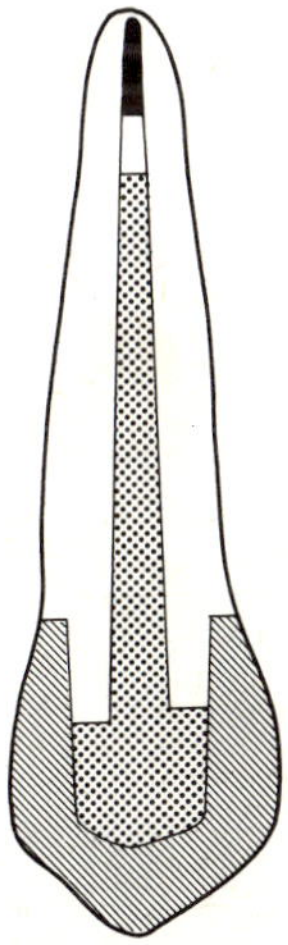

Fig. 6.64. *Post crown preparation |3. The maximum tooth tissue has been retained and the tooth restored to a full crown preparation by means of a post-core unit.*

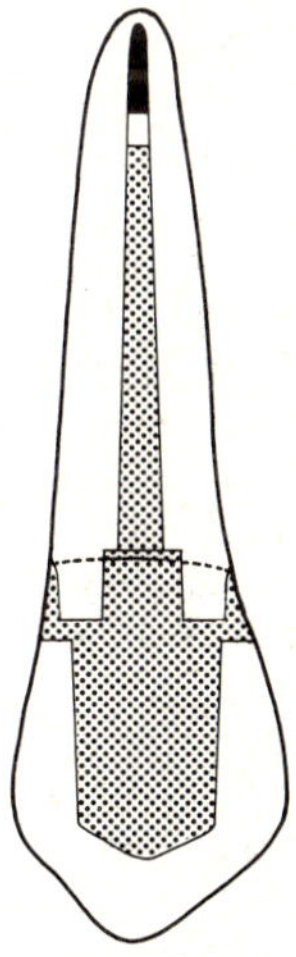

Fig. 6.65. *Post crown preparation for a bridge retainer. Note maximum length of post, countersink to prevent rotation, and full collar cervically.*

gold at the cervical margin. The collar directly increases retention by acting in a similar manner to the MOD, the collar being near-parallel to and opposing the post. It is also, in effect, a small full crown.

Where a collar is used then this will, if correctly prepared, effectively counteract any rotational forces but if this is omitted or it is shallow, then an eccentric countersink should be cut into the root face between 2–3·5 mm deep, depending on the tooth involved. Unfortunately, however, whereas this strengthens the junction between the post and the core, it tends to weaken the root at the one point where maximum strength is required.

An alternative is to use 1 or 2 pins parallel and lingual to the post.

Post Crown Techniques

The wide variety of techniques suggested for the construction of post crowns indicates only too well the problems experienced by the profession with this restoration in the past. It should always be constructed in 2 units, the post combined with the core, and the crown.

The post/core unit may be fabricated either by:

a. Casting it as one unit.

b. Casting a core onto a prefabricated post.

c. Using a prefabricated post/core unit.

Cast Post/Core Units. These are usually cast in a type 4 hard gold. They have the advantage of complete flexibility of design; it being possible to make the post exactly fit the root canal, providing there are no undercuts, whatever its shape or size. Moreover the post and core together with collar are one integral unit.

They are of particular value when the root canal is large or irregular in shape as for instance when caries has occurred. Their disadvantages are:

a. It may be difficult to obtain an accurate impression of the root either by direct or indirect means and to duplicate this in the laboratory is often no simple matter. One method of overcoming this is by employing standardized plastic pins such as 'Endowels'* corresponding in diameter to the reamers employed. They may be used in conjunction with a direct or indirect technique and burn out quite easily in the furnace prior to casting.

b. Cast gold, particularly when used in fine section, for instance for constructing posts for lower incisors, tends to be weak and may fracture. An alternative is to use a base metal for casting but here difficulties with accuracy of fit are likely to occur.

Prefabricated Posts with Cast Cores. By using a prefabricated post together with matched drills so that it exactly fits the root canals the necessity for taking an accurate impression of the majority of the canal is avoided; however, this presupposes that the root canal is of relatively standard size and does not taper too strongly. Generally speaking the post is likely to fit accurately in the apical two-thirds but may well be too small coronally. To overcome this, provide a sound junction between the core and the post and counteract any rotational force an eccentric countersink up to 3·5 mm deep is cut in the root face around the root canal. Thus when the gold core is cast it will reinforce the coronal part of the post.

A system such as that just mentioned has been described by Harty and Leggett (1972). A nickel-cobalt-chromium post† is used, the diameter varying from 1·1 to 1·5 mm. A twist drill of slightly larger diameter than the posts is employed to enlarge the root canal until a length of the Wiptam wire is an easy fit within the canal. An overall impression is then taken with the wire in situ. Prior to casting the impression the post is 'sleeved' with a length of stainless-steel tube to facilitate its removal.

After the model is prepared a length of wire is cut to a suitable size and that part onto which the core is to be cast is roughened to make certain of a good bond between the core and post.

The advantages of this technique are that it is inexpensive and simple to

* Star Dental Manufacturing Co. Inc., Conshohocken, Pa., USA.

† Wiptam Nickel-chromium Clasp Wire. Fried, Krupp, Essen, Germany.

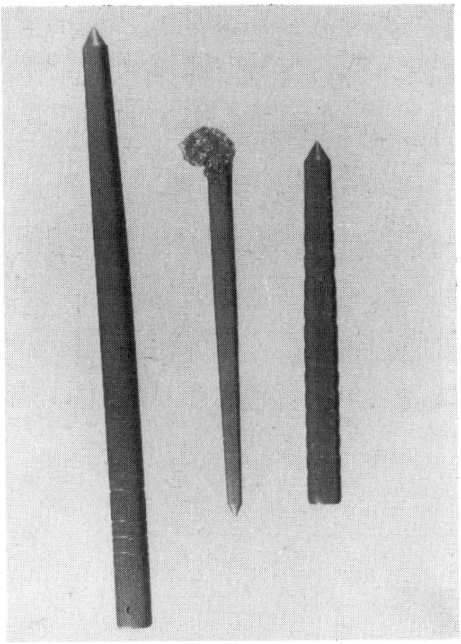

Fig. 6.66. *P.D. tapered smooth and roughened plastic pins for impressions and patterns for cast post crowns. The head of the centre pin has been heated and distorted to improve retention in the impression.*

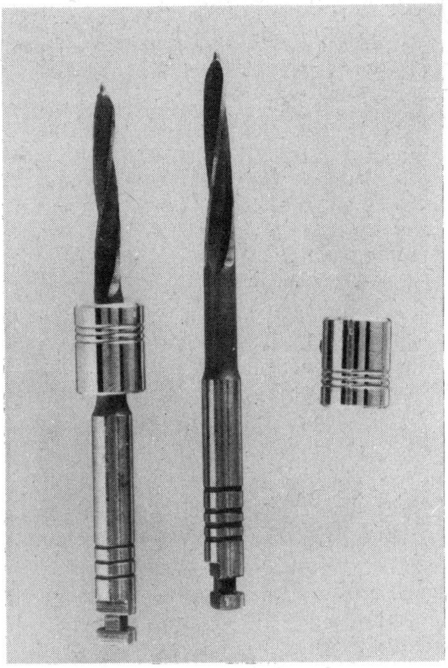

Fig. 6.67. *Drills complete with depth limiting sleeve which match the P.D. plastic impression pins and also the prefabricated metal posts.*

employ; moreover the fit of the post is determined from the outset. A disadvantage is that the post is parallel-sided whereas roots and root canals taper, which can on occasions give rise to problems so far as fit is concerned and could mean with a thin root that the chances of a lateral perforation are increased.

An alternative is to use prefabricated tapered posts such as the stainless steel ones manufactured by P.D.* They also supply smooth tapered plastic pins with matched drills which may be used for impression taking (*Figs.* 6.66, 6.67). These can, if required, be substituted by roughened plastic pins prior to casting in the laboratory. A refinement which will assist in the complete seating of the post during cementation is the provision in it of longitudinal grooves.†

Prefabricated Post/core Units. The basic advantage of prefabricated post/core units such as the Charlton‡ is that they may be cemented into the root canal at the first visit and an overall impression taken of what then, in effect, becomes a porcelain jacket crown preparation. This saves time and expense and simplifies the impression technique; however, the core of a post crown should always be as close to the ideal shape for supporting a porcelain jacket crown as possible and this it is very seldom possible to achieve with a standard post/core unit. To try to

* Produits Dentaires, Vevey, Switzerland and Union Broach Corporation, New York, NY, USA.

† Epox. American Consolidated Mfg Co. Inc., Philadelphia, USA.

‡ Percy J. Clark, Wiltshire, England and Unitek Corporation, Montovia, California, USA.

overcome this problem plastic post/core units have been marketed, the cores of which may be modified in the laboratory prior to casting. It would seem likely that the best results will usually be obtained by employing either a plastic or a prefabricated metal post onto which the core is waxed up and cast, thus achieving the optimal shape for it.

Screw Posts. An alternative to the conventional cast of prefabricated post/core unit is the Kurer screw post system in which retention is provided not by the cement but mainly by the thread of the post. The root canal is first enlarged with a reamer and then threaded with a tap. A countersink is now prepared in the root face for the post/core unit so that it will fit the tooth tissue accurately. An antirotational device is provided by placing an amalgam or composite filling into a cavity cut in both the core and the root face.

The disadvantage of this technique is that a standard core is used which has to be shaped to a suitable form to receive the crown and unfortunately in the majority of cases an ideal shape cannot be achieved.

The Three-quarter Pinlay

The design of this is similar to the three-quarter crown except that pins are substituted for the mesial and distal rails (*Fig*. 6.68). A further one or two pins are also incorporated at the cingulum and a short thick one may be employed near the incisal edge. To provide maximum strength a gold incisal edge is usually provided (*Fig*. 6.68). However, this may be omitted for aesthetic reasons and an incisal bevel prepared instead, thus almost eliminating any display of gold.

When using pinlays it must always be remembered that the retention the pins provide is relatively limited and that it is desirable that the crowns of the teeth being prepared are thick labiopalatally and of reasonable length. Moreover the castings must be rigid otherwise, should flexion occur, they will become unseated but may still be held in place by one or more of the pins and thus rapid caries will occur.

A 'step' is always provided to give an

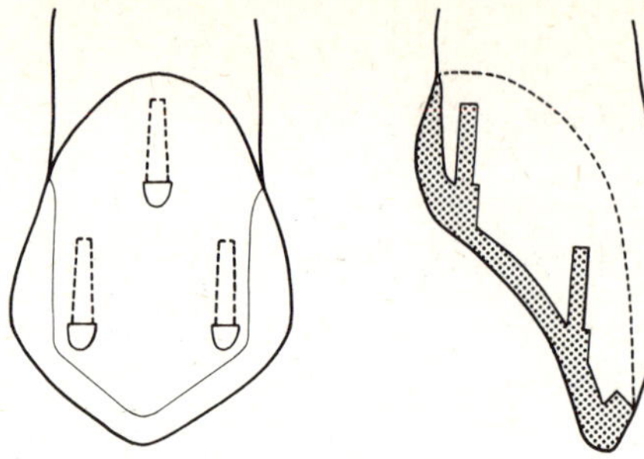

Fig. 6.68. *The three-quarter pinledge. Note countersink to increase thickness of gold in the region of the pin.*

increase in the thickness of gold at the junction of the pin with the rest of the casting.

The Alignment of Multiple Pinlays

Although the pinholes drilled in one or possibly two retainers may be aligned by eye so as to give a common line of insertion it would be practically impossible to do so where large numbers of pins are involved. There are two main ways of overcoming this, either directly by using a paralleling device in the mouth or indirectly on the model in the laboratory (McCormack, 1976).

Direct Technique

The first device described to enable multiple parallel pinholes to be drilled in the mouth was the Pontostructor, which was designed by Karlström in 1941.

Like most subsequent developments, it makes use of a plate which is firmly anchored to the teeth not being prepared and to which is attached a swivelling adjustable arm with a sheath at one end which controls the angulation of the bur. It is so devised that in whichever direction the handpiece is moved the long axis of the drill remains constant.

The difficulty with the Pontostructor is that it is rather complex and difficult to use. Its bulk is also a disadvantage and often prevents its application in the posterior region. A further complication

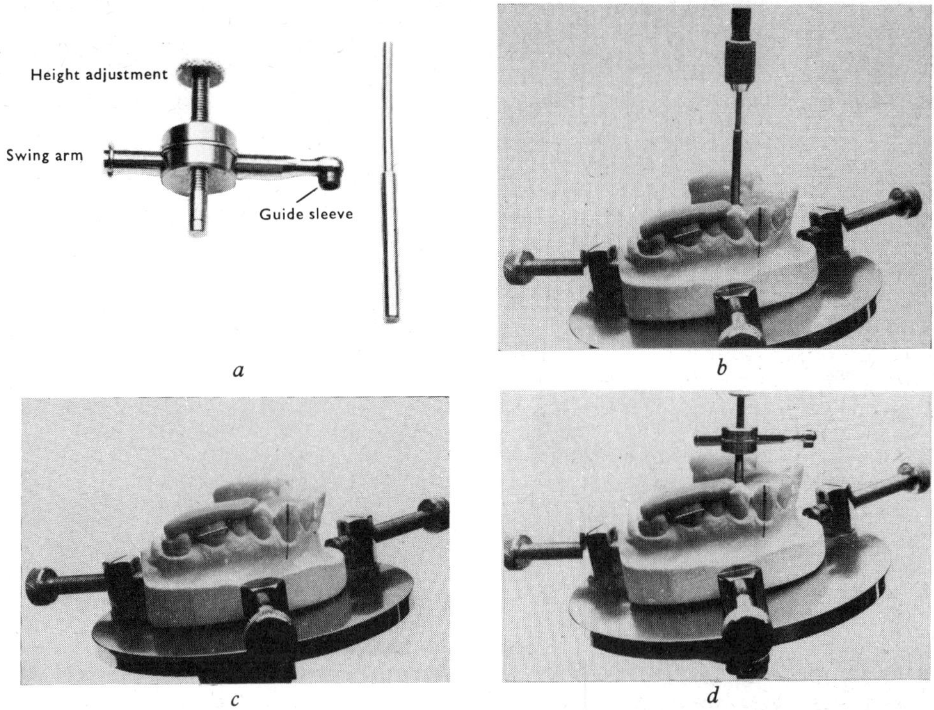

Fig. 6.69. *The P.P. Paralleling Instrument. a, The basic instrument consisting of height adjustment screw, swing arm, guide sleeve and, on the right, mounting mandrel for the base support. b, The base plate is constructed, the model mounted on the parallelometer, and the correct alignment determined from the model and radiographs. c, The base support is positioned with the mounting mandrel and fixed in place with self-curing acrylic. d, The paralleling instrument mounted on its base support.*

is its relatively large and rigid metal base which sometimes proves difficult to fit into the palate.

Because of these difficulties simpler and more adaptable devices have now come on to the market. Examples of these are the P.P. developed by Göransson (*Fig.* 6.69) and the Prec-in-Dent devised by Karlström (1971). This latter will be described in more detail so as to illustrate the general design principles and use of a paralleling device.

Prec-in-Dent. This, like most other paralleling instruments, is retained in the mouth with a self-curing acrylic or a heat-moulded plate (*Fig.* 6.70*b*). Incorporated in this is a special disposable plastic base which is connected to the remainder of the instrument by means of a ball joint (*Fig.* 6.70*a*), thus permitting the angulation to be adjusted to that most suitable for any particular case. It also incorporates a locking pin which fixes the angulation of the device once the correct setting has been determined. This is actuated by a locking bar.

Attachments are available for both conventional and high-speed handpieces (*Fig.* 6.70*e*) and a swinging arm is incorporated so as to permit pin holes to be drilled at various levels without having to adjust it.

Technique. First the plastic base is ground until it fits easily into the palate. A self-curing acrylic or thermoplastic base is now laid down on the model. This should generally overlay the occlusal

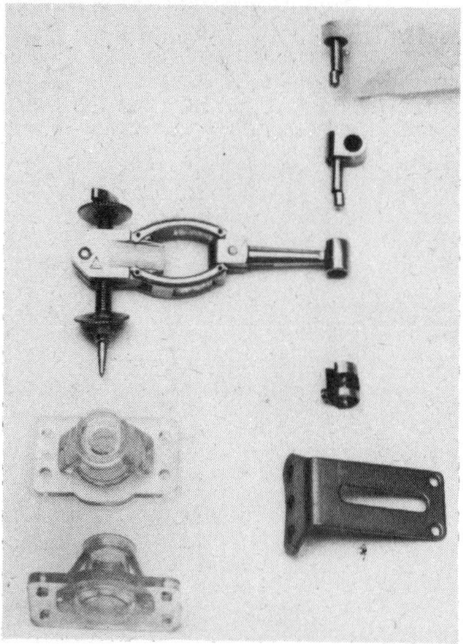

a

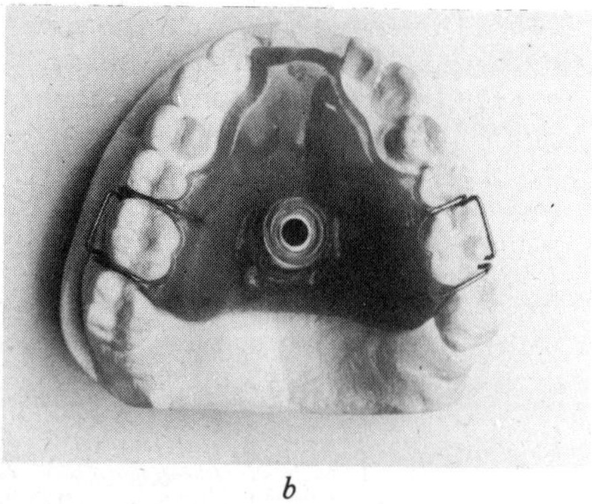

b

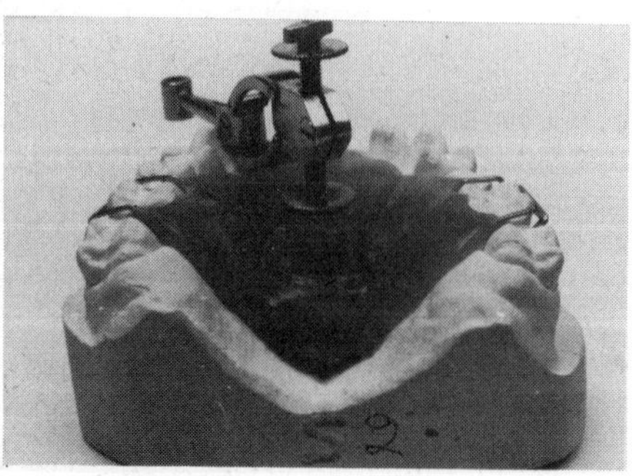

c

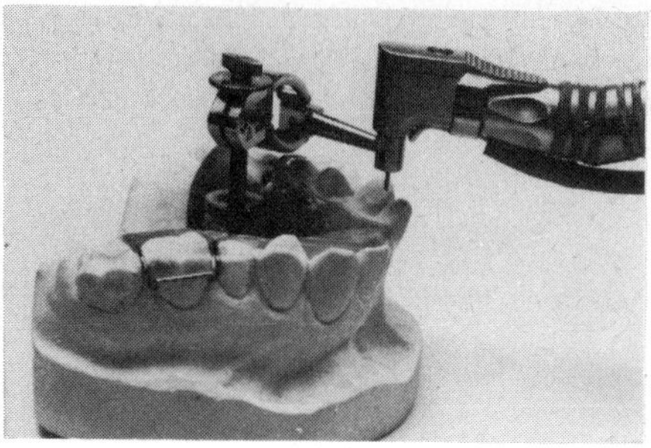

d

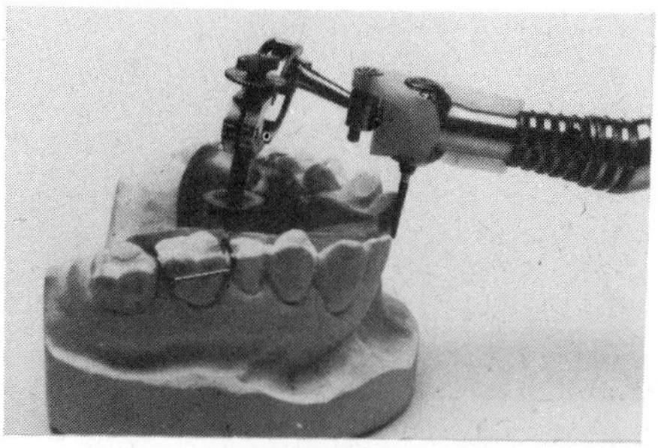

e

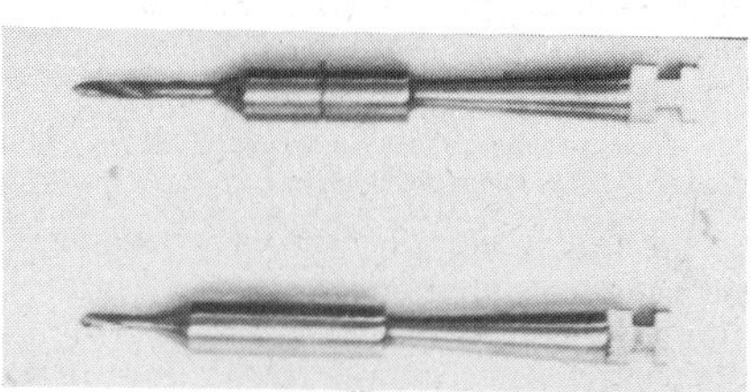

f

Fig. 6.70. *The Prec-in-Dent Paralleling Instrument. a, The kit consists of plastic mounts to which the floating arm is fixed. Attachments for horizontal use and a high-speed handpiece are also shown. b, The plastic mount fitted to the base plate. Clasps are incorporated to increase stability. Where possible, occlusal coverage should also be provided. c, The instrument mounted on its base plate. The locking pin at the top is turned to fix the angulation. d, A right-angle handpiece being used with the special drill shown in f. e, The adaptor for the high-speed handpiece in position. f, Special drills with a tapered shank are employed so that the handpiece may be moved without disturbing the angulation of the drill.*

surfaces of the teeth but be kept well clear of those that are to be prepared. If necessary, clasps may be incorporated in it for additional stability. The disposable plastic unit is now fitted on to the base plate (*Fig*. 6.70*b*). Its position is not critical but ideally it should be in the midline a little cervical to and parallel with the occlusal surfaces of the teeth.

When the acrylic has set, the appliance is removed from the model, trimmed and polished. The actual paralleling device is now fixed to the base plate by means of a ball joint and locking disc which permits the angulation to be varied.

The correct alignment for the pinlays may now be determined either in the mouth or on the model by studying the angulation of the teeth and, from X-rays, the size and shape of the pulps. After assessing the correct angulation the parallelometer may be positively locked in this position by turning the locking bar until the locking pin is driven into the plastic base below the ball joint (*Fig*. 6.70*c*). The pinhole created will subsequently permit accurate relocation of the angulation should the instrument have to be disturbed for any reason.

The parallelometer is now ready for use. It is not usually required for the initial preparation of the teeth which is carried out freehand, first with an airotor and then with low-speed instrumentation. However, its use is essential for drilling the pinholes and is often also of value for aligning several box preparations or getting these parallel with the pin holes.

After the ledges for the pins have been cut, starting points are made on these with a half-round bur. The parallelometer should now be fitted into position. To reduce any chance of it moving during use it is advisable to use a little quick setting zinc oxide and eugenol cement to locate it positively.

The handpiece, complete with a twist drill of appropriate size and length, is now inserted into the guide sleeve and the pinholes prepared (*Fig*. 6.70*d*). The PR drills advocated possess a tapered shank which allows the handpiece to move relative to the drill without affecting the angulation of the pinhole being cut (*Fig*. 6.70*f*). This is highly desirable as it is almost impossible to hold a handpiece at exactly the same angulation for any length of time.

The floating arm will usually provide sufficient adjustment for drilling most pinholes. However, if required, the height of the arm can be varied by an adjusting wheel. This alters the vertical level of the arm by 0·5 mm for each complete turn. If necessary this can be used as a guide for the depth of penetration of the drill; but the use of a drill such as the Spirco, which, because it incorporates a stop, will only drill to a known depth, is to be preferred.

The rest of the technique is similar to that already described when discussing pinledge preparations and impressions earlier in the chapter. Should it prove necessary to drill parallel horizontal pin holes an attachment is available for this purpose.

Further Paralleling Devices. Many other paralleling devices are available. Some use a revolving disc and others have a guide pin which is inserted into the first pinhole cut. An arm is attached to this which will direct the drill down the second pinhole parallel with the initial hole drilled.

Probably the simplest of all methods is to drill the initial pinhole, insert a plastic pin in it and then, using this as a guide, cut the second pinhole. This can be repeated until all the pinholes are drilled.

Indirect Multiple Pin Alignment

In practice most paralleling devices used in the mouth work tolerably well but their bulk makes their application difficult in the posterior region. The other difficulty is that however well manufactured they always tend to develop some play in their joints which leads to inaccuracies. An alternative to the alignment of multiple pinholes in the mouth is to carry out this procedure indirectly, drilling the holes first on a model in the laboratory, prefabricating the pinlays, and then using a template to drill corresponding holes in the natural

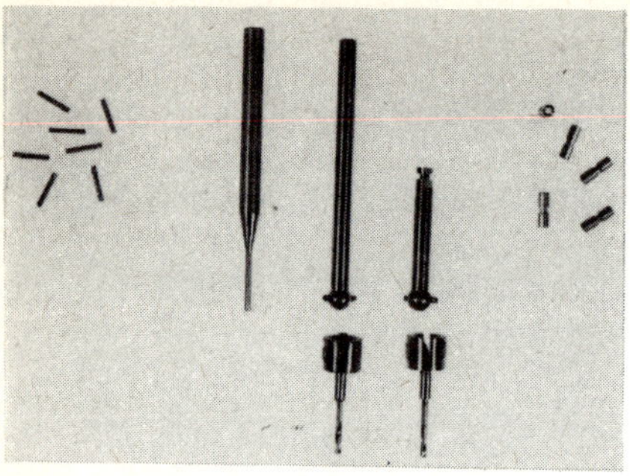

Fig. 6.71. *The Ney parallel-pin kit consists of knurled iridioplatinum pins of different thicknesses and lengths, drill bushings and their mounting mandrel and twist drills in two sizes which may be used in right-angle or straight handpieces.*

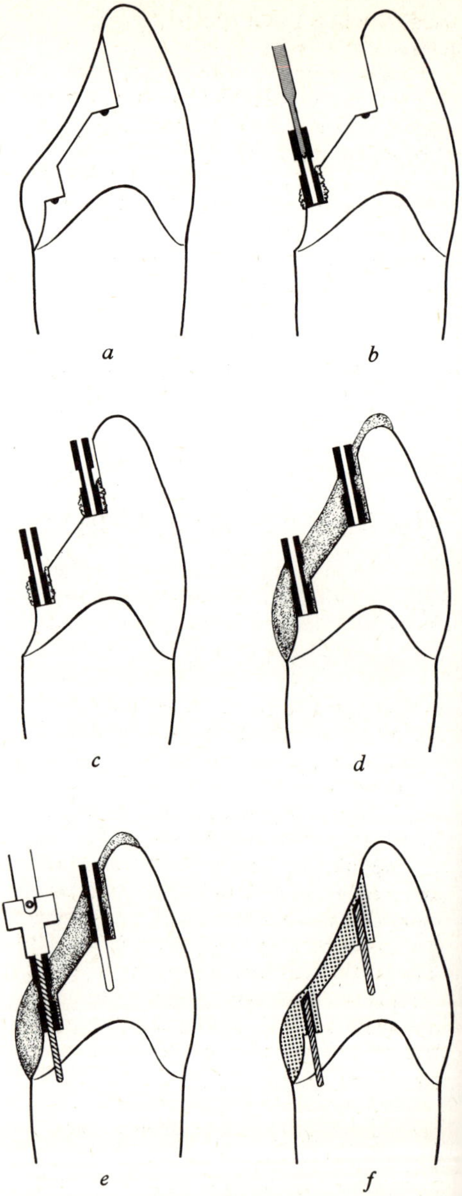

Fig. 6.72. *Indirect multiple-pin alignment (the Ney technique). a, The pinledge preparation. Starting points for the pinholes are made in the mouth with a half-round bur. b, A drill bushing being positioned on the duplicate model with the (paralleling) mandrel and fixed in place with a little wax. c, The drill bushings are all located parallel to each other by means of the mandrel and parallelometer. d, The template is made by joining the drill bushings together with acrylic and then extending this over the incisal edges of the teeth. e, The pinholes are now cut in the master model with a drill of standard length; it is the bushing which determines the depth of the pinhole. f, The completed casting incorporating iridioplatinum pins.*

teeth. A kit for this purpose is marketed by J. M. Ney & Co.* (*Fig*. 6.71).

The pinledge preparations are performed in the usual manner in the mouth. Steps are provided for the pinholes and starting points marked on these with a half-round bur (*Fig*. 6.72*a*). However, the actual pinholes are not prepared at this stage. An impression is then taken and two stone models are cast, a master on which the actual bridge will be constructed and a duplicate which is

* J. M. Ney & Co., Hartford, Connecticut, USA.

used for the construction of a drilling template.

This is mounted on a parallelometer and the correct angulation decided on for the pins. This will be determined not only by the angulation of the abutment teeth but also by the position and size of the pulps of the teeth which will have been assessed from the X-rays. The length and thickness of pins required must be decided at the same time.

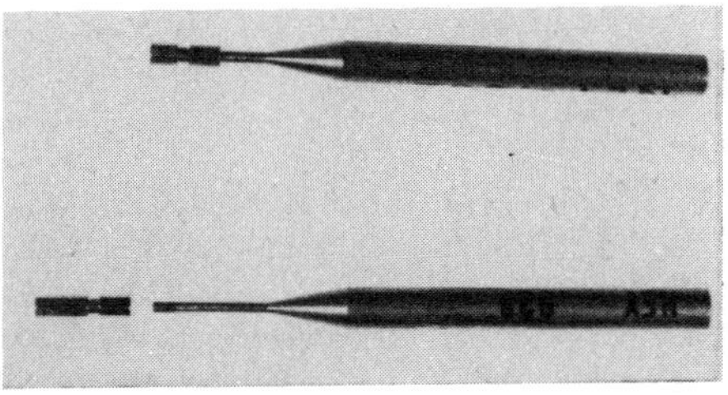

Fig. 6.73. *Mandrel used for paralleling the bushes on the duplicate model.*

Drill bushings are now positioned on the model at the site of each pinhole by means of a special mandrel mounted in the parallelometer (*Fig*. 6.73). As each one is placed it is lightly fixed with a little sticky wax (*Fig*. 6.72*b*).

Five different lengths of drill bushing are used in conjunction with a standard length drill. This thus gives five different lengths of pinhole (*Figs*. 6.74, 6.75). The longer the bush the shorter the hole.

After all the bushings have been mounted (*Fig*. 6.72*c*) they are positively located to each other and also to the teeth by flowing self-curing acrylic over and around them. However, care must be taken not to occlude the holes in the bushes. The acrylic is now built up until it is sufficiently thick to provide a rigid drilling template (*Fig*. 6.72*d*).

This is removed from the model and trimmed. The acrylic is cut through at the incisal edge in several places so that it is possible to see that it is always fully seated.

It is now returned to the duplicate model on the parallelometer and the special mandrel is used to check that all the drill bushings are still parallel to each other.

The template is next transferred to the master model and, providing that it is fully seated, the pinholes are drilled in the dies (*Fig*. 6.72*e*). This is done by hand using the matching twist drills and making certain that the pin holes are carefully cleaned out.

Knurled parallel-sided iridioplatinum pins are now placed in the pinholes, a little oil being used to help to centre them. If a twist drill of 0·7 mm has been used then the size of pin required will be 0·6 mm and if one 0·8 mm in diameter was employed then a pin of 0·7 mm is indicated.

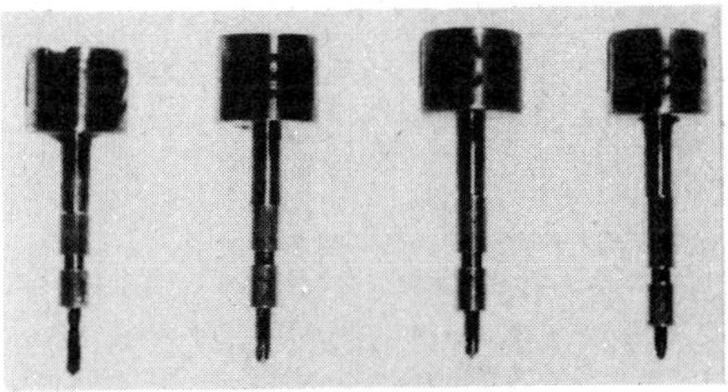

Fig. 6.74. *A standard length drill is used in conjunction with bushings of different length. The shorter the bushing the deeper the pinhole cut.*

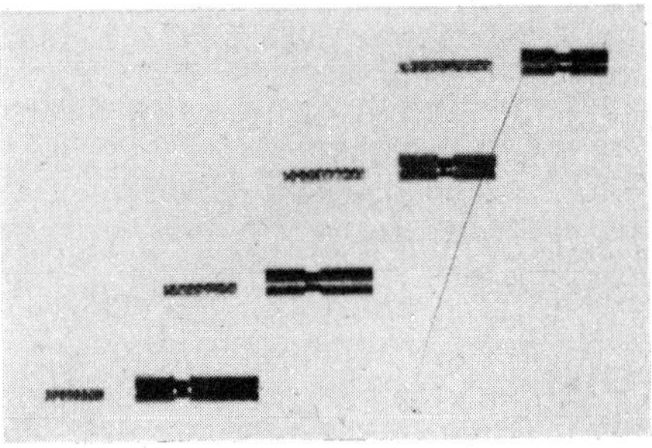

Fig. 6.75. *Drill bushings alongside their matching iridioplatinum pins. The shorter the pin required the longer the bushing used.*

The pins should protrude from the pinholes about 1·5 mm so as to give them a firm anchorage to the wax pattern.

Some authorities prefer at this stage to

join all the pins together with self-curing acrylic, so as to be able to check their angulation by removing them 'as one' prior to completing the wax-up. If this is done then the acrylic must be kept well clear of the margins of the preparations.

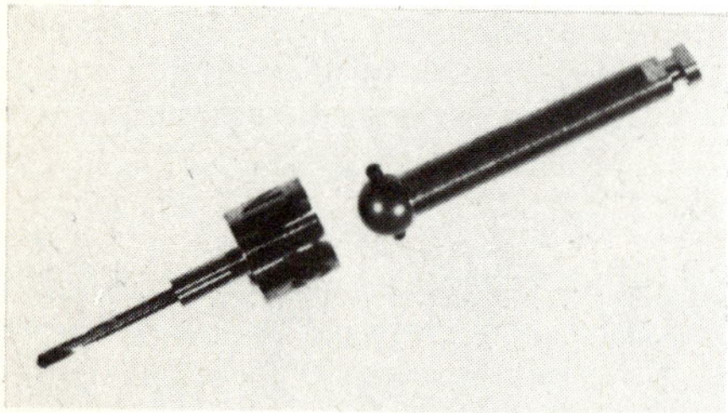

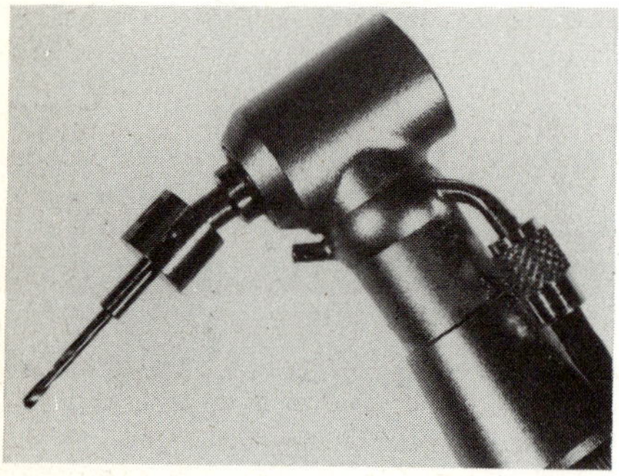

Fig. 6.76. *The drills used incorporate a universal joint which allows the handpiece to be moved without affecting their angulation.*

The bridge is now completed ready for fitting (*Fig.* 6.72*f*) in the mouth. At this stage the abutment teeth are carefully cleaned and the acrylic bushing template is inserted into the mouth. To be certain that it will not move during use it may be fixed in place with a little zinc oxide and eugenol cement.

The correct drill for each pinhole is now placed in the handpiece. Each incorporates a universal joint so that the angulation of the handpiece may vary without affecting the drill (*Fig.* 6.76). It is important that the initial preparation should be taken through to dentine, otherwise difficulty will be experienced in penetrating the enamel with the twist drills. They must be run slowly because any heat generated will soften the acrylic around the bushing and allow it to move. It is, of course, essential that the drill be inserted right up to its stop on each occasion.

The pinholes are now all carefully cleaned out and the bridge tried in. If all is satisfactory then it can be cemented using a slow setting mix of zinc phosphate cement. This should be worked up the pinholes with a spiral root-canal filling instrument.

■ Minor Retainers

a. Three-quarter and Full Crowns

When either of these restorations are

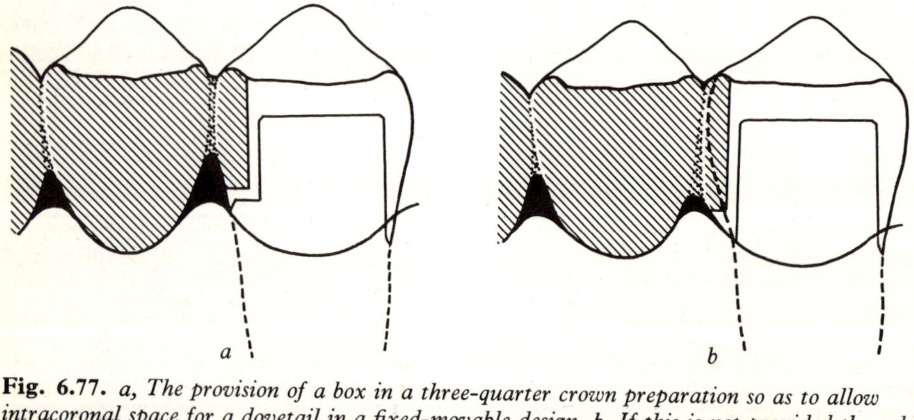

Fig. 6.77. *a, The provision of a box in a three-quarter crown preparation so as to allow intracoronal space for a dovetail in a fixed-movable design. b, If this is not provided the gold will have to be extended at the cervical margin and this will result in loss of the interproximal embrasures and food packing.*

used as minor retainers the preparation is similar to that already described. The only modification required is the provision of a box to house the dovetail intracoronally (*Fig.* 6.77*a*). If this is not done the contour of the retainer will be poor (*Fig.* 6.77*b*), encouraging plaque retention and thus periodontal breakdown.

b. Selberg Modification of the Three-quarter Crown

This restoration is most commonly employed on upper anteriors, particularly the canine, and avoids the destruction of one of the contacts, normally the mesial, thus preventing any undue display of gold (*Fig.* 6.78). Likewise the incisal edge is not involved. It is more retentive than the Class III inlay and yet aesthetically as pleasing.

The preparation is commenced half-way between the cingulum and the mesial contact and extended through the distal contact. If used as a minor retainer a box is normally incorporated at this point to house the dovetail. Retention is provided in part with pins. The preparation is capable of considerable modification to suit the particular requirements of any one tooth or bridge design.

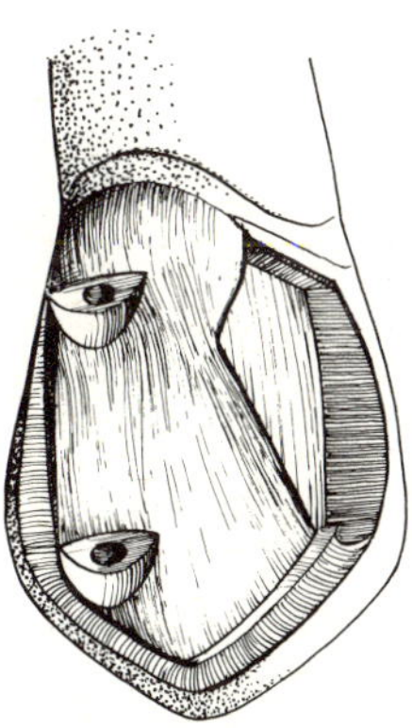

Fig. 6.78. *Selberg modification of the three-quarter crown, shown here with a distal box which is required for its use as a minor retainer.*

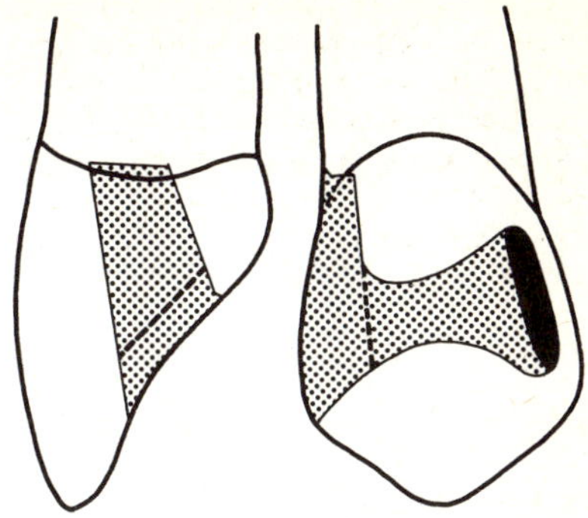

Fig. 6.79. *Class III inlay preparation for a minor retainer. Note mesial countersink to increase retention, and distal box to house the dovetail.*

c. Class III Incisal Withdrawal Inlay

When a Class III inlay is used as a minor retainer it has to have an incisal line of withdrawal to provide a box roughly parallel with the angulation of the major retainer, so that a dovetail may be housed intracoronally (*Fig.* 6.79).

Care must be taken to obtain good retention from the lock. A mesial countersink is usually provided, to create, in effect, a preparation akin to an MOD. Alternatively a pin may be employed, but it is doubtful if it will provide as much retention.

The preparation should be bevelled on the cervical margin of the lock otherwise the enamel prisms will break down at this point and result in a faulty margin. However, only a minimum of tooth tissue must be removed or retention will be lost.

It cannot be emphasized too strongly that this preparation should only be employed for the minor retainer of a bridge where the operator is certain of adequate retention, which implies a larger and more fully erupted tooth than the average. Should cementation failure occur the inlay will be retained in place by the rail, and rapid caries will ensue.

d. Class II Inlay

The Class II inlay used as a minor retainer is similar to the standard preparation. However, it is important to make certain that the box is large enough

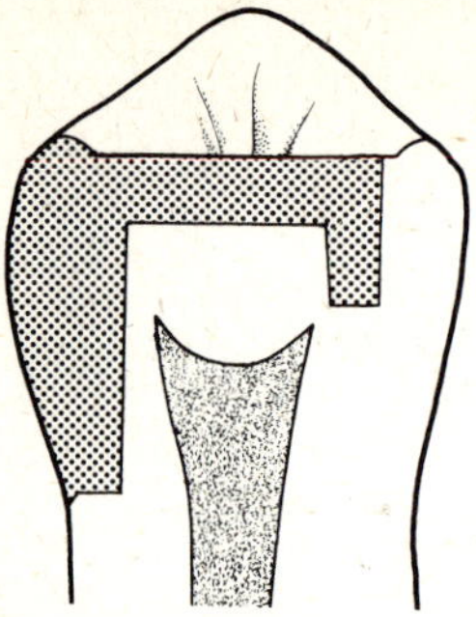

Fig. 6.80. *Class II inlay with countersink in the lock to increase retention.*

to house the dovetail intracoronally and still allow sufficient gold for a really rigid casting. Similar remarks apply to the MOD.

To increase retention of the MO or DO gold inlay a countersink is usually provided at the end of the lock as shown in *Fig.* 6.80. Alternatively, a pin may be incorporated in the casting. To provide the maximum of retention a system of vertical non-parallel pin fixation may be employed.

Despite all that has been written on bridge retainers in this chapter it must be stated in conclusion that there are so many variable factors, not only with regard to the patient's dentition and cooperation but also the operator's ability, that no firm rules can apply in any specific case. The only certainty is that it must always be correct, when in doubt, to make certain of retention by providing too much rather than too little.

Bibliography

Baum L. and Contino R. (1970) Ten years experience with cast pin restorations. *Dent. Clin. North Am.* **14,** 14.

Clyde J. S. and Sharkey S. W. (1978) The pin ledge crown. A reappraisal. *Br. Dent. J.* **144,** 239.

Courtade G. L. (1970) Methods for pin splinting the lower anterior teeth. *Dent. Clin. North Am.* **14,** 3.

Cross W. G. (1971) A modification of a horizontal non-parallel screw splint. *Br. Dent. J.* **130,** 442.

Goransson P. (1967) The P.P. parallel pin instrument. A. B. Svenska Instrument Co. Stockholm.

Hannah C. M. (1973) Prefabricated post and core patterns. *J. Prosthet. Dent.* **30,** 37.

Harty F. J. and Leggett L. J. (1972) A post crown technique using a nickel-cobalt-chromium post. *Br. Dent. J.* **132,** 394.

Jørgensen K. D. (1955) The relationship between retention and convergence angles in cemented veneer crowns. *Acta Odontol. Scand.* **13,** 35.

Karlström G. (1968) Parallel pins and fixed partial dentures. *J. Prosthet. Dent.* **19,** 613.

Karlström G. (1971) A paralleling instrument for the guidance of pin channels and high speed preparations. *J. Prosthet. Dent.* **19,** 613.

Kurer H. G., Combe E. C. and Grant A. A. (1977) Factors influencing the retention of dowels. *J. Prosthet. Dent.* **38,** 515.

Lorey R. E. and Myers G. E. (1968) The retentive qualities of bridge retainers. *J. Am. Dent. Assoc.* **76,** 568.

Lovdahl P. E. and Nicholls J. I. (1977) Pin-retained amalgam cores *vs* cast-gold dowel cores. *J. Prosthet. Dent.* **38,** 507.

McCormack J. M. (1967) Paralleling in conservative dentistry. 2: The pin sleeve method of constructing multipin crowns. *Br. Dent. J.* **123,** 397.

McCormack J. (1976) Mechanical methods of paralleling pinholes. *Dent. Update* **3,** 75.

McCormack J. (1976) The clinical use of parallel sided pins. *Dent. Update* **3,** 129.

Nickolls E. (1963) The restoration of root-filled teeth. *Dent. Practnr Dent. Rec.* **13,** 459.

Roberts D. H. (1967) The use of the three-quarter crown in standard and modified form in bridge work. *Br. Dent. J.* **122,** 430.

Roberts D. H. (1970) The failure of retainers in bridge protheses. *Br. Dent. J.* **128,** 117.

Roberts D. H. (1970) The relationship between age and the failure rate of bridge protheses. *Br. Dent. J.* **128,** 175.

Sced I. R. and McLean J. W. (1972) The strength of metal/ceramic bonds with base metals containing chromium. *Br. Dent. J.* **132,** 232.

Shillingburg H. T., Hobo S. and Fisher D. W. (1974) *Preparations for Cast Gold Restorations*. Berlin and Chicago, Buch-und Zeitschriften-Verlag, 'Die Quintessenz'.

Smith C. L. (1970) Prefabricated parallel pin castings. *Dent. Clin. North Am.* **14,** 31.

Standlee J. P., Collard E. W. and Caputo A. A. (1970) Dentinal defects caused by some twist drills and retentive pins. *J. Prosthet. Dent.* **24,** 185.

Thompson A. (1967) Paralleling in conservative dentistry. *Br. Dent. J.* **123,** 328.

Weine F. S. et al. (1973) The use of standardised tapered plastic pins in post and core fabrication. *J. Prosthet. Dent.* **29,** 542.

Weissman B. (1965) A non-parallel universal horizontal pin splint. *J. Prosthet. Dent.* **15,** 339.

Winstanley R. B. (1971) Pin retained amalgam restorations. *Br. Dent. J.* **130,** 327.

7

ANTERIOR BRIDGES

Requirements of an Anterior Bridge
Indications for Use
Fixed-fixed Bridges
General Technique for Anterior Bridges
The Anterior Fixed-movable Bridge

The main reason for placing an anterior bridge is to improve a patient's appearance, and this consideration must always be kept to the forefront during its design and construction. The other principal purposes are to correct any speech defects caused by the missing tooth and to maintain an orthodontic result. A fixed bridge will always do this more efficiently than a removable prosthesis because of its positive stabilization of the teeth and the fact that it cannot be left out by the patient.

There are two main types of anterior bridge, fixed-fixed and fixed-movable. Besides these the cantilever and spring cantilever designs may be used in this region, but these will be considered separately as their design is entirely different.

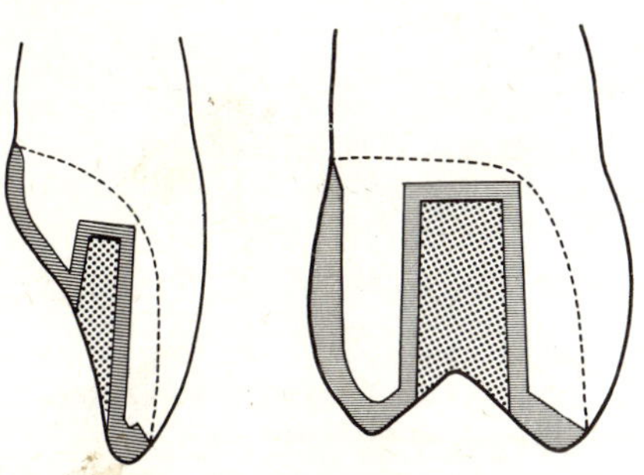

Fig. 7.1. *It is more difficult to provide a satisfactory intracoronal dovetail in anterior retainers because of their sloping lingual surfaces.*

Whereas in the posterior region the bridge most commonly employed in short-span cases is a fixed-movable one, in the anterior region the fixed-fixed designs are often to be preferred. There are several reasons for this:

1. It is more difficult to provide a good dovetail with which to lock the two parts of the bridge together positively (*Fig.* 7.1). This is because of the general morphology of the anterior teeth and in particular the lack of width labiolingually.
2. Because of the curvature of the arch and the direction of the forces applied, appreciably more stress is placed on the connectors in this region.
3. Where the teeth on either side are restored with full crowns adequate retention will be available for a fixed-fixed bridge and the complication of a joint can be dispensed with. This is particularly desirable with the bonded porcelains which are now used for the majority of anterior fixed-fixed bridges.

REQUIREMENTS OF AN ANTERIOR BRIDGE

■ Aesthetics

The main requirement of an anterior bridge, as already mentioned, is a good appearance and thus the labial aspect of the pontic must be aesthetically pleasing. This should also be taken into account when designing the retainers.

Ideally no gold should be visible on the labial aspect of the bridge. However, if this is unavoidable it should be kept to the minimum compatible with providing sufficient protection for the facing or strength for the retainers. The labial shoulder should usually be finished *just* subgingival to avoid showing the margin of the preparation. However, if the necks of the teeth are not displayed during smiling the finish may be supragingival, if other factors do not contraindicate it. Lingually the margin should generally be supragingival, the extent of this varying with the length and shape of the clinical crown and the degree of retention required.

INDICATIONS FOR USE

The anterior fixed bridge has several specific advantages over the removable prosthesis. Its stability is of great value, particularly when speaking. This obviously applies especially to those who earn their living by speech, such as teachers, actors, and singers. It is also of material help to musicians playing wind instruments. The psychological as well as strictly practical benefits to be gained by the fixed prosthesis are considerable.

It has the further advantage that its bulk is far less than any alternative form of prosthesis, except possibly an implant, and more nearly corresponds to the teeth it replaces. This again assists good elocution.

Where the anterior teeth are badly positioned or rotated, possibly due to early tooth loss or congenital absence, then a fixed bridge will usually produce the best aesthetic result (*Fig.* 7.2). By crowning the teeth to be used as abutments they and the teeth being replaced can be arranged so as to produce the optimum in aesthetics. This would not be possible with a removable prosthesis.

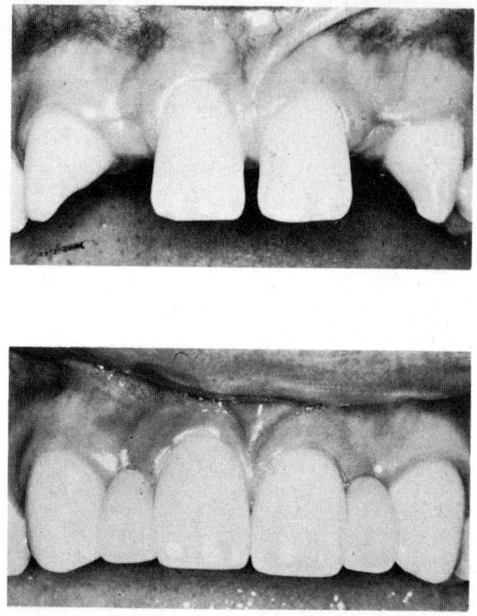

Fig. 7.2. *Congenital absence of 2|2 and poorly formed 3|3 treated by fixed-fixed metal-ceramic bridges.*
(By courtesy of Mr R. D. N. Atkinson.)

FIXED-FIXED BRIDGES

■ Abutments

The choice of abutments for various bridge designs has already been mentioned in Chapter 6. Usually if any one incisor is missing then the use of the teeth on either side will be adequate. However, if a canine is missing it may prove necessary to involve the central as well as the lateral mesially. An alternative to this would be a cantilever bridge supported by both the premolars distally.

If the two centrals have been lost both the lateral and the canine will usually be required as abutments because the root surface area of the lateral on its own would be inadequate. Where a central and lateral on the same side need replacement the use of the canine and central as abutments will usually prove sufficient, but each case requires individual assessment.

Retainers

Probably the most popular retainer for the anterior fixed-fixed bridge is the bonded full crown. This has the advantage that there will be no display of gold labially and that it is often possible to construct the bridge in one unit using similar materials for both pontic and retainers.

The pinledge preparation may also be employed, although care must always be taken to make certain that the castings have adequate retention and in particular are sufficiently rigid.

The three-quarter crown and three-quarter pinlay both have the disadvantage that an incisal edge of gold is displayed. Unless the clinical crowns of the teeth are rather longer than normal the three-quarter crown scarcely provides sufficient retention and is liable to cementation failure, particularly if used on the lateral.

When a post crown has to be employed, every effort must be made to obtain maximum retention, using a gold collar around the whole of the root face and keeping the post as long as possible. A separate full crown is then used as a retainer over this.

Pontics

A. Form

The form of the anterior pontic is largely governed by aesthetic requirements, whereas in the posterior region the dictates of hygiene are more important. Thus with the anterior pontic the labial morphology chosen will be that which will produce the best aesthetic result. However, it can be made a little thinner labiolingually than the tooth it replaces so as to make it more easily cleanable.

Where there has been appreciable loss of tissue in the pontic area, but not so much that soft-tissue replacement is necessitated by a removable prosthesis, the neck of the pontic may be curved in labially. This will enable the clinical margin of the pontic to be at the same level as the neighbouring teeth and it will also avoid covering too much of the mucoperiosteum (*Fig*. 7.3). However, the degree to which this can be done depends to some extent on the smile line. Where necessary a little soft tissue may be replaced by baking pink porcelain on to the pontic cervically.

If a lot of soft tissue has been lost a removable prosthesis, possibly precision retained, is indicated.

B. Type

The choice of pontic depends mainly on the aesthetic requirements of the patient and the materials used for the construction of the retainers. Thus if bonded full crowns are chosen the pontics will also usually be made of the same material. However, if three-quarter crowns or pinledges are employed and some incisal

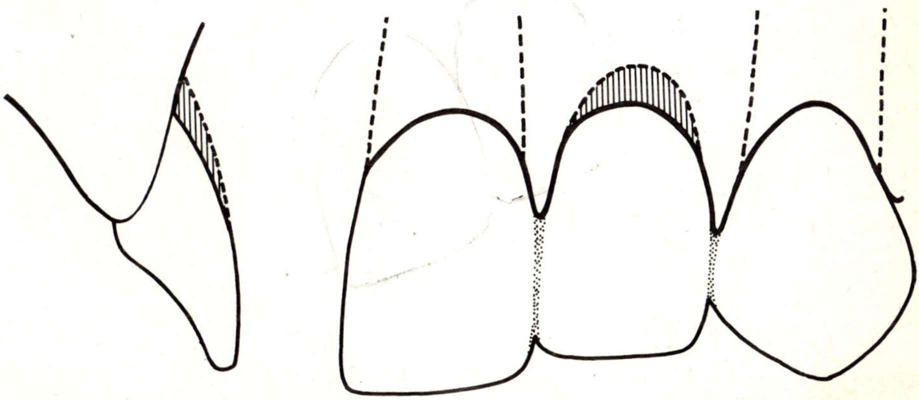

Fig. 7.3. *By curving the labial aspect of the pontic in at the cervical margin, its gingival contour can be made to match that of the neighbouring teeth.*

gold is displayed because of this, a manufactured facing such as the long-pin (*see Fig*. 5.9, p. 72) or reverse pin pontic may be employed. When the pinledge has been designed to avoid any incisal gold a bonded porcelain pontic is indicated.

■ Materials employed

Acrylic alone is not a satisfactory material for fixed bridges; however, if combined with gold some of its defects can be eliminated. Thus gold can be placed on the palatal aspect to prevent wear and over-eruption in this region. Similarly the fit and tissue contact can be of gold to reduce gingival irritation. However, even then the life of the bridge will still be limited to 5–7 years because of the discoloration and wear of the acrylic.

Where gold and porcelain are employed separate porcelain facings may be used or the material fused to gold. With the former which are now used relatively rarely, protection of the porcelain is required incisally unless the bite is favourable. The use of the porcelain bonded to gold materials probably provides the strongest of all bridges. They are therefore particularly useful in all cases where the bite is heavy or close. Their only disadvantage is that sometimes the life of the bridge may be limited by the relatively soft gold which, in the case of a heavy bite, can be worn through in 7–10 years. To overcome this a lingual shoulder may be provided (*see Fig*. 6.52, p. 110) and the porcelain extended to this to protect the gold.

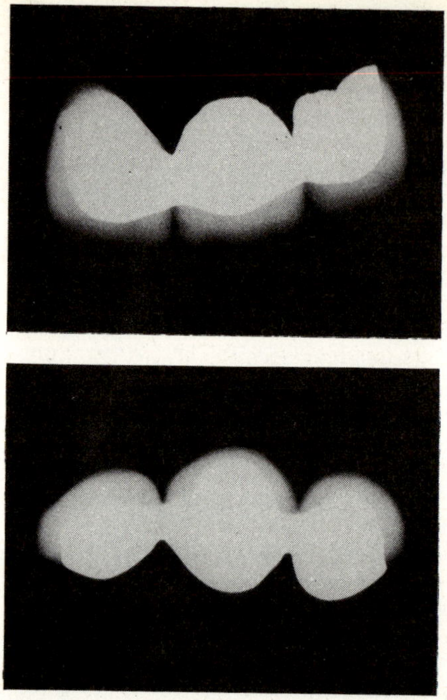

Fig. 7.4. *The thickness of the metal subframe may be checked by x-raying the bridge in two different planes using an intra-oral x-ray and a standard exposure.*

■ Types of Anterior Fixed-fixed Bridge

The three main types, all employing full crowns, which will be discussed here are:

1. The porcelain bonded to gold bridge.
2. Porcelain jacket crowns over a gold subframe.
3. The all-porcelain bridge.

Porcelain bonded to Gold Bridge

This is the most adaptable of all anterior bridges. It provides good strength, satisfactory aesthetics, has a porcelain to tissue fit surface, and is very reliable. Its only disadvantage is that it is not always possible to achieve a completely satisfactory aesthetic result. In the case of the incisors, particularly those being used as abutments, it is difficult to obtain sufficient space for an adequate thickness of both gold and porcelain, the reduction of labial enamel required being of the order of 1·5 mm. This is especially true with the young patient and is accentuated if the crowns are thin labiolingually.

The problem is at its worst in the lower anterior region as the maximum possible space that can be provided is limited by the distance between the pulp of the abutment tooth and the occluding surface of the upper incisors (*Fig*. 6.48, p. 108). This applies in particular to the patient with a Class II, division 2 malocclusion.

A point to be guarded against is the provision of wide embrasures and a good appearance of separation between the teeth at the expense of the interproximal metal (*Fig*. 5.3, p. 70). This may well result in its fracture and necessitate a remake.

The strength and thickness of the metal may easily be checked prior to cementation by taking occlusal and labial x-rays of the bridge, using a standard exposure (*Fig*. 7.4).

It is usually desirable to employ a one-piece casting for the bridge as this will avoid any solder joints. However, if soldering has to be carried out then it is best to do it after the individual components have been manufactured. To minimize any thermal shock it is safest to carry this out in the furnace. The disadvantage of soldering the gold components together before applying the porcelain is that the solder joints may move at the glaze stage because of the close proximity of the melt points of the gold solder and the porcelain.

Porcelain Jacket Crowns over a Gold Subframe

This type of bridge is described in Chapter 5 (*see Fig*. 5.15, p. 75). It has the advantage that a somewhat better aesthetic result can sometimes be achieved than with the bonded porcelains. This is particularly true where the lighter shades have to be employed. Its disadvantage is the fragility of the porcelain jacket crowns which is accentuated by the weakness created in them by the solder joints of the subframe.

Its only other disadvantage is that the lower position of the solder joints tends to be unhygienic and may, when they are visible, mar the aesthetics. For all these reasons this type of bridge is seldom employed nowadays.

To improve the overall aesthetic result the gold subframe on the upper part of the labial aspect may be omitted so as to prevent the gold shadowing through at this point and also to enable a greater thickness of porcelain to be provided.

The All-porcelain Bridge

Where a simple two-unit cantilever bridge is being employed then an all-porcelain design often proves adequate. However, in the case of a fixed-fixed bridge far greater stresses are imposed on the material used in its construction. This is because it is held rigidly at either end and any force applied to one retainer must be transmitted, via the pontic, to the other one. This will be resisted by the periodontal membrane of the tooth involved and thus if the material of which the bridge is constructed is weak it will fail.

In the past fixed-fixed anterior bridges made entirely or almost entirely of porcelain have not been used to any great extent as they have a high failure rate. Various methods of reinforcement such as the use of platinum gauze and wire have been employed but have not proved entirely satisfactory. However, with the advent of the stronger aluminous porcelains there has been a renewed interest in this type of bridge.

Advantages and Disadvantages

The all-porcelain bridge has many advantages including an excellent aesthetic result, good soft-tissue tolerance, and relatively low laboratory costs, possibly only one-half those of the bonded materials.

However, the fit obtainable with porcelain is not as good as that attained with gold and bridges made entirely of this material are far more likely to fracture than those made of porcelain bonded to gold. They are definitely unsuitable for use in the posterior or lower anterior regions or in any case where the occlusion is at all unfavourable.

The only other disadvantage of the all-porcelain bridge is that a palatal shoulder has to be provided on the abutment teeth thus resulting in further loss of tooth tissue. This is not necessary with a bonded full crown.

Methods of Reinforcement

There are many ways in which these bridges may be reinforced. Thus a high-strength material containing up to 50 per cent of fused alumina can be used for the core and the palatal aspect of the crowns and pontics. This is approximately 80 per cent stronger than the ordinary porcelains. The rest of the material used for building up the labial and incisal aspects can also incorporate alumina crystals but the amount has to be reduced so as to achieve a satisfactory aesthetic result.

Finally, rods or sheets of pure alumina (*Fig.* 7.5), which are about nine times stronger than pure porcelain, can be incorporated in the bridge on its palatal aspect.

One of the chief problems of constructing an all-porcelain fixed-fixed bridge is the marked contraction of the material which takes place on firing which makes it difficult to maintain the correct relationship between the two retainers. This may be overcome by:

a. A slow build-up of the core material and the completion of this before the rest of the porcelain powders are applied.

b. By making the bridge in separate units and then joining these together either with a low fusing porcelain or rods of pure alumina. The latter method is to be preferred because of the greater strength obtainable.

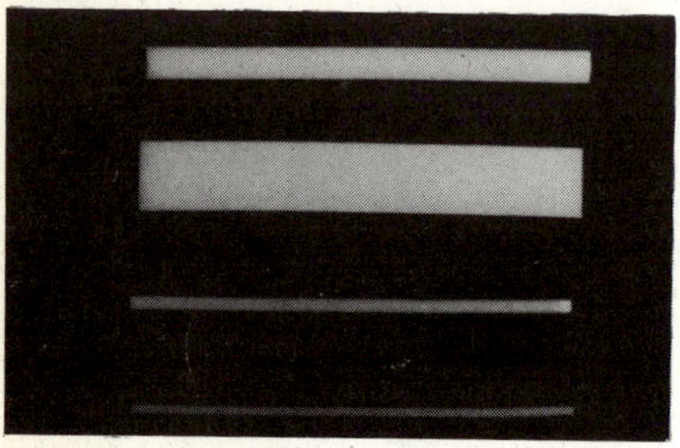

Fig. 7.5. *Rods and sheets of pure alumina used for reinforcing porcelain bridges.*

Technique. After the abutment crowns and the pontic have been made, slots are cut into these to allow for the seating of the alumina rods. They are approximately 3–4 mm long and 1·5 mm in diameter and should be positioned so that they pass through the contact point (*Fig.* 7.6).

The bridge components are now waxed together and a refractory model cast to them to maintain their correct relationship during firing. The rods are fused into position in the slots, using dentine powders. This must be carried out in several firings to make certain that the slots are completely filled with porcelain and the joint will be strong.

c. Rod span method. An alternative to the previous two methods is to use the

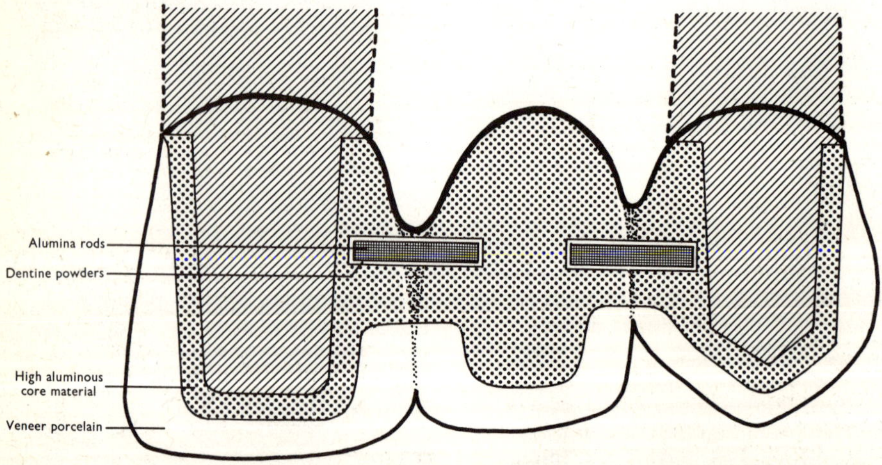

Fig. 7.6. *An upper anterior bridge built up in separate units and then joined by alumina rods baked into place with low fusing porcelain.*

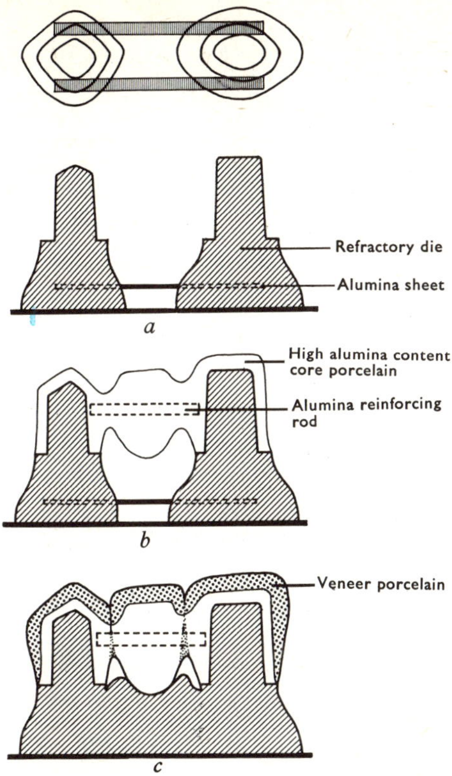

Fig. 7.7. *Rod-span technique for an upper anterior all-porcelain bridge. a, Individual dies are poured up in a refractory material and joined together with two strips of pure alumina b, The cores are built up with a porcelain with a high alumina content. The pure alumina reinforcing rod is then ground to fit between them and fused into place. After this, the main build-up is carried out with aluminous porcelain. c, The final veneers of dentine and enamel are applied and the correct tissue contact established on the master model.*

'rod span' technique, whereby an oval rod of pure alumina is incorporated in the bridge. To control dimensional changes during its firing a refractory model has to be used.

Technique. Both a master stone or silver-plated model and a refractory model are required for this technique. The latter may be obtained either from the original impression or by means of duplication. The advantage of the latter method is that the dies are trimmed first on the master cast and this will be copied on the duplicate.

The refractory model is prepared by pouring the material into each of the abutment regions of the impression separately and then joining these together by embedding a rod or sheet of pure alumina in them. Thus when set the separate abutment dies should be linked by the alumina sheet (*Fig.* 7.7*a*).

The platinum foils are now laid down on the master model and the cores built up making certain that the porcelain extends right down to and involves the whole of the width of the shoulder.

The core crowns are now transferred to the refractory model and an alumina rod is cut to fit between them. This is now fused in place with high fusing core material and then the bridge is once again offered to the master model to check location.

The main build-up of the bridge is now completed on the master model using the core material with a high alumina content (*Fig.* 7.7*b*). However, firing is still carried out on the refractory model. One millimetre of clearance is left over the entire labial surface to allow for the final veneers of dentine and enamel. When these have been built up the foils are removed, the margins checked on the master model, and the bridge glazed (*Fig.* 7.7*c*). As this is carried out at 900°C there is no chance of distortion of the bridge as the fusing point of the core mass is some 200°C higher.

The bridge is now ready for trying in the mouth.

GENERAL TECHNIQUE FOR ANTERIOR BRIDGES

The technique for the construction of an anterior bridge is similar to that described later for bridges in general. However, because of the higher aesthetic requirements it is usually desirable to have a try-in when two or more teeth are being replaced. For the same reason a good temporary bridge is always required and thus it is often best to have one made in the laboratory of heat-cured acrylic.

■ Possible Difficulties

Lack of Pontic Width

Where there has been some loss of space and orthodontics is contraindicated this may be compensated by: *a*, Discing the teeth next to the abutments. Thus if 1| is being replaced using 2|1 as abutment the mesial aspects of 3|2 would be reduced a little. *b*, By reducing the size of the abutment crowns, for instance on |1 when 1| is being replaced, not only will more space be created for the pontic but it will not need to be so wide in order to match the smaller |1. *c*, By increasing the curvature of the arch and moving the incisors labially a little.

Tilted and Rotated Teeth

Where the abutment teeth are misplaced it is usually desirable that they should be corrected. There is little point in having an aesthetically pleasing pontic if the appearance of the abutments in poor.

Where the teeth are very badly positioned, orthodontics may be indicated prior to placing the bridge (*a*) to correct the position of the teeth and improve their appearance, (*b*) to simplify their preparation and avoid the necessity for devitalization or even the risk of an exposure.

If the misplacement of the teeth is only moderate this can usually be overcome by using a full crown to change their external morphology. Should devitalization prove to be necessary then as much tooth tissue should be preserved as possible so as to give maximum retention for the post crown.

THE ANTERIOR FIXED-MOVABLE BRIDGE

The anterior fixed-movable bridge may be used to replace either the upper lateral or occasionally the central. However, it cannot usually be employed to replace the maxillary canine as the adjoining teeth would be inadequate as abutments; neither is it often a suitable design for replacing the lower anterior teeth because of their small size and the difficulty of housing a satisfactory dovetail intracoronally.

In the majority of instances an upper lateral may be replaced by a cantilever bridge using the canine as the abutment. However, occasionally it may be felt that some additional support is required from the central. This can be achieved by placing a *strong* incisal withdrawal Class III inlay with mesial countersink in the central (*Fig.* 7.8) or, possibly safer, a three-quarter crown or pinlay, and cutting a slot in this to support the dovetail fixed to the pontic.

A similar design may very occasionally be employed when replacing the central, but in this instance the other central is used as the major and the lateral as the minor retainer.

Where the teeth on either side of the gap need crowning then a fixed-fixed design is to be preferred. An exception to this is if one of the retainers cannot be made as retentive as would be ideal. A typical example is a post crown which lacks retention, possibly because of previous caries in the root face and canal.

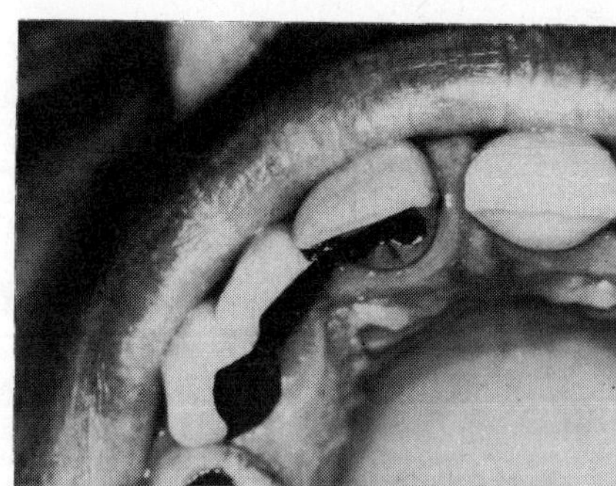

Fig. 7.8. *A fixed-movable bridge at 3–1|. By using this design only a light retainer, a Class III inlay, is needed on 1| and the tooth's natural labial and mesial surface can be preserved.*

In this instance the chance of the post becoming uncemented will be greatly reduced if a fixed-movable design is employed instead of fixed-fixed and the post crown is made the minor retainer.

A further advantage of the fixed-movable bridge is that problems of alignment may be overcome more easily as the angle of insertion of the retainers do not have to be identical.

■ Abutments and Retainers

It is usually desirable to replace only one tooth with an anterior fixed-movable bridge incorporating a conventional laboratory-made dovetail. If the span is longer than this a fixed-fixed design should usually be resorted to, or the dovetail replaced by a precision retainer (attachment). When fully seated the two parts of this lock together so positively that the design must be considered to be fixed-fixed. This will necessitate a stronger retainer.

Major Retainers

The bonded or faced full crown, the three-quarter crown, three-quarter pinlay and pinledge are all satisfactory major retainers for a fixed-movable bridge. The bonded full crown has the advantage that there will be no display of gold and that the pontic can be made of the same material.

Minor Retainers

A good Class III inlay, reinforced with pins or a mesial countersink, may occasionally be used as a minor retainer and this should not result in any visible gold. However, a more retentive preparation is nearly always indicated. A box must be incorporated in the preparation to enable the dovetail to be housed intracoronally and have a line of withdrawal fairly close to that of the major retainer. In practice it is not always easy to accommodate the dovetail when the tooth lacks width labiopalatally. An alternative is to use a Selberg or a three-quarter crown, but this latter does involve some gold showing incisally. In both cases the preparation will have to be modified to incorporate the dovetail intracoronally. Where the tooth has to be

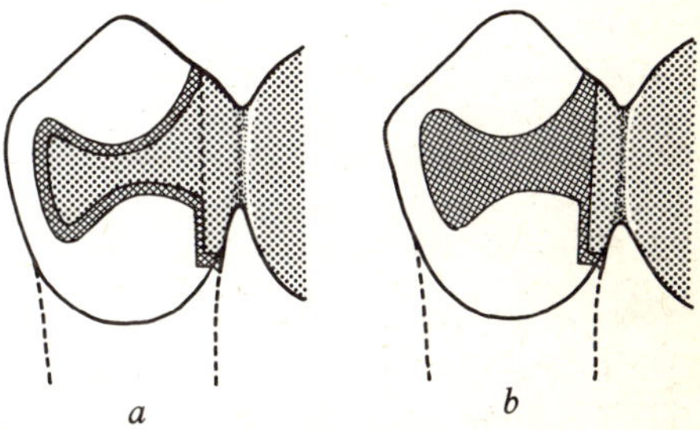

Fig. 7.9. *a, A modified dovetail in which an additional shallow lock is extended over the palatal surface of the retainer. b, Conventional anterior dovetail.*

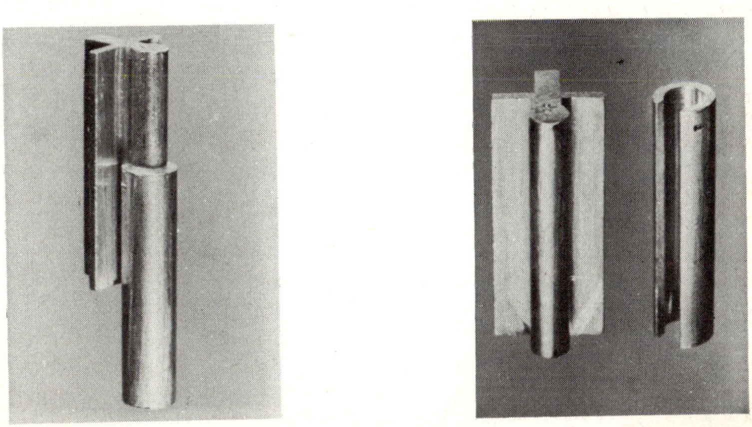

Fig. 7.10. *A precision attachment suitable for use in the anterior region.*

restored with a full crown this will of necessity be the retainer employed. However, in this case a fixed-fixed design will usually be indicated.

■ The Connector

The conventional laboratory-made dovetail and slot is satisfactory where only one tooth is to be replaced and the minor abutment is reasonably wide labiopalatally (*Fig.* 7.9*b*). However, if there is any doubt regarding the adequacy of the dovetail then a 'double dovetail' such as that shown in *Fig.* 7.9*a* may be used. If more positive location still is required and space allows, a precision retainer may be incorporated in the design (*Fig.* 7.10) but then both bridge retainers must be strong as similar retention is required to that needed for a fixed-fixed bridge which usually implies the provision of full crowns.

It must be remembered that if the dovetail is made of a metal–ceramic gold then it should be made a little thicker to compensate for its lack of strength. Furthermore the margins of the slot (*Fig.* 8.2, p. 143) should be entirely of gold otherwise crack propagation may occur in the porcelain.

Bibliography

McLean J. W. (1967) The alumina reinforced porcelain jacket crown. *J. Am. Dent. Assoc.* 75, 621.
De Trey's Aluminous Porcelain Technique Book. Issued by the Amalgamated Dental Co.

8

POSTERIOR BRIDGES

Types of Posterior Bridge Prostheses
Posterior Fixed-fixed Bridges
Fixed-movable Bridges . Connectors
Pontics used in Posterior Bridge Prostheses

The main purposes of posterior bridge prostheses are to increase masticatory efficiency, prevent drift or over-eruption of the teeth, and make functional those which would otherwise be unopposed. The remaining principal reason is aesthetics, which usually applies only in the case of a missing premolar. Other factors have already been discussed elsewhere in this book.

There is never any justification for placing a bridge in the posterior region of the mouth unless there is a definite indication for its presence. Thus, if the standing teeth are in a stable position, the periodontal condition has been unaffected by the tooth loss, and there has been no over-eruption of an opposing tooth, probably because it is still partially functional, then a bridge should not be placed unless the patient specifically requests it on the grounds of reduced masticatory efficiency or aesthetics.

It must be remembered that the construction of any bridge necessitates the mutilation of one or more teeth. Furthermore the finishing margins of any restorations, however well executed, will inevitably increase the degree of plaque retention, particularly if the teeth used as abutments were previously sound and unrestored.

In instances where the proposed abutments need extensive restoration, then the placing of a bridge, provided these teeth are suitable for this purpose, is far more justifiable.

It should also be borne in mind that any bridge, however perfect, is liable to fail at some stage and that when it does so the abutment teeth may be adversely affected. Thus by placing a bridge unnecessarily one may be shortening rather than increasing the life of the patient's dentition. All too often a small single-unit posterior replacement is seen which has failed after a few years, possibly due to bad design or execution, and this had resulted in further tooth loss and what has then become the necessity of constructing a relatively long-span and difficult bridge to redeem a mutilated mouth.

TYPES OF POSTERIOR BRIDGE PROSTHESES

There are two main types of posterior bridge, *fixed-fixed,* in which all the components are rigidly joined together, and *fixed-movable,* in which the bridge consists of two parts connected to each other by such means as a dovetail and slot. This allows limited movement of the two parts of the bridge relative to each other in one plane only, usually the vertical. It also permits the two or more retainers to have entirely different lines of insertion, thus making more retentive preparations possible with less destruction of tooth tissue (*see Fig*. 6.4*a, b*, p. 84).

Where it is considered essential to place a fixed-fixed bridge in a case where the axial inclinations of the two abutment teeth are widely divergent, the *telescopic* or *double full crown technique* may be employed (*see Fig*. 6.4*c*, p. 84). This initially involves placing a simple full crown on one of the abutment teeth, the external surface of which has a similar angulation to the preparation on the second abutment. After this a conventional fixed-fixed bridge can be placed.

Two main variations of the fixed-movable design are the fixed semi-movable bridge in which the vertical movement of a fixed-movable bridge is severely limited, and the incorporation of precision retainers in the prosthesis.

POSTERIOR FIXED-FIXED BRIDGES

These have the advantage that the abutment teeth are rigidly splinted together and thus the stresses of mastication are always relatively evenly distributed between them. This is particularly valuable when the periodontal condition is suspect, as the splinting effect may often appreciably increase the life of the abutment teeth. It is also of assistance in long-span cases, for instance from the canine to the second molar, where it is desirable to spread the load as evenly as possible.

Full occlusal coverage of the abutment teeth is always desirable in fixed-fixed bridge prostheses. If this is not carried out cementation failure is liable to occur. This is because when masticatory forces are applied to an unprotected cusp then the tooth will literally be bitten down from the inlay which is rigidly held in place via the pontic to the second retainer (*see Fig*. 6.43, p. 104). *Fig*. 6.44, p. 104, illustrates just such a case in which an MOD gold inlay has become uncemented. A further reason for always using full occlusal coverage is to prevent cuspal fracture, particularly in a non-vital tooth.

In a fixed-fixed bridge far more stress is thrown on the cement bond between the retainer and the abutment tooth than in a fixed-movable design. This is because the design prevents the independent natural movement of each of the abutment teeth. Inevitably the castings and solder joints will also be more highly stressed and therefore more likely to flex or fail. Even the slightest movement of any part of the retainer, frequently the slice or box adjoining the pontic, will result in failure of the cement as this is a rigid material. Thus in time the casting will become partly or completely uncemented.

It will be seen (*see Fig*. 6.12, p. 90) that the failure rate of the three-quarter crown when used with fixed-fixed bridges is three times as high as in the fixed-movable type. Thus, unless it is possible to be certain that they will provide adequate retention, a full crown should be resorted to. This is often completely acceptable in the posterior region as aesthetics, particularly on a molar, usually presents no problem.

The reason for extreme caution when deciding on a suitable retainer is the disastrous results of cemention failure in a fixed-fixed bridge. Caries is extremely rapid, an exposure usually resulting within a few months. Even within 3–4 weeks there will be generalized decalcification of the prepared surface of the abutment. The reason for the rapid caries is that plaque rapidly forms on the abutment beneath the retainer and it is impossible for normal oral hygiene to dislodge it. Unfortunately no pain is generally experienced until a considerable time after the pulp is exposed. This is probably because the pulp is protected from masticatory forces by the occlusal gold.

It is important to bear in mind that the longer the span the greater will be the stress imposed on the solder joint and interproximal metal and indeed the structure in general. Thus the longer the span the stronger must the metal sub-

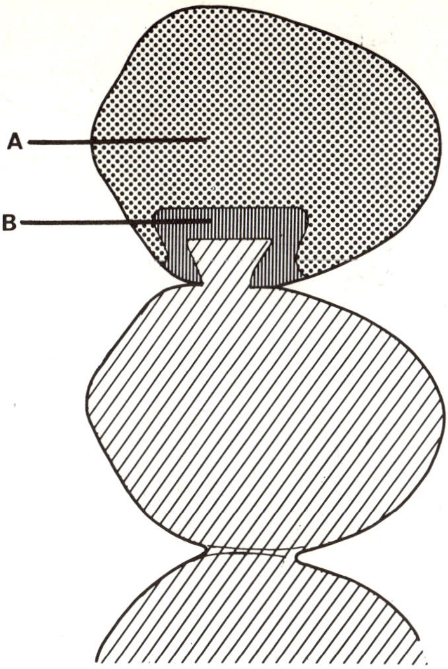

Fig. 8.2. *If a dovetail is cut in a bonded porcelain crown then it must be entirely in gold* (B) *and surrounded by an adequate thickness of the metal, otherwise crack propagation may occur in the porcelain* (A).

moderately long, but it is desirable to avoid a fixed-fixed bridge, for instance because of unfavourable angulation of the abutment teeth or difficulty in providing adequate retention in one of them, then a fixed-semimovable design may be employed. This type is similar to a fixed-movable bridge but the relative movement as between the two components is far more restricted. It is only just sufficient to break the stress as between the two parts of the bridge and decrease the liability to cementation failure. Because of the very limited movement of the two bridge retainers relative to each other the abutment teeth have to be prepared with the same line of insertion as for a fixed-fixed design and the bridge placed in one unit. The only exception to this is the use of the Vale sliding bar (*Fig*. 8.3) in which the bridge is constructed and cemented in two components as for a fixed-movable design and after this a horizontal bar or bolt is slid from the pontic into the minor retainer, thus locking the two components together.

Another and probably the commonest connector used in fixed-semimovable bridge prostheses is the covered dovetail. In this a conventional fixed-movable

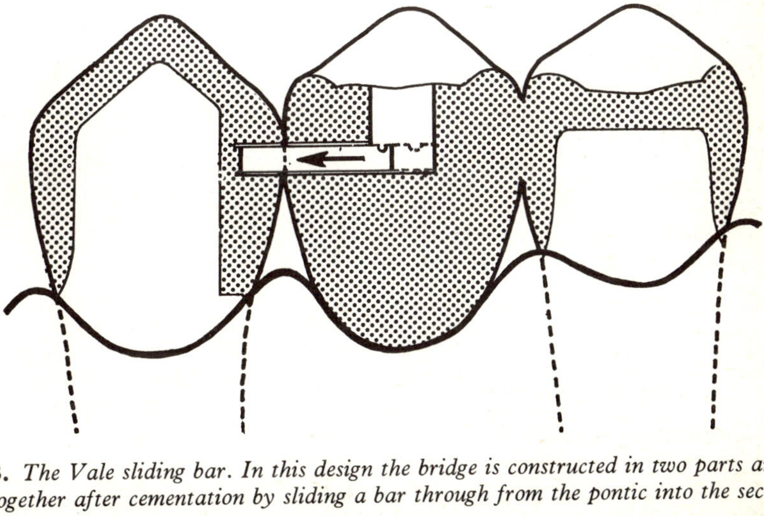

Fig. 8.3. *The Vale sliding bar. In this design the bridge is constructed in two parts and locked together after cementation by sliding a bar through from the pontic into the second retainer.*

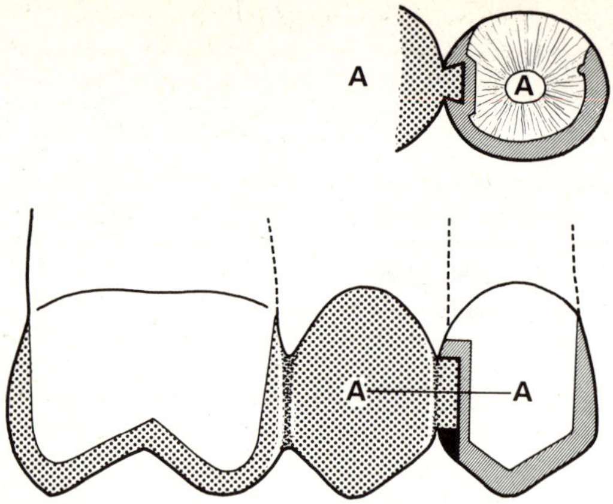

Fig. 8.4. *The covered dovetail. A conventional dovetail is prepared and then the top of this removed and soldered to the top of the slot in the minor retainer, thus severely limiting vertical movement.*

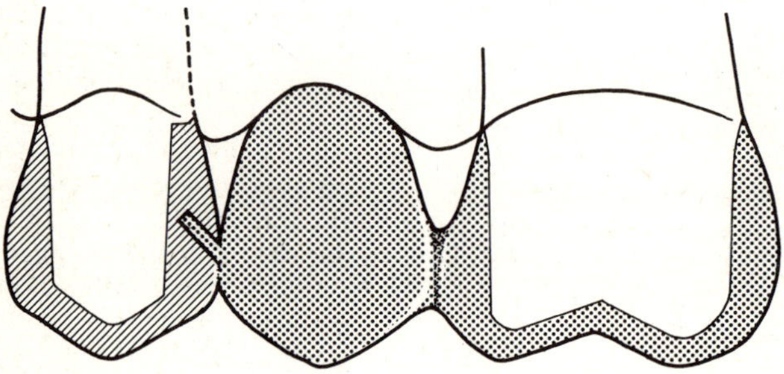

Fig. 8.5. *The 45° pin. The two components of a fixed-movable bridge may be joined by a 45° pin which will limit vertical movement.*

bridge is constructed and then the top of the dovetail is cut off and soldered to the top of the slot in the minor retainer, thus severely limiting the degree of vertical movement available (*Fig.* 8.4). The only disadvantages of this method are that it does result in a weaker dovetail than in a fixed-movable design and that the laboratory procedures are more complex.

A third method used which achieves a somewhat similar result to the covered dovetail is the use of a 30° (or possibly 45°) pin (*Fig.* 8.5). As can be seen from the diagram, this will severely restrict both vertical and horizontal movement between the two retainers. Lastly a ball and socket type of junction may be employed.

■ Incorporation of Precision Retainers

Instead of using the conventional dovetail and slot made in the laboratory for a fixed-movable bridge a precision retainer may be incorporated in the design. However, the frictional fit of these devices is very high. This is because both male and female components are usually individually machined to very fine limits. Thus the bridge becomes virtually fixed-fixed once both sections are cemented into place. Because of this, equal retention is required from both retainers. One of the advantages of incorporating a precision retainer in posterior bridges is that whilst retaining the advantages of a fixed-fixed bridge the necessity of aligning the two or more preparations is greatly reduced. This will result in less reduction of tooth tissue and more retentive preparations, and decreases the risk of pulpal exposure.

The preparation housing the precision retainer requires a much deeper box than would be the case with a conventional dovetail and thus unless the crown of the tooth is fairly large and well erupted and the pulp small then it may be impossible to accommodate them intracoronally.

To provide a completely rigid junction between the two parts of the bridge a screw may be passed through the two components of the precision retainer after the bridge has been cemented in place, thus preventing all movement.

PONTICS USED IN POSTERIOR BRIDGE PROSTHESES

Where there is adequate space and aesthetics is of no consequence, a sanitary pontic is satisfactory (*see Fig*. 5.20, p. 78). However, when the space is limited it should not be used as there will be inadequate clearance between it and the soft tissues for satisfactory cleaning. This will result in food stagnation and tissue irritation, the gingivae proliferating up until they are in firm contact with the undersurface of the pontic. At this stage the pontic becomes most unsanitary and a complete remake of the bridge is indicated.

Where the occlusion is close a pontic fabricated from bonded porcelain is the type of choice and is indeed the most suitable type for general use in the posterior region because of its extreme flexibility of design and the ability to have porcelain next to the tissues and, where necessary, occlusally. However, where occlusal porcelain is provided care must be taken to keep this to an even thickness and well supported by the underlying gold, particularly on the cusps. The porcelain should never be allowed to exceed a thickness of 1·5 mm, otherwise its strength rapidly decreases and cuspal fracture is liable to occur.

In instances where only minimal space is available for a pontic and both the bonded and sanitary designs are contra-indicated then an all gold pontic may be employed.

9

THE CANTILEVER BRIDGE

Advantages . Indications and Contraindications . Specific Uses
Incorporation of the Cantilever Bridge with other Designs
Maintenance

In this design the pontic is 'cantilevered' out from one side of the abutment tooth and obtains support from that one side only. To gain additional support two adjacent abutment teeth may sometimes be used or cantilevered pontics may be incorporated in other bridge designs. Although somewhat limited in application, it is one of the most useful and reliable of all designs. In surveys of bridge work carried out at the Eastman Dental Hospital over a ten-year period it proved to have a lower failure rate than any other type.

ADVANTAGES

The main advantage of the cantilever bridge is the simplicity of its design, which not only accounts for its reliability but also results in a relatively short chairside time and low laboratory fees. Other advantages are the excellent aesthetics which can be provided, particularly if an all-porcelain bridge is used, and the ease with which it can be kept clean by the patient.

INDICATIONS AND CONTRAINDICATIONS

Its main indication is in the anterior region where only relatively limited occlusal stresses are likely to be applied to the pontic. In the posterior region simple cantilever designs employing only one abutment must be used with care if overloading is to be avoided. In instances where it is considered to be the most suitable replacement for a posterior tooth, two abutments are often required. A particular use of this design in the posterior region is the stabilization of the occlusion, for instance when the lower second and third molars are missing and over-eruption of the upper second molar with a consequent derangement of the occlusion, is liable to take place. In these instances all that is often required is a small cantilevered extension passing distally from a three-quarter or a full crown on the first molar.

Contrary to possible expectations, it is extremely rare to see rotation of an anterior cantilever bridge occurring. Over a series of several hundred cases the only times on which this has been noted are when there has been a generalized periodontal breakdown with drifting and mobility of several other teeth. The reason why rotation does not occur is that it is the muscular balance between lips, cheek and tongue which determines the stable position of any tooth and likewise of any pontic. Occlusal forces are of a very intermittent nature and, provided the pontic is not in traumatic occlusion in centric, lateral or protrusive excursions, will have no tendency to move it.

SPECIFIC USES

■ Replacement of Upper Lateral

The commonest use of the cantilever bridge is in the replacement of an upper lateral using the canine as the sole abutment. This design is particularly good because there is the nearly ideal condition of a very strong abutment tooth carrying a relatively small pontic.

Occasionally where a central has to be crowned, and the lateral on the same side is missing, then, if all the local factors are favourable, the central may be used as the abutment tooth and an all-porcelain bridge placed.

One advantage of this type is that where there is a lack of space this can be 'evened out' by reducing the width of the neighbouring central a little, making the jacket crown acting as retainer smaller also, and finally overcoming any lack of space by overlapping the lateral pontic a little over the canine.

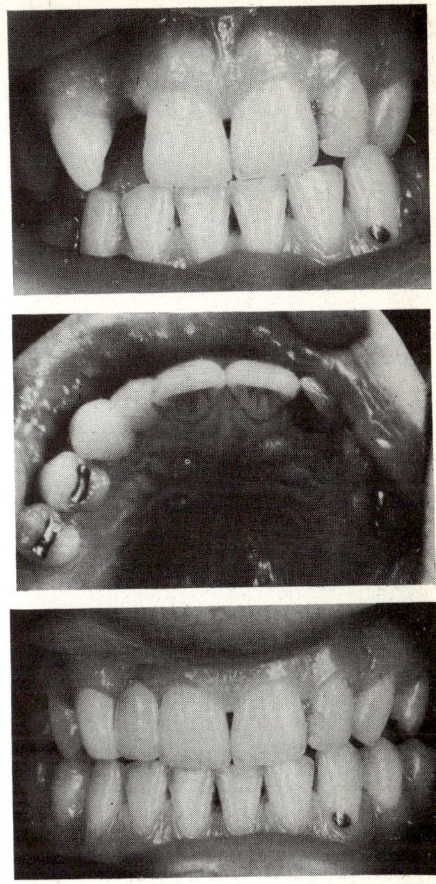

Fig. 9.1. *An all-porcelain bridge at 32|. Because of the smooth, highly glazed surface of the pontic it can overlap the neighbouring tooth without any risk of caries and thus produce a better aesthetic result.*

Retainer and Pontic

The choice of retainer and pontic types varies very much depending on the condition of the canine and the age, sex and aesthetic requirements of the patient. The simplest design incorporates the use of a gold three-quarter crown or three-quarter pinlay on the canine and a bonded or possibly a long-pin pontic. However, a three-quarter crown or pinlay may not provide sufficient retention if the crown of the abutment tooth is short and the occlusion unfavourable. In these instances, resort must be made to the bonded full crown.

Where aesthetics is of prime importance, and particularly when the canine requires a full crown restoration, then an all-porcelain bridge may be employed (*Fig*. 9.1). This can be used in all cases where a porcelain jacket crown would be considered a satisfactory replacement for the canine, disregarding the fact that it will also be employed as a retainer. The liability of the porcelain to fracture is no greater than that of a single crown in similar circumstances. The pontic is made of solid porcelain and is, therefore, extremely unlikely to break. Likewise it is rare for the junction between the pontic and the retainer to fail.

This bridge is one of the most satisfying that can be placed. It requires no more chairside time than a simple jacket, and provides as good an aesthetic result as that achieved by any other bridge design. It is exceptionally easy for the patient to keep clean and the pontic to tissue contact is entirely porcelain, giving rise to the absolute minimum of gingival irritation.

Where the occlusion is heavy a bonded porcelain restoration must be used. However, this has two disadvantages:

a. The material is far more costly and time consuming in the laboratory than porcelain alone.

b. It is doubtful if the aesthetic results achieved will be as good as with an all-porcelain bridge, except possibly in the older patient when darker shades are being employed (*Fig.* 9.2).

Thus, even in the case of a fairly heavy occlusion, it may be reasonable to use an all-porcelain bridge in the first instance, warning the patient that there is an increased risk of failure but pointing out the advantages. If the orginal model is kept and is undamaged, or a duplicate is made, then should the bridge fail, another one constructed in bonded porcelain can always be made with the minimum of inconvenience to the patient.

Some authorities prefer to build the bridge as two separate units and then join these together afterwards with a low fusing porcelain, possibly reinforced by rods or discs of pure alumina. The advantage of this is the natural appearance of separation between the teeth. However, it does result in a weaker bridge than if it is built up as one unit.

■ Replacement of the Upper Canine

The canine is one of the most difficult teeth to replace by a bridge. The stresses this tooth has to carry are great and it is often impossible to avoid placing the pontic is such a position that it will carry the full force of the occlusion in lateral excursions. The other problem is that only a poor abutment tooth, the lateral, is available mesially and that even the first premolar is by no means a strong abutment.

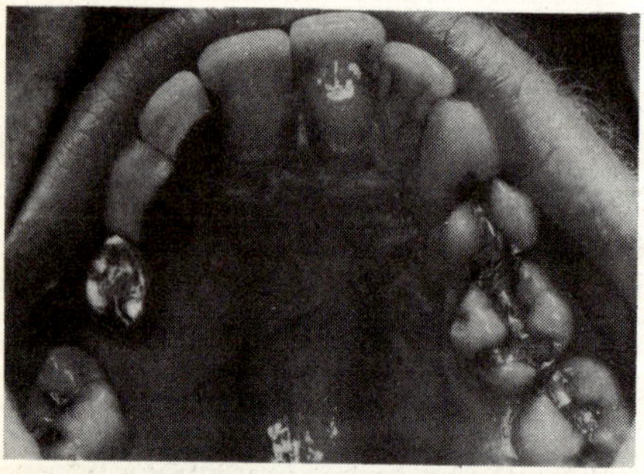

Fig. 9.2. *A metal-ceramic cantilever bridge replacing* 2⌋.

Because the lateral is usually best avoided the most satisfactory method of replacing the canine is by a cantilever bridge coming forward from the first and second premolars. It is only on rare occasions that a single premolar will be of sufficient strength to carry a canine pontic.

Three-quarter crowns are usually the retainers of choice, providing that the clinical crowns are of adequate length to secure good retention. If they are short, bonded crowns will generally be required. However, the full crown has the disadvantage over the three-quarter crown in that it necessitates a far greater degree of tooth tissue reduction and is more likely to result in gingival irritation, particularly at the buccal margin, which would not normally be involved by a three-quarter crown. The advantage of using a bonded full crown as the retainer is that it prevents the small display of gold at the incisal edge which is unavoidable with a gold three-quarter crown.

When three-quarter crowns are used as retainers, a bonded pontic is usually employed (*Fig.* 9.3) but a long pin may also be used.

A porcelain jacket type pontic is not particularly suitable as it is very prone to fracture (*Fig.* 9.4). This is because of the heavy occlusion in this region and the inherent weakness of this pontic when used with cantilever and fixed-fixed bridges (*Fig.* 5.15*b*, p. 75).

■ Replacement of Upper Central

Very occasionally, where the occlusion is favourable, the root surface area high, and the periodontal condition good, and particularly if there has been some loss of space, one central may be cantilevered from the other. Two such cases have

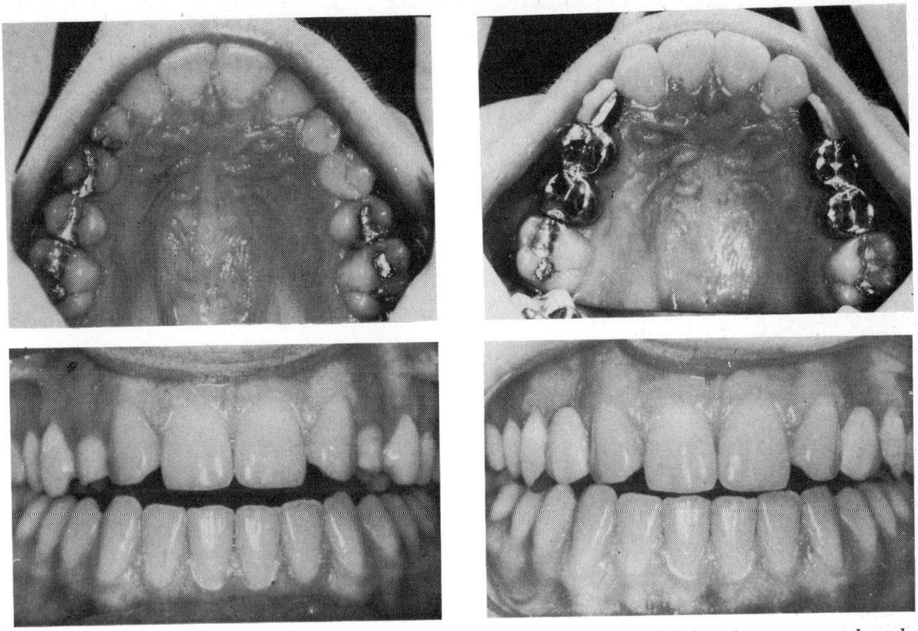

Fig. 9.3. *Loose retained $\underline{c|c}$ replaced by cantilever bridges. Bonded pontics were employed and gold three-quarter crowns used as retainers. Note minimal display of gold due to its correct bevelling.*
(By courtesy of D. N. Atkinson.)

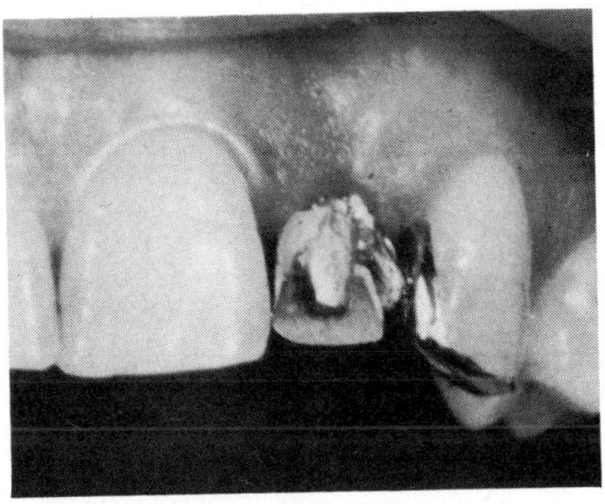

Fig. 9.4. *A fractured porcelain jacket-type pontic at $\underline{|2}$. The solder joint inevitably causes a weakness in the pontic.*

been seen which were still completely satisfactory after 18 and 30 years respectively. Because of the light occlusion an all-porcelain bridge is nearly always possible and best.

Although, as stated previously, rotation is a very rare occurrence with a cantilever bridge, in these circumstances it is desirable to give the central a little extra support because of its rounded root form and relatively low root surface area. This can be achieved quite simply by slightly overlapping the neighbouring lateral and in effect creating a slot, which, of course, must have the same line of insertion as the retainer. Providing the porcelain is well glazed, there is very little risk of this giving rise to caries. This is probably the only occasion on which it is justified to obtain some degree of support from a tooth by covering it, even to a limited extent, without first placing a restoration in it. The practice of putting a gold rest on an unprepared and unprotected tooth is to be deprecated.

■ Replacement of Posterior Teeth

Where a tooth on one side of a bounded saddle is unsuitable as a bridge abutment then a cantilever design may be considered. For instance the first premolar may be cantilevered from the second premolar and first molar joined together and on occasions the second premolar may be cantilevered from just the first molar, particularly if there has been some closing of the space to be restored.

The restoration of the unbounded saddle area, for instance the lower first or second molars where no distal abutment exists, is always a difficult problem. A small unilateral or even bilateral partial lower denture is often unsatisfactory and poorly tolerated by the patient. Similarly there may be contraindications to a precison-retained prosthesis, for instance because of inadequate space and crown length. Other alternatives are an implant, possibly coupled to a fixed-fixed bridge or a cantilever bridge.

Of these the latter is quite often to be preferred. It must be remembered that it is frequently unnecessary to replace all the missing teeth and thus if all the lower molars on one side are missing the replacement of just the first molar by a cantilever design employing full crowns on both premolars as retainers may be all that is required. This will be better tolerated by the patient than a partial denture and providing the occlusion is correct and the patient's oral hygiene is good little sign of overloading is likely to occur.

Thus cantilever designs may be employed in the posterior region but it must be remembered that where possible a conventional fixed-fixed or fixed-movable bridge is usually to be preferred.

INCORPORATION OF THE CANTILEVER BRIDGE WITH OTHER DESIGNS

In many instances a cantilever bridge can be used in conjunction with fixed-fixed designs. However, it must be borne in mind that an additional load will be placed on the abutment teeth, particularly the one next to the cantilevered pontic, and that cementation failure and periodontal overloading are more likely to occur unless great care is taken in the design and execution of the bridge (*see Fig*. 19.8, p. 253).

An example of the compound bridge mentioned above would be a fixed-fixed design running from the upper canine to the second premolar, replacing the first premolar and with the lateral cantilevered from the canine mesially. In this bridge a full crown would be indicated for the canine and possibly the second premolar also.

Whereas with periodontally sound teeth very high stresses will be applied to the retainers, the cementing media, and indeed the whole structure of the bridge if excessive cantilevering of pontics is carried out, should the teeth be mobile due to advanced bone loss then the stresses applied to the bridge will be drastically reduced as the whole structure including the roots of the abutment teeth, will be able to move, to some degree in unison, when a load is placed on them.

It is thus practical in some cases of advanced periodontal disease to employ successfully quite extensive cantilever designs; with only a small risk of failure and indeed it is often indicated to stabilize the occlusion and prevent over-eruption and further breakdown of the periodontium.

MAINTENANCE

The patient should be instructed in the use of dental floss to clean the undersurface of the pontic (*see Fig*. 5.6, p. 71). Interdens are desirable for use around the abutments, particularly if more than one has been employed.

Bibliography

Henderson D., Blevins W. R., Wesley R. C. and Seward T. (1970) The cantilever types of posterior fixed partial dentures: laboratory study. *J. Prosthet. Dent.* **24**, 47.

10

THE SPRING BRIDGE

Indications for Use . Contraindications . Advantages . Disadvantages
Design . Abutments and Retainers . Pontic . Labial Gumwork . The Bar
Fitting of the Bridge . Routine Maintenance
Yearly Checks of Bridge: Points to Watch
The Lower Spring Bridge

The spring bridge is probably the most controversial of all types and is still by no means widely accepted. However, it has many desirable features. A posterior tooth is generally used as the abutment when replacing an upper incisor, thus avoiding the mutilation of what may be two sound anterior teeth. An excellent aesthetic result is readily achieved and the clinical time required is relatively short.

The basic principle of the spring bridge is the carrying of the pontic by a tooth not immediately related to it and connected to it by a flexible palatal bar—hence the name 'spring' bridge. The essential feature of the design is that the pontic is principally tissue borne, the abutment tooth merely retaining the prosthesis in place. Thus the bar must be of sufficient flexibility to allow it to be pressed on to and gain support from the mucoperiosteum during mastication.

The tissues in the lower arch are incapable of giving this support and thus a spring bridge in its true meaning cannot be constructed in this region. If one is used the bar has to be made sufficiently rigid to prevent any appreciable pressure being transmitted to the underlying mucosa, otherwise ulceration will occur. The design thus becomes, in effect, a straight cantilever bridge.

INDICATIONS FOR USE

■ A. Where Aesthetics is of Prime Importance

The aesthetic results obtained with a spring bridge are fully comparable with those achieved with a porcelain jacket crown, which is generally the pontic of choice. The abutment employed is usually a posterior tooth and thus there will be little visible gold.

■ B. Where the Teeth on Either Side of the Space are Unsuitable as Abutments

This may be (i) Because it is not considered justifiable to cut into two sound anterior teeth; (ii) Because the retainers would have insufficient retention; (iii) Because too much gold would be shown, or (iv) Because their root surface area or periodontal condition renders them unable to carry the additional load.

■ C. Where a Diastema is Necessary on one or both Sides of the Pontic (*Fig.* 10.1)

In this instance a 'spring' is the only possible type of bridge, as with other designs the pontic usually has to be

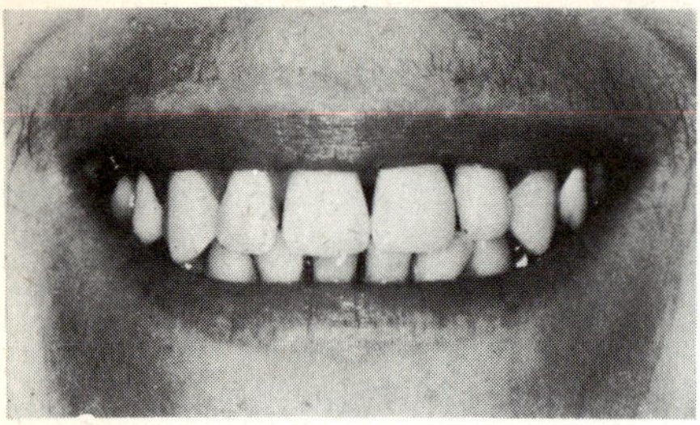

Fig. 10.1. *Spring bridge replacing 1|. Note the natural aesthetic result achieved by being able to provide a diastema distal to the pontic.*

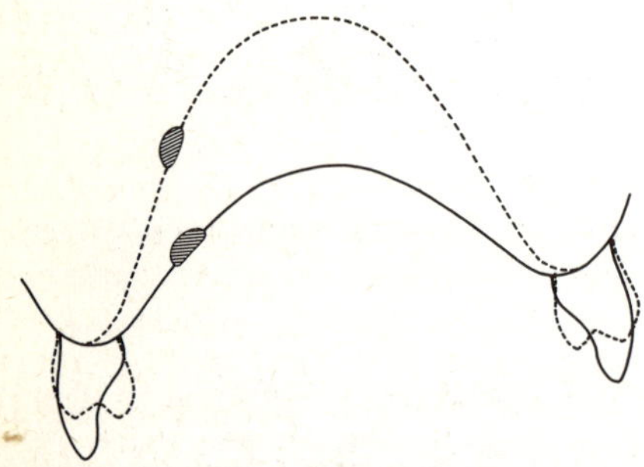

Fig. 10.2. *The farther back a spring bridge is placed the steeper the angulation of the palate and the less tissue support which will be obtained. Molar cross-section is shown in dotted outline, canine cross-section in solid.*

directly connected to the neighbouring teeth.

CONTRAINDICATIONS

1. In young patients where the clinical crowns are short and unlikely to provide adequate retention.

2. When the teeth on either side of the space need crowning and are thus the retainers of choice.

3. When a lower tooth has to be replaced.

4. Where the shape of the palate is unfavourable. The steeper its sides the less the resistance it will be able to give to any vertical force applied. Similarly the farther back in the arch the bar is placed the less satisfactory the result will be because of the steeper angulation of the palate in this region (*Fig*. 10.2). The bar is also more likely to be noticed by the patient.

5. Where there is appreciable soft tissue loss which must be made good.

6. When the proposed abutment tooth is unopposed or lacking a mesial or distal contact, in which case it might move after the bridge is placed. It must be remembered that any movement of the abutment tooth is magnified many times at the pontic.

ADVANTAGES

1. An excellent aesthetic result is readily obtained and only a short chairside time is required.

2. The design is well accepted by the patient. Indeed, out of over 500 spring bridges fitted at the Eastman Dental Hospital not one has had to be removed because the patient could not tolerate it.

3. The failure rate is low and even when this does occur the adverse consequences are minimal.

DISADVANTAGES

Occasionally the bar may become permanently bent (*Fig*. 10.3), when it moves upwards and labially, or it may fracture due either to accidental trauma or fatigue. In the latter case, if the bar is made of gold this usually occurs after 4–5 years.

2. The theoretical and practical considerations of the design need to be fully understood not only by the operator but also by the technician if a satisfactory result is to be achieved. For this reason the stages in the construction of a spring bridge are illustrated in some detail (*Figs*. 10.4, 10.5, 10.12–10.19).

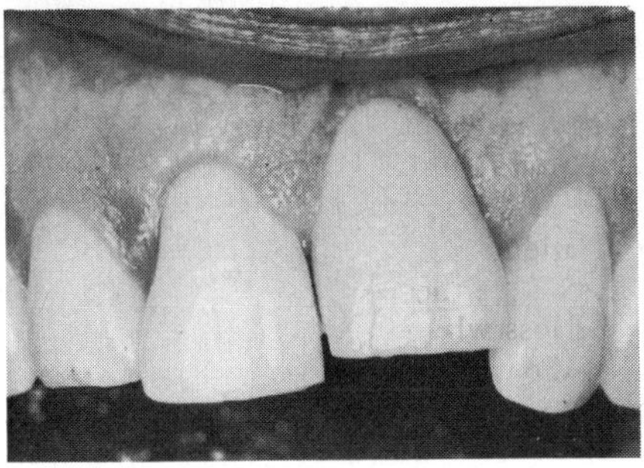

Fig. 10.3. *Spring bridge replacing |1 in which the pontic has become depressed due to bending of the bar.*

DESIGN

This bridge is frequently the ideal replacement when an upper central is missing (*Figs.* 10.4, 10.5). It is also often of value in replacing the lateral and can occasionally be used to advantage for the canine.

It is readily incorporated in other bridge designs, an example being shown in *Fig.* 11.1, p. 163.

ABUTMENTS AND RETAINERS

When either of the upper central incisors is being replaced the tooth generally indicated as the abutment is the first premolar. If, however, there is any doubt as to the ability of this tooth to carry the load both premolars may be used. The premolar is used in preference to the canine, despite its somewhat smaller root surface area, because of the greater degree of retention available and because a more favourable line is achieved for the bar.

When the lateral is being replaced the second as opposed to the first premolar is to be preferred as the abutment, providing its root surface area is adequate. This is because it will increase the length and improve the angulation of the bar. When a bar is too short its rigidity is increased and cementation failure or periodontal overloading may occur. If the bend of the bar is too acute it will tend to trap food.

Occasionally when the premolars are unsuitable as abutment teeth the first molar may be employed. This is especially likely to occur if the tooth to be replaced is a lateral or canine and loss of the second premolar has resulted in mesial drift of the first molar.

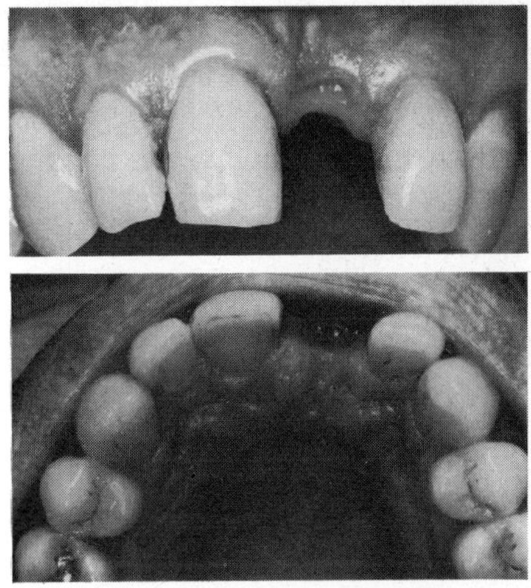

Fig. 10.4. *Patient suitable for spring bridge. Note relatively sound anterior teeth, well-erupted |4 and favourable angulation of palate.*

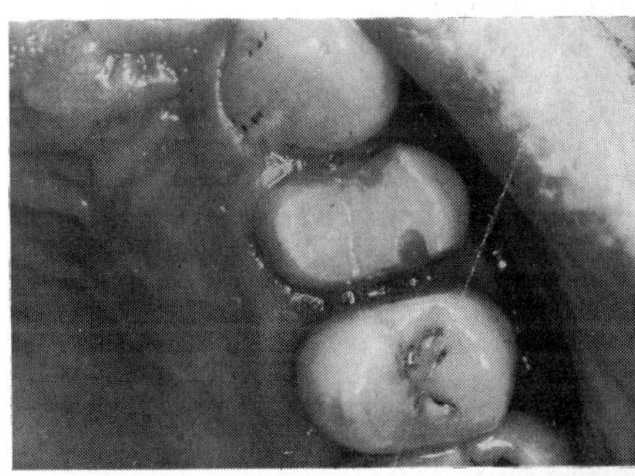

Fig. 10.5. *|4 preparation. Note curve of mesial slice to avoid any display of gold and curve of distal slice, where gold will not be seen, to improve retention.*

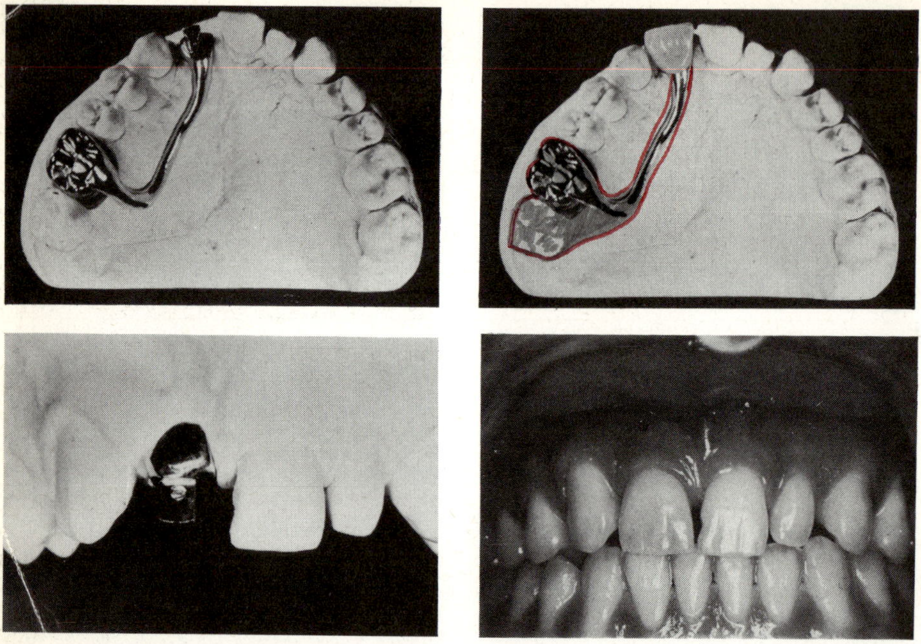

Fig. 10.6. *A spring bridge with removable pontic section which is held in place by a precision retainer with a 'ball catch' on its palatal aspect (the Hüser).*
(By courtesy of R. Valentine.)

The retainer of choice, provided adequate retention can be achieved, is the three-quarter crown (*Fig*. 10.5), as it destroys less tooth tissue than the full crown, preserves the natural buccal façade of the tooth and because of its shorter cervical margin, is less likely to cause plaque retention.

If it is essential to use a canine as the abutment and a three-quarter crown is indicated, double slots may be employed to increase the retention available. Alternatively, particularly if the condition of the canine justifies it, a full crown may be desirable.

■ Double Retainers

When double retainers are used it must always be remembered that the degree of retention is only equal to that of the weakest retainer. Using two abutments decreases the load on the periodontal tissues of any one tooth but increases the chance of cementation failure of either retainer. Thus it is undesirable to pair the canine and first premolar, particularly if the crowns are short and three-quarter crowns are used. The retainer on the canine, being far weaker than that on the premolar, is likely to become uncemented but will continue to be held in place and as a result rapid caries will occur beneath it (*see Fig*. 19.13, p. 255).

When two retainers are used the bar should be taken from the more posterior one, as in this way any force which may be transmitted to the second retainer will be of a compressive nature and therefore cementation failure is less likely to occur. The direction of the force applied to the periodontium will also be more favourable.

PONTIC

The pontic usually indicated is a porcelain jacket crown placed over a gold

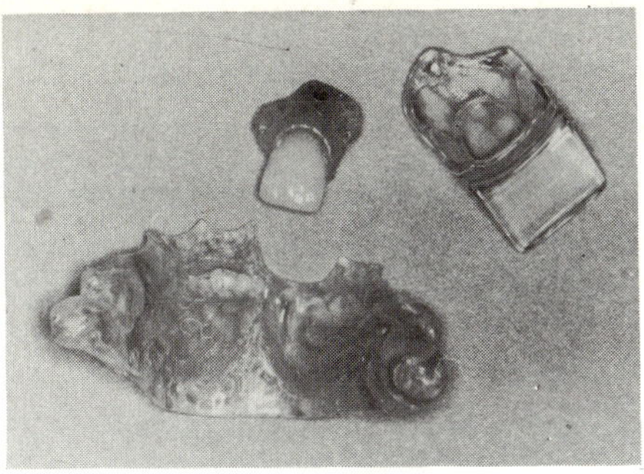

Fig. 10.7. *The pontic has a tube incorporated in it to permit the pin of the special tool to lock onto it and remove it. Below is the bite guard used to immobilize the bar.*

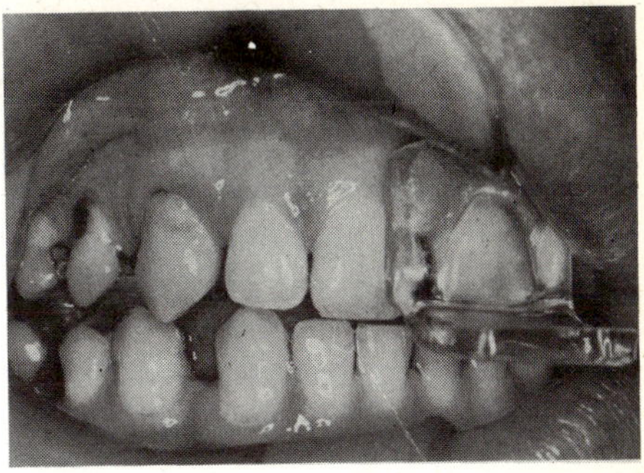

Fig. 10.8. *Bite guard and tool for removing pontic in position.*

core (*see Fig*. 5.18, p. 77). This type of pontic is particularly well suited to the spring bridge because it produces an excellent aesthetic result and at the same time is unlikely to fracture because the flexible bar cushions the effect of any impact. An all-porcelain to tissue contact is desirable on the labial aspect.

The golds used in metal-ceramic restorations are not suitable for the bar of the spring bridge because of their relatively poor elasticity. The pontic can, however, be constructed of one of these materials and soldered to a bar made of hard gold. This is of value where the occlusion is very close, as in a Class II, division 2 malocclusion.

At the present time the nickel-chrome alloy is used only for the bar and core and this is soldered to a gold three-quarter crown because of the better fit obtainable and the more favourable wear characteristics of gold, i.e. its rate of wear more nearly approaches that of tooth tissue. A separate porcelain jacket type pontic is cemented to the core.

LABIAL GUMWORK

This may occasionally become necessary when marked recession of the alveolus has occurred, although a removable prosthesis is usually indicated in these cases. However, if any gumwork is incorporated it should be kept to an absolute minimum to avoid food trapping and should always be made of porcelain. An alternative in these instances is to make the pontic section removable, when it can be made of acrylic. This may be achieved by using a precision retainer such as a Hüser (*Fig*. 10.6).

To avoid damage to the bar during removal of the pontic an acrylic plate is inserted by the patient on which he can bite (*Fig*. 10.7). This fits over and immobilizes the bar. A tool is also provided to engage a steel sleeve in the removable section and simplify its removal (*Fig*. 10.8).

THE BAR

The factors to be considered in the design of the bar are:

a. The line to be followed.

b. The degree to which it should be let into the tissues.

c. Its shape and surface area.

d. Its degree of flexibility.

■ A. Line to be Followed

This depends on the tooth to be replaced, the abutment chosen, and the shape of the palate (*Fig*. 10.9).

It is important that the bar be kept well away from the gingival margins to avoid food being trapped between the teeth and the bar. If two spring bridges are to be placed their bars must be kept fairly well apart for the same reason (*Fig.* 10.10). The bars of separate spring bridges should never be joined otherwise the design will, in effect, be converted into a fixed-fixed one. This will limit independent movement and cementation failure is likely to ensue (*Fig.* 10.11). The bend of the bar must not be too acute otherwise food may become trapped in this region. Furthermore the liability of the bar to fracture is increased.

It is best to run the bar between rather than across the rugae so that the patient notices it as little as possible. It should run straight back from the pontic to the bend. This is the part which is tissue bearing and absorbs the majority of the

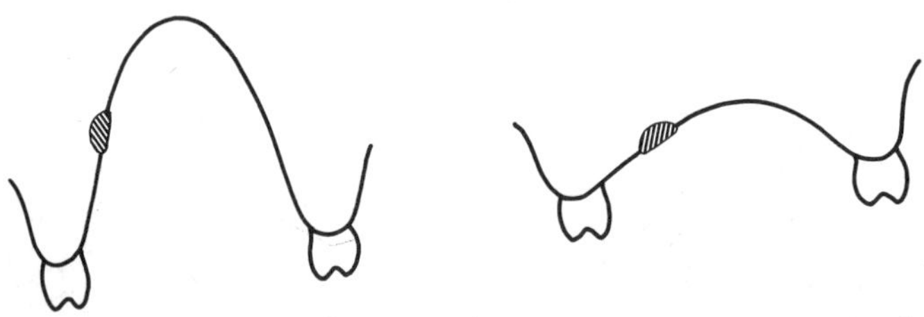

Fig. 10.9. *The steeper the angulation of the palate the less tissue support obtained and the less suitable the case for a spring bridge.*

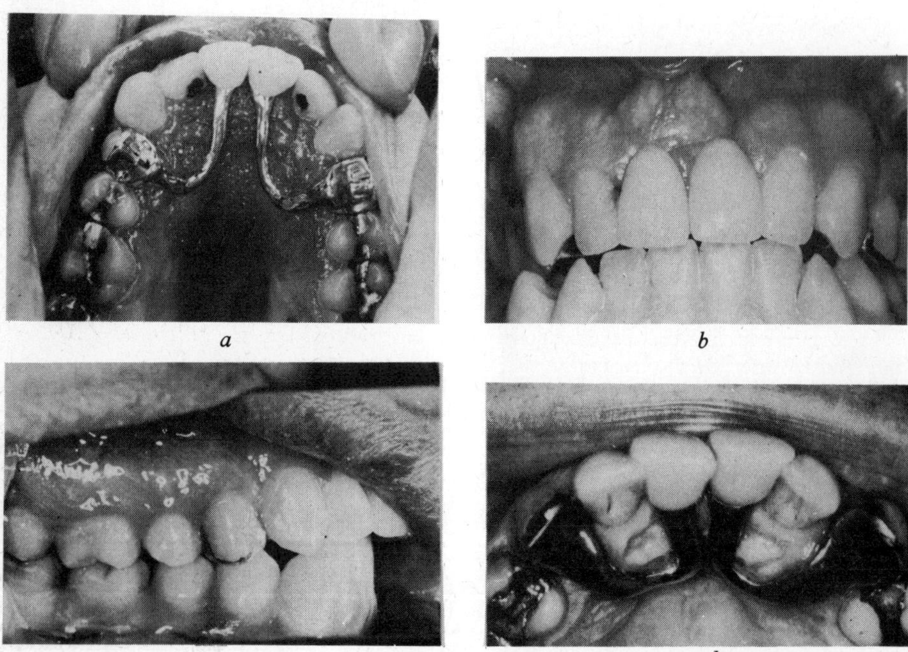

a b c d

Fig. 10.10. *a, b, and c, Spring bridges replacing* 1|1. *Note that the bars are kept well clear of each other and also the gingival margins of the standing teeth. The mesial slice of the three-quarter crown on* 4| *is curved to minimize any display of gold. d, Spring bridges in which the bars are too close together, which will give rise to food-packing and gingival irritation.*

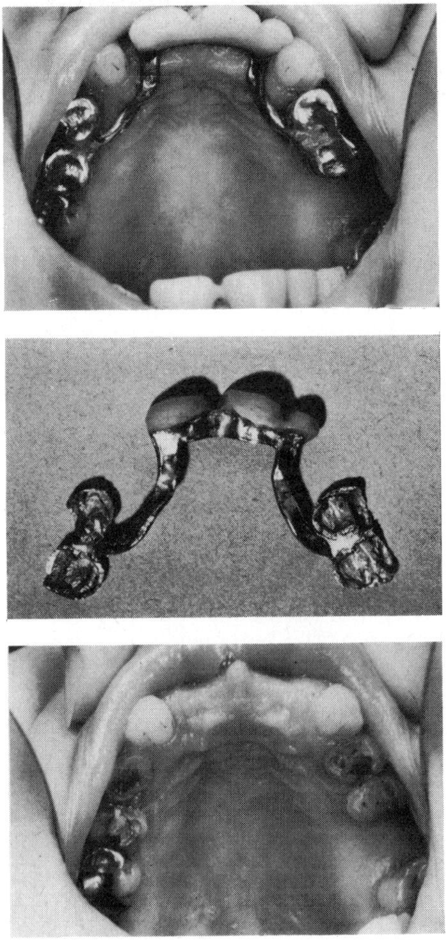

Fig. 10.11. *If two spring bridges are joined together the design, in effect, becomes fixed-fixed, movement is limited, and cementation failure may occur.*

forces of mastication. The line of a typical bar is as shown in *Fig.* 2.29. p. 27.

■ B. Letting the Bar into the Tissue

The palate should be palpated with the large end of a ball burnisher so that the firmness of the tissues at any one point can then be estimated and recorded on the model and the bar let in to the appropriate depth (*Figs.* 10.12*a, b,* 10.15).

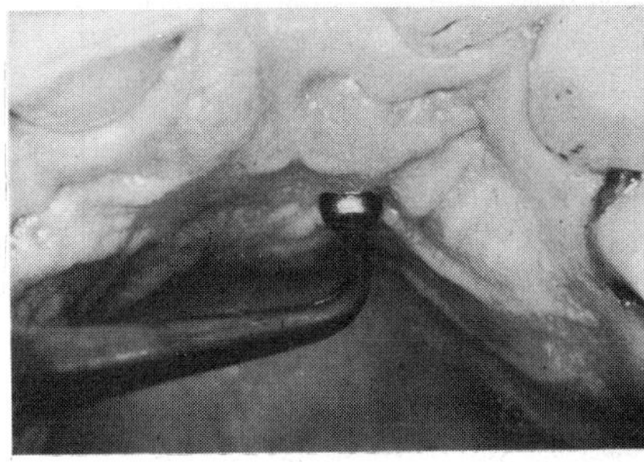

a

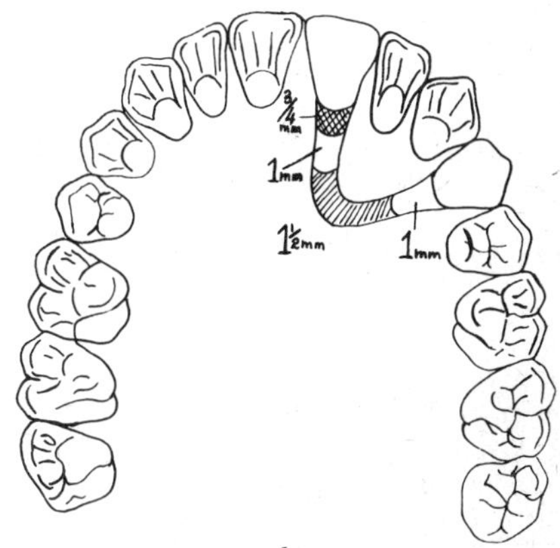

b

Fig. 10.12. *a, The palate is palpated with the large end of a ball burnisher to assess the resilience of the palate. b, This information is then recorded on a stone model which is subsequently used as a guide for grooving out the final model to the correct depth (see Fig.* 10.15*b*).

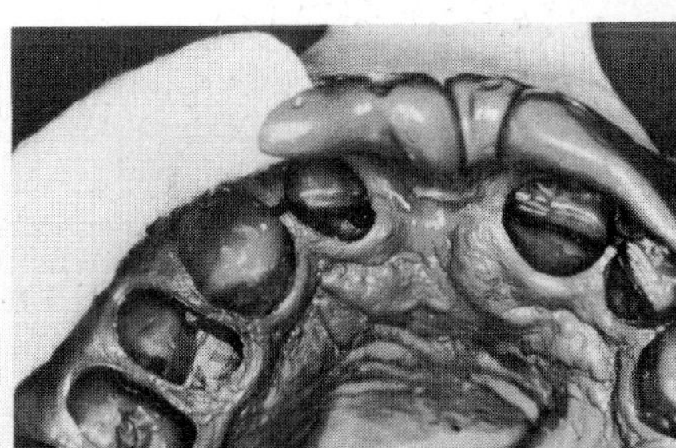

Fig. 10.13. *Impression recording the preparation, all the occlusal surfaces and the palate in the region of the bar.*

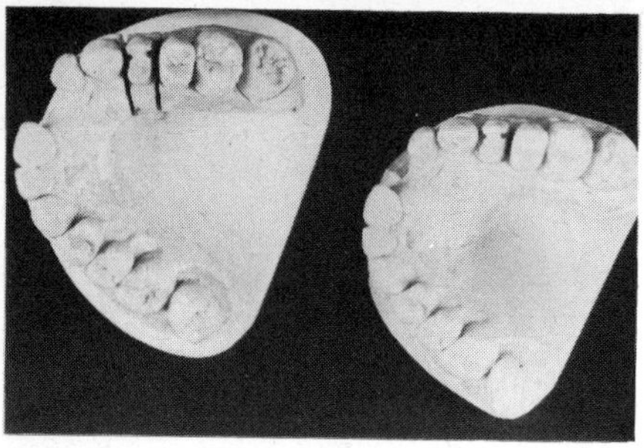

Fig. 10.14. *Two models are poured from the impression, a sectioned one on which the three-quarter crown is waxed up and an unsectioned one on which the bridge is completed.*

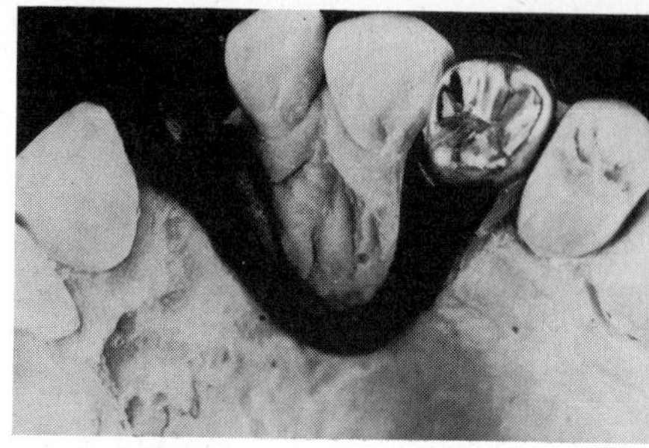

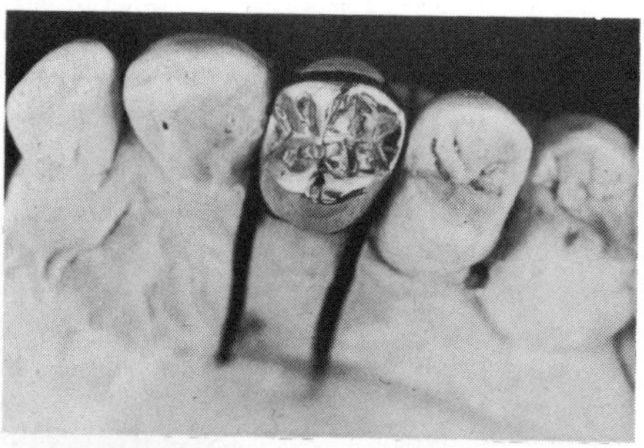

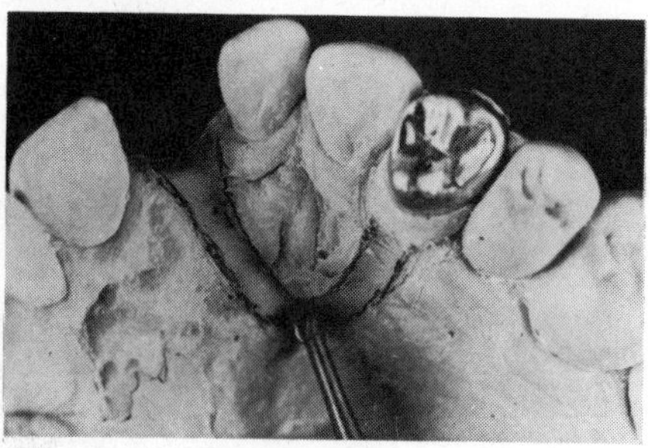

Fig. 10.15. *The three-quarter crown is waxed up, cast, finished and then transferred to the unsplit model which is grooved to take the bar.*

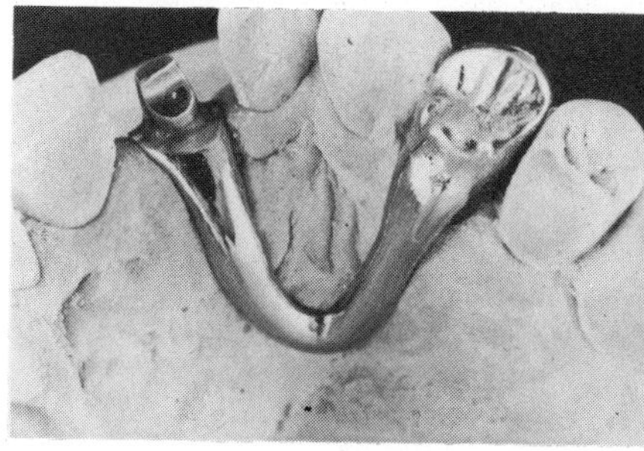

Fig. 10.16. *The bar, complete with core is now waxed up, cast and soldered to the three-quarter crown.*

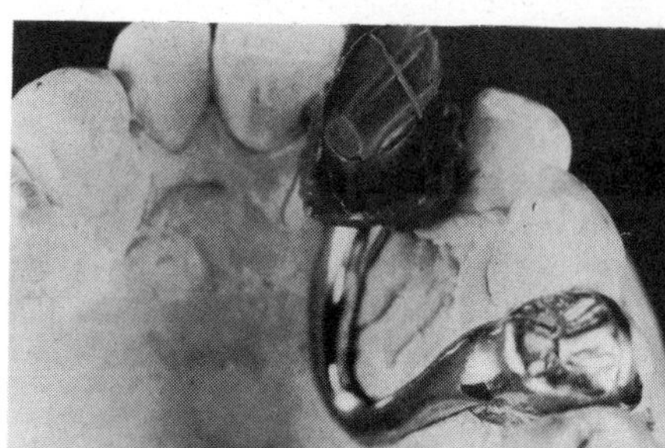

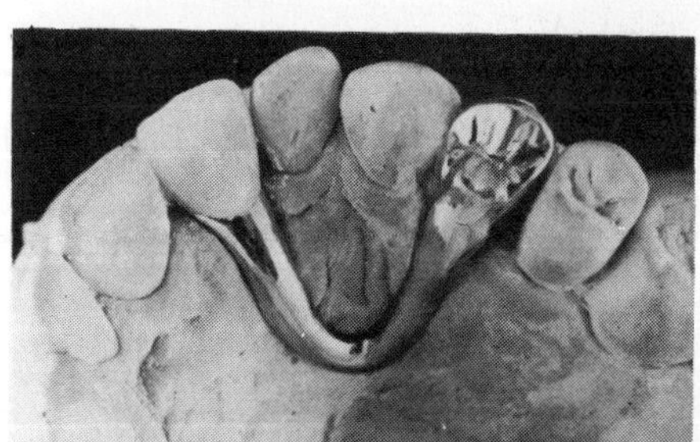

Fig. 10.17. *An impression is taken of the core so that a separate die may be made on which the foil is laid down and onto which the core mass is baked prior to transferring it back to the unsplit model for completion.*

■ B. The Bar

This should be checked carefully to see that there are no signs of a fracture commencing which nearly always takes place at the bend. Occasionally tearing occurs at the solder joint. This is particularly likely to happen if a nickel-chrome bar is joined to a gold retainer and the correct soldering technique has not been employed. Thus it is essential that in these cases a nickel-chrome flux such as 'Oxynon' should always be used.

Should the bar bend the pontic will move labially and upwards (*see Fig*. 10.3) and if this is slight it is best accepted. Should it occur soon after the bridge is placed and then apparently stabilizes a new pontic may be placed but only after investigating the occlusion first to see why the bar bent in the first instance. In all other instances the only solution is a remake with a bar of better design.

■ C. Periodontal Condition of the Abutment Tooth

This should always be checked:

a. By recording and comparing it from year to year to make certain that no signs of overloading are present.

b. By comparing the periodontal condition of the abutment tooth with that of the same tooth on the other side of the arch to see if any periodontal breakdown is local or general.

If the tooth shows signs of overloading, which is rare, the bridge should be remade, either using a different abutment, incorporating a second one in the existing design, or using a different type of bridge.

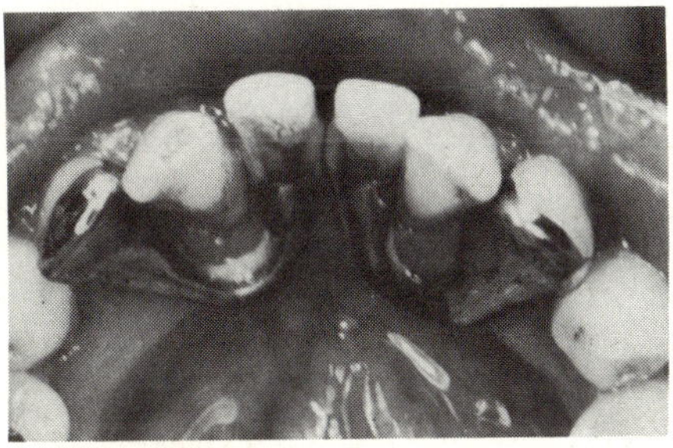

Fig. 10.22. *Calculus deposits on, and food packing around, two lower spring bridges.*

THE LOWER SPRING BRIDGE

This is not a very satisfactory bridge design and should rarely be employed. It must be remembered that it is not a true spring bridge, as little movement can be permitted in the bar and only minimal tissue support will be obtained.

■ Its Main Disadvantages are

a. It is often difficult to achieve adequate retention from any lower tooth which is likely to be used as an abutment.

b. The direction of the occlusal forces is the reverse of that in the upper jaw and this, coupled with the shape of the lower alveolus, means that the tissue support gained is minimal.

c. The mucosa overlying the lower ridge is thin and tolerates pressure badly. Thus quite a few lower spring bridges have to be removed because of ulceration beneath them. This occurrence is extremely rare in the upper arch.

d. Deposits of calculus around the bar make it difficult to keep clean (*Fig*. 10.22).

e. The line of the bar is of necessity fairly near the gingival margins of the teeth.

■ Precautions in Construction of a Lower Spring Bridge.

In a lower bridge the bar should not be let into the tissues at all for the reasons already explained and very little movement should be permitted, otherwise irritation of the mucosa will occur.

All the other design features are similar to those for the upper bridge.

Bibliography

Jeffrey I. W. M. (1975) The biomechanics of the spring cantilever bridge. Ph.D. Thesis. University of Dundee.
Thompson A. R. F. (1943) Notes on dental conservation. *Guy's Hosp. Gaz.* 57, 44.

11

COMPOUND BRIDGES

Advantages . Fixed-fixed and Spring Bridges
Fixed-fixed and Cantilever Bridges
Fixed-fixed and Fixed-movable Bridges

Quite often no one bridge type will suffice as a satisfactory replacement for several missing teeth. However, by combining two or more different types (a compound bridge) the problem can usually be overcome.

ADVANTAGES

One of the main advantages of a compound prosthesis is that it enables a relatively complex bridge to be broken down into several smaller units. Thus, should a failure occur or repair work be necessitated at any time, only a small part of the whole bridge will have to be disturbed.

The following example may make this point clearer. The ⌊45 7 require replacement and the prognosis for ⌊8 is somewhat doubtful. Thus rather than make the whole bridge fixed-fixed, the distal part comprising ⌊7 pontic and ⌊8 retainer is joined to the anterior section by means of a dovetail. Should ⌊8 require extraction at a later date then the main part of the bridge will not be disturbed.

A further advantage of compounding different bridge types is that it simplifies the construction of the prosthesis:

a. By enabling it to be made in several short rather than two or three long visits, thus putting far less strain on both the patient and the operator. It may also simplify the clinical procedures, for instance by avoiding the necessity of taking an accurate impression of 7–8 teeth all at the same time.

b. By permitting the construction of a bridge where the unfavourable angulation of the abutment teeth would prevent a conventional fixed-fixed design being used. It will also avoid any undue destruction of tooth tissue and even devitalization which might be required if all the abutment preparations had to be parallel.

FIXED-FIXED AND SPRING BRIDGES

A design which may prove of value is the combination of a posterior fixed-fixed bridge and a spring bridge (*Fig.* 11.1).

⌊3 F.C. ⌊45 pontics ⌊6 — Fixed-fixed

¾-crown with distal slot ⌊7 pontic ⌊8 ¾-crown — Fixed-movable

Providing the prosthesis is correctly designed it should not result in overloading of the abutment teeth as the pontic of the spring section of the bridge will be largely tissue borne.

Where this combination is used the bar should usually be taken off the distal retainer. In this way any force transmitted to the second retainer will be of a favourable compressive nature. If the bar is fixed to the anterior retainer, when pressure is applied to the pontic a 'see-sawing' effect may be created and a decementing force applied to the second retainer.

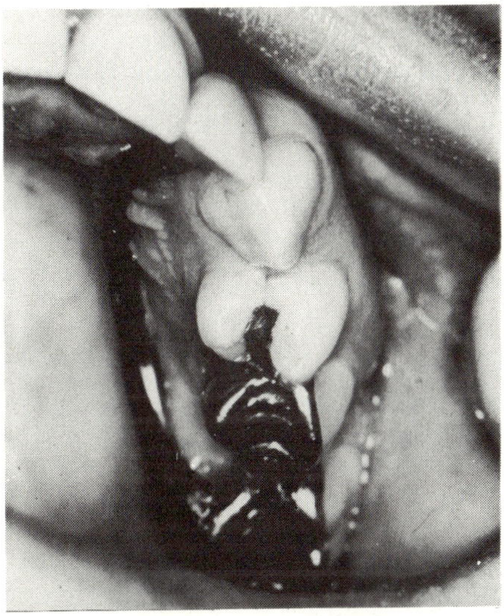

Fig. 11.1. *Fixed-fixed and spring bridges being combined to replace |2 6. There is only a small all-gold pontic at |6.*

FIXED-FIXED AND CANTILEVER BRIDGES

Fixed-fixed and cantilever bridges may also on occasions be satisfactorily combined (*Fig.* 11.2). Whereas the amount of cantilevering permissible from a single abutment is strictly limited, particularly if its root surface area is low, far more extensive cantilevering may be carried out if there are multiple abutments. Thus only a small distal cantilever could safely be extended from an upper second premolar but if this was part of a larger bridge involving, say, 3 1|1 3 5 as abutments then the distal extension could be much more extensive. However, it must be remembered that the strain imposed on the structure of the bridge, and particularly the distal aspect of the second premolar, will be considerably increased and thus the bridge should be strengthened accordingly.

It should also be borne in mind that the more stable the abutment(s) the more stress that will be placed on the bridge and the more mobile the teeth the lower the maximum occlusal load which the patient can apply to the prosthesis and thus the less likely structural or cementation failure is to occur. The most unfavourable situation arises when one

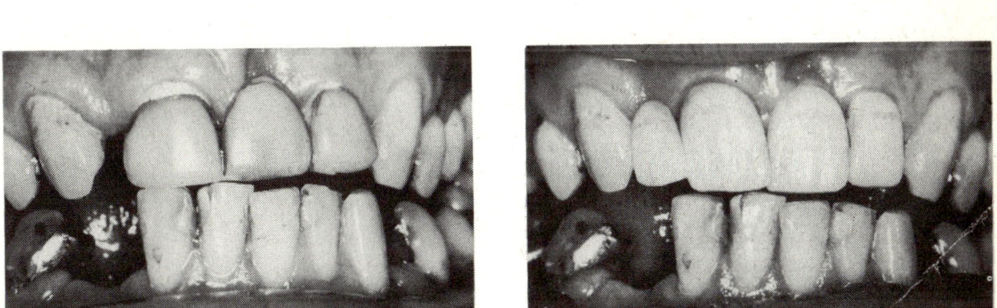

Fig. 11.2. *Missing 2| and a three-unit acrylic bridge being replaced by a four-unit bonded bridge, which is a combination of fixed-fixed and cantilever designs. Note characterization of porcelain to match 3|. The lower arch has still to be restored.*
(By courtesy of Mr D. N. Atkinson.)

abutment is firm and all the others are highly mobile. Care must be taken not to overload the abutment tooth from which the cantilever is carried particularly when only 2 abutments are used. Thus it would be quite permissible to cantilever an upper lateral from a fixed-fixed bridge extending from the canine to the second premolar as the canine is a powerful abutment and the lateral is a relatively small tooth. However, it would generally not be satisfactory to cantilever a first premolar from a fixed-fixed bridge extending from the second premolar to the third molar. Overloading of the periodontium of the former tooth would be likely to occur (*see Fig*. 19.8, p. 253) because of its small root surface area.

FIXED-FIXED AND FIXED-MOVABLE BRIDGES

A combination of fixed-fixed and fixed-movable bridges has many advantages: (1) All the retainers do not have to have the same line of insertion and withdrawal, thus simplifying preparations and conserving tooth tissue; (2) In the case of the minor retainers, lighter preparations may be used; (3) Should the fixed-fixed section of the bridge fail and have to be removed then usually the minor retainer may be left in situ.

A simple combination of fixed-fixed and fixed-movable bridges is shown in *Fig*. 11.3.

A more complex combination of bridge types is that shown in *Fig*. 11.4. In effect there are three bridges, one in the anterior region from the upper left canine to the upper right canine and two posterior bridges, each extending from the first premolar to the first molar. The anterior bridge is joined to the posterior bridges by means of dovetails and slots on the distal aspects of the canines. Thus it will gain support from them and this will tend to prevent the labial drift which is liable to occur in later life, particularly if there is any periodontal breakdown or

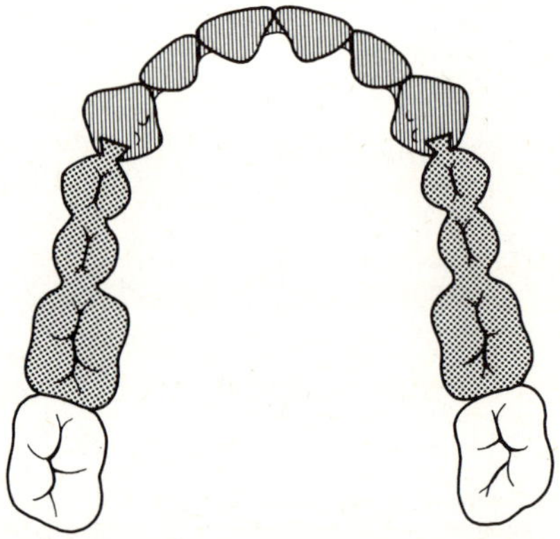

Fig. 11.4. *An anterior fixed-fixed bridge being linked to two posterior fixed-fixed bridges by dovetails.*

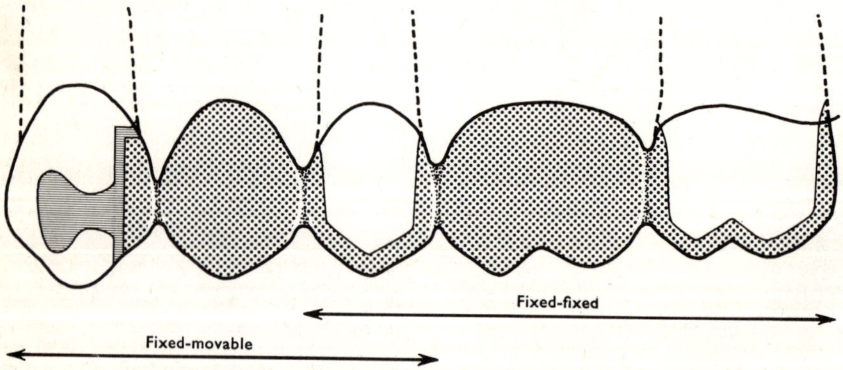

Fig. 11.3. *A combination of fixed-fixed and fixed-movable bridges. By using this design, the retainer in the canine can have a different line of insertion to those on the other teeth. Likewise, it does not have to be so retentive.*

posterior occlusal collapse. If either of the posterior bridges requires remaking at a later date, due to pontic failure or further tooth loss, it will not disturb the anterior bridge. Similarly, if the anterior bridge has to be removed, this can be done without disturbing the posterior bridges, by merely removing the dovetails from the anterior aspect of the retainers in the first premolars. If it is desirable to remake the anterior bridge it is possible to relink it to the posterior bridges by cutting slots in the mesial aspects of the retainers on the first premolars and incorporating dovetails in the new anterior bridge. However, the initial design and preparation of the retainers on the 4|4 will have to incorporate mesial boxes to house the slots.

Precision retainers are of particular use in compound bridge prostheses as they usually permit the separation of two or more components. The screw devices are especially valuable in this respect as they enable the operator to insert the various components with entirely different lines of insertion and then to lock them together (*Fig*. 12.8, p. 171). A further advantage is that they can be separated at any time should one of the components require repair.

The use of precision retainers in fixed bridge prostheses is discussed in greater detail in the next chapter.

12

THE USE OF PRECISION RETAINERS IN FIXED BRIDGE PROSTHESES*

Alignment of Abutments
Continuity of Treatment
Providing a Removable Prosthesis
Reducing the Strain on One or More Abutment Teeth
Stabilizing a Full Lower Prosthesis

Although precision retainers, or precision attachments as some people prefer to term them, have been employed since the beginning of the century, it is only in the past 10–15 years that they have come into general use. This is largely due to the extremely fine tolerance of which modern machine tools are now capable and the wide range of retainers which have recently been designed by dental surgeons, particularly in Switzerland and in the USA.

The use of the term 'precision retainer' implies a partly or wholly machined device consisting of male and female components which is used in restorative dentistry to retain removable or semi-removable prostheses. They may also on occasions be incorporated in fixed bridges.

Both components are usually individually machined to very fine limits (*Fig.* 12.1) so that they fit each other far more

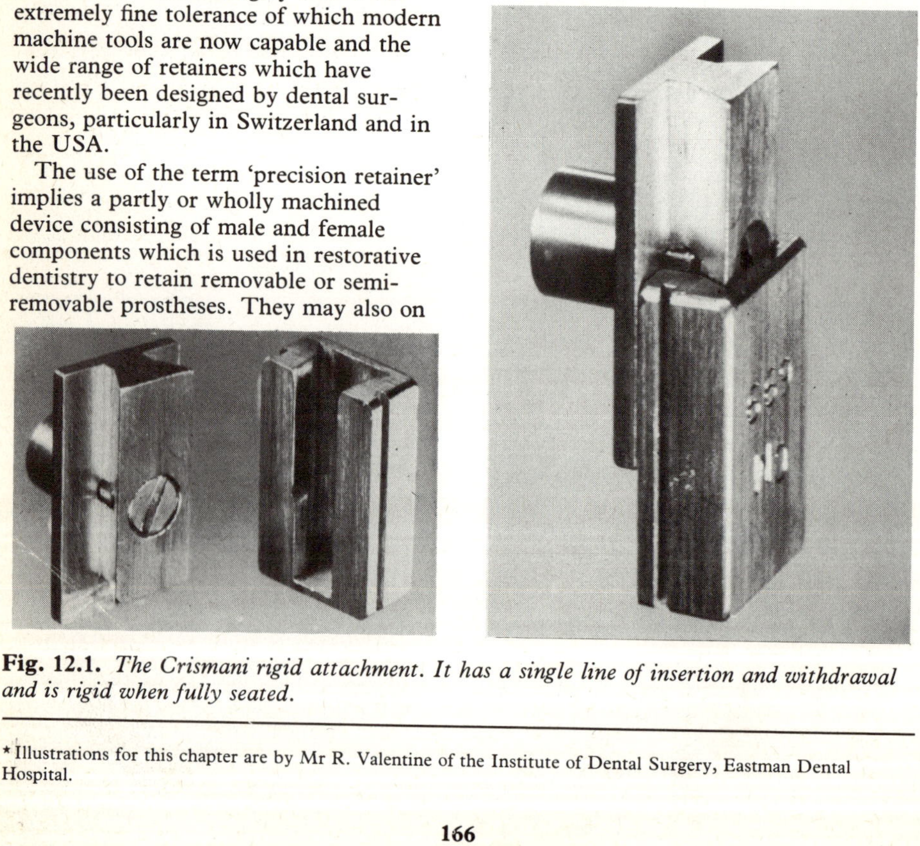

Fig. 12.1. *The Crismani rigid attachment. It has a single line of insertion and withdrawal and is rigid when fully seated.*

* Illustrations for this chapter are by Mr R. Valentine of the Institute of Dental Surgery, Eastman Dental Hospital.

accurately than the conventional dovetail and slot made in the laboratory.

The majority of precision retainers are factory made. However, there is also a wide range which may be milled in the laboratory by the technician (*Fig.* 12.2) using a parallelometer. Steiger and Boitel (1959) designed many of these, of which the best known example is the CSP (Channel, Shoulder, Pin).

Probably the most important factor to be remembered when considering the use of precision retainers is their size. Although they look small it is surprising how often there is insufficient space to accommodate them, particularly if they have to be housed intracoronally (*see Fig.* 2.25, p. 23). Quite drastic reduction of tooth tissue, including the provision of a deep box, is nearly always necessary and this cannot be achieved on small teeth, particularly anteriors and those with short clinical crowns. The size of the pulp is a further limiting factor.

The only safe method is to assess each case individually on the models, doing a trial preparation and seeing from this if it is possible to house the precision retainer one requires to use.

Because of the very considerable demands made on retention by most precision-retained prostheses, full crowns are nearly always indicated.

The classification for precision retainers (*below*) which is based on the use to which they are put has been devised at

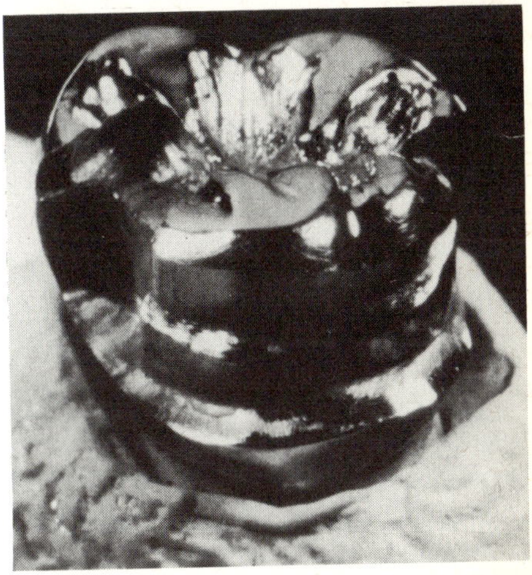

Fig. 12.2. *A laboratory-milled rigid attachment based on the CSP as conceived by Steiger.*

Rigid retainers	Rigid attachments (on vital teeth)	Adjustable	Chayes McCollum Stern Crismani
		Non-adjustable	Beyeler C & M 643
	Rigid anchorages (non-vital teeth)	All adjustable	Eccentric Bona Gerber
Movable retainers	Movable attachments (on vital teeth)		Dalbo Crismani
	Stress breakers (for partial dentures)		Gerber hinge Ancorvis hinge
	Movable anchorages (non-vital teeth)		Bona Dolder bar Andrews bar
Auxiliary devices	Activators		Ipsoclip
	Latches, bolts, screws		Schubiger Hruska

the Institute of Dental Surgery by Mr R. Valentine in collaboration with other colleagues in this field.

In fixed bridge work it is primarily the rigid retainers and auxiliary devices such as the screws which are of value. The ways in which they can help in the design and construction of a basically fixed bridge include the following:

1. In overcoming problems of alignment.
2. Providing for possible future loss of one or more of the abutment teeth.
3. Providing a prosthesis which is removable (*a*) by the patient or (*b*) by the operator.
4. Reducing the stress on one or more of the abutment teeth.
5. Stabilizing a full lower prosthesis.

1. ALIGNMENT OF ABUTMENTS

Where it is impossible or undesirable to prepare two or more abutment teeth so that the castings have a common line of withdrawal, for example in cases of tilting or rotation, the simplest solution frequently is to use a fixed-movable bridge incorporating a dovetail and slot. However, if the span is long or the periodontal condition is doubtful then the benefits of fixed splinting may be required. This can often be provided by the use of precision retainers. The two components of these fit together so accurately that for all practical purposes, once fully seated in the mouth, the bridge will be completely rigid.

An example of this is shown in *Fig.* 12.3, suitable retainers to use in this case being the Beyeler, rigid Crismani, Stern or Chayes. On rare occasions where alignment problems are severe, it may be necessary to use precision retainers in the abutments at both ends of the pontic area.

2. CONTINUITY OF TREATMENT

Where the prognosis of one of the abutment teeth is suspect this should always, as far as possible, be taken into consideration when planning the prosthesis. One of the easiest ways of doing this is by the incorporation of a precision retainer in the design. This will allow the failed abutment to be removed without disturbing the other castings.

An example of this is the incorporation of a rigid Crismani (*Fig.* 12.4) in the distal aspect of the second premolar as

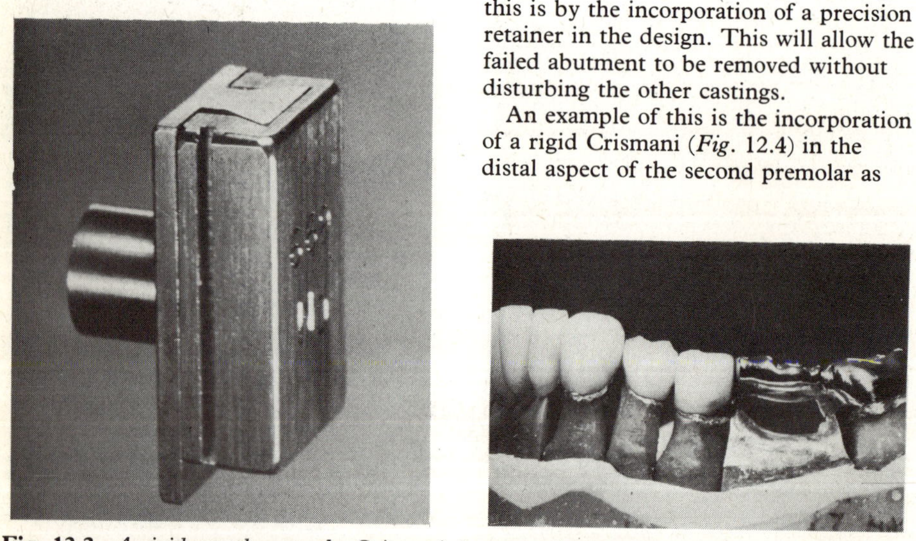

Fig. 12.3. *A rigid attachment, the Crismani, here seen incorporated in the mesial retainer of a bridge to allow different lines of insertion for the two castings but still provide the benefits of a fixed-fixed design.*

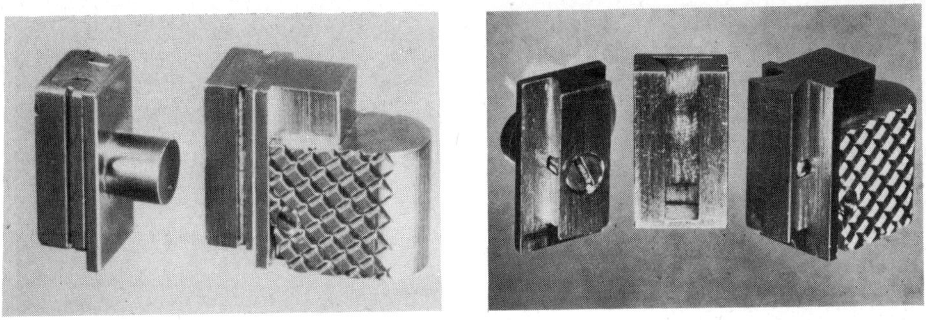

Fig. 12.4. *The matrices of the corresponding rigid and movable Crismani attachments are identical in size and thus the patrices are interchangeable.*

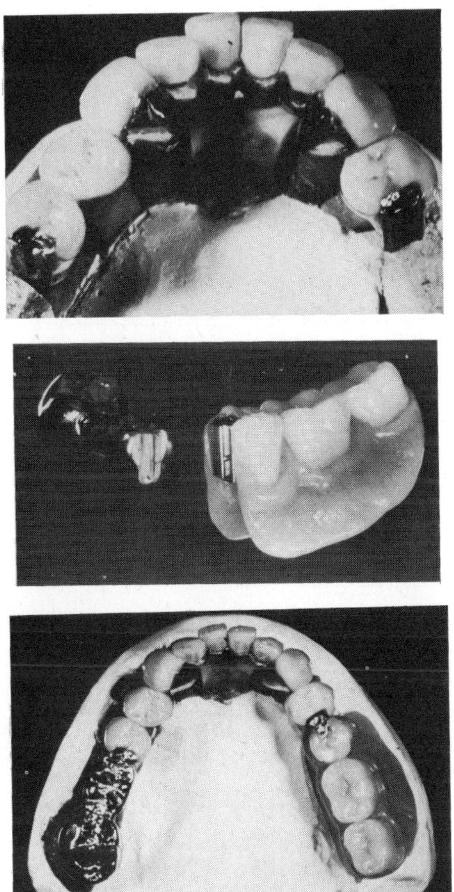

Fig. 12.5. *A free-end saddle prosthesis and a fixed bridge, both incorporating a Crismani patrix, the former movable, the latter rigid.*

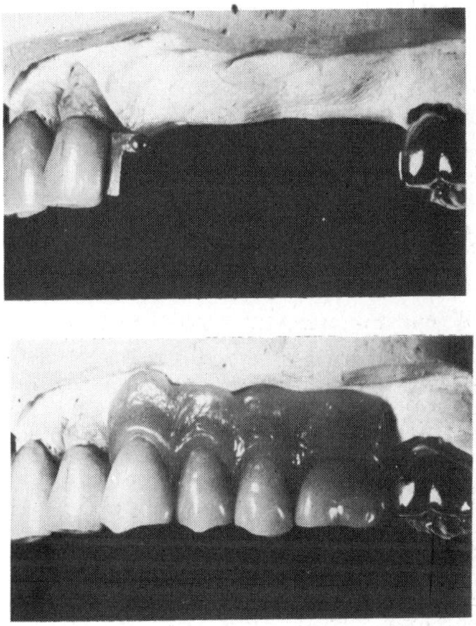

Fig. 12.6. *A removable precision-retained prosthesis with a Dalbo mesially and a Stern attachment distally.*

shown in *Fig.* 12.5. If at a later stage the distal abutment is lost this can be removed together with the pontics. This will not disturb the mesial retainers and subsequently a free end saddle can be placed, fitting a movable Crismani into the female portion of the rigid Crismani already present in the premolar. A further example using a Dalbo in the distal aspect of the canine, with all the upper anterior teeth crowned and splinted together, is shown in *Fig.* 12.6.

An alternative method of achieving the same results, particularly in extensive bridges, is the use of the auxiliary devices.

3. PROVIDING A REMOVABLE PROSTHESIS

This may be achieved by making it removable (*a*) by the patient or (*b*) by the operator.

■ A. Removable by the Patient

Where there is considerable soft tissue loss which must be made good this will usually necessitate a fully removable prosthesis such as a chrome-cobalt denture. An alternative is to incorporate one or more precision retainers into a bridge which allows the pontic or saddle area to be removed by the patient.

Examples of this are the use of the Dolder or Andrews bars and laboratory-milled bars (*Fig.* 12.7) which use devices such as the Ipsoclip to retain the removable section in place.

■ B. Removable by Operator

If for any reason it may be desirable to remove a bridge at some time subsequent to cementation, this can be made possible by the incorporation in the design of screws (*Fig.* 12.8) or latches.

Examples of why this may become necessary are:

i. The doubtful prognosis of one of the abutment teeth, which has already been discussed.

ii. To simplify the treatment of any caries which may occur at the margins of the castings.

iii. To assist periodontal surgery.

iv. To replace the pontics. This is usually necessary after 5–7 years if they are made of acrylic because of the discoloration and wear.

4. REDUCING THE STRAIN ON ONE OR MORE ABUTMENT TEETH

This may be desirable for a number of reasons, one of the main ones being when it has not been possible to achieve

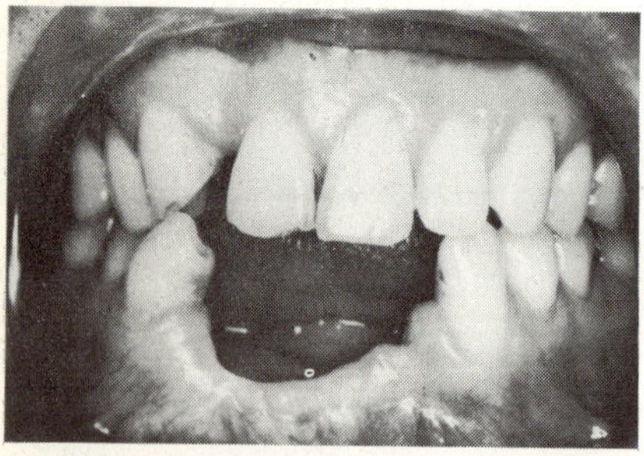

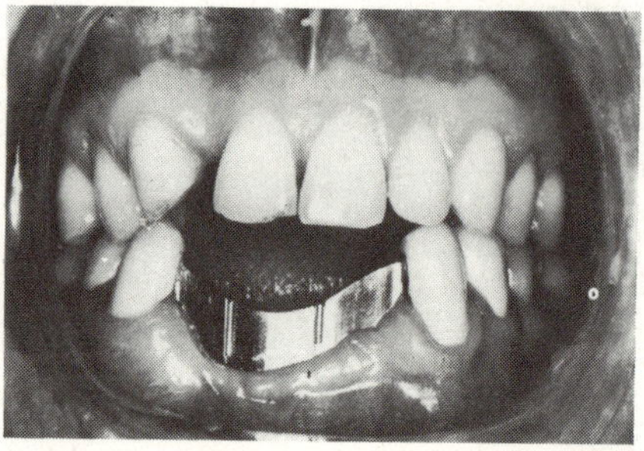

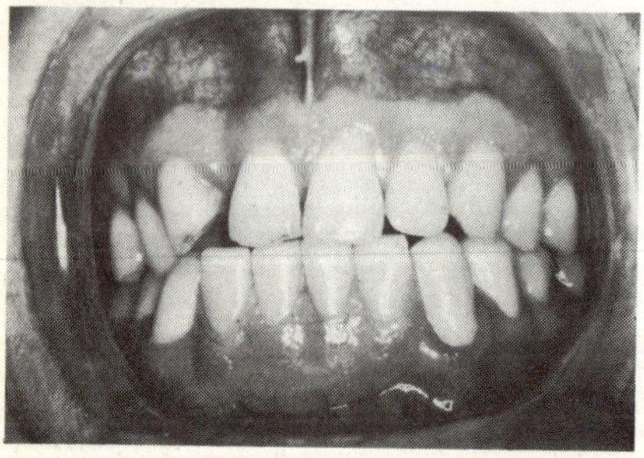

Fig. 12.7. *A patient with considerable anterior soft tissue loss.* 54|34 *were prepared for bonded full crowns and these were used to support a laboratory milled bar. This has locating grooves and a ball catch (the Ipsoclip) to retain the final prosthesis, which is removable by the patient.*

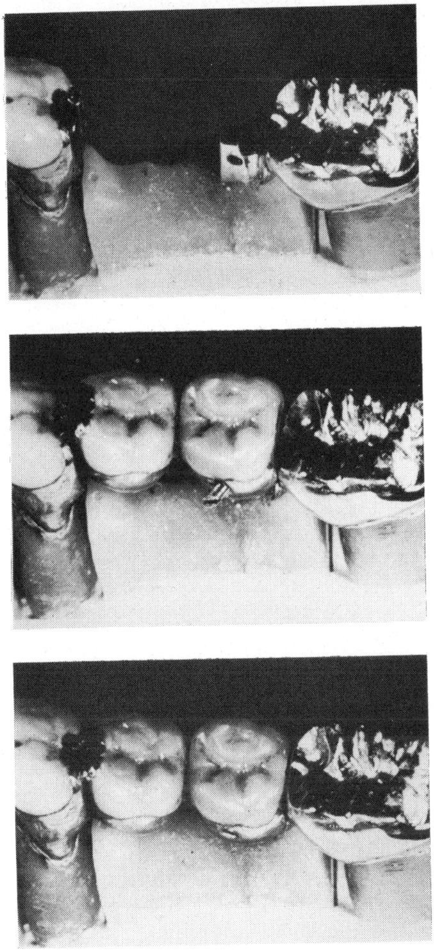

Fig. 12.8. *A prosthesis which can be removed by the dental surgeon by means of a screw. Mesially a rigid Crismani is incorporated in the design.*

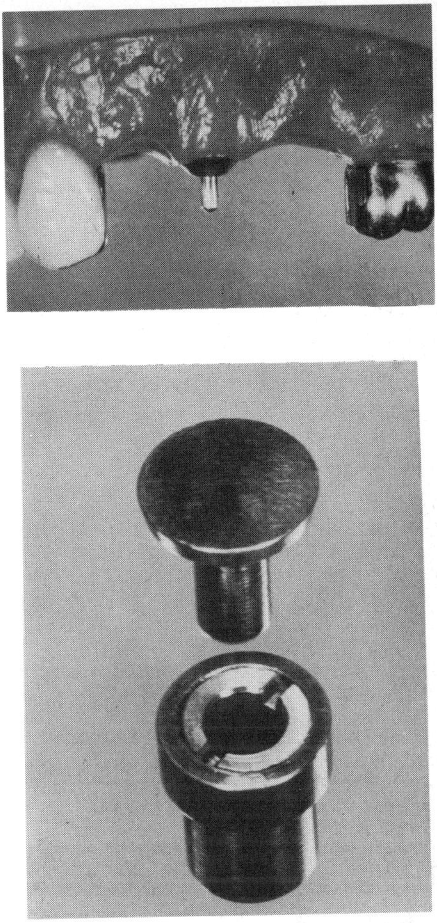

Fig. 12.9. *A removable prosthesis replacing the first premolar and first molar. A Gmür has been fixed to the root cap on the second premolar, thus reducing the chance of cementation failure of the casting.*

adequate retention on one of the abutment teeth. This is particularly liable to occur with the non-vital tooth which has a short or bifurcated root canal rendered even more unfavourable by caries.

In the example shown (*Fig.* 12.9) the post crown on the premolar lacked retention and thus it would have been likely to have come uncemented if the bridge had been made fixed-fixed. By incorporating a Gmür in the design the decementing force on this tooth is greatly decreased as it is no longer rigidly fixed to the other abutments.

5. STABILIZING A FULL LOWER PROSTHESIS

Several different types of precision retainer have been devised to stabilize the apparent full denture. These are soldered to root caps which must have good

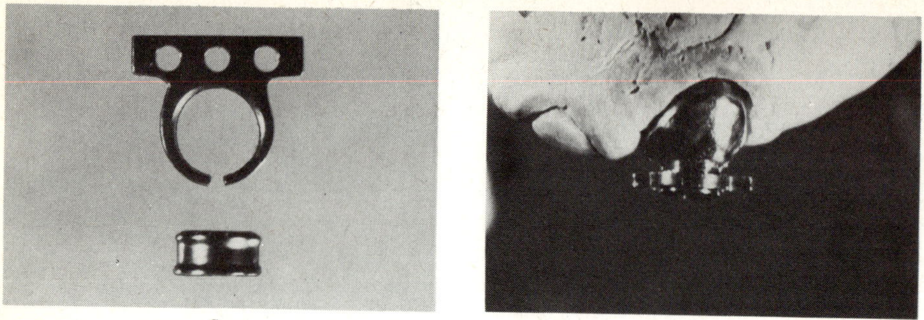

a *b*

Fig. 12.10. *a, The Eccentric or Rotherman precision retainer (attachment). Note the deep slot in the patrix which permits vertical movement of the prosthesis. b, The root cap should follow, so far as possible, the natural contour of the ridge.*

retention otherwise they will become uncemented when the prosthesis is removed by the patient.

Probably the simplest to use and also the one which requires least space is the Eccentric (Rotherman). These are designed to stabilize the prosthesis but allow sufficient vertical movement (note wide groove in the patrix, *Fig.* 12.10*a*) to ensure that it is entirely tissue borne. The patrix is soldered to the root cap (*Fig.* 12.10*b*) and the matrix is incorporated in the denture. Two Eccentrics will provide all the stability which is required for the majority of full lower dentures. (*See Fig.* 2.20*a, b,* p. 19.)

The foregoing is only a brief outline of the possible ways in which precision retainers may assist in the design of a fixed bridge prosthesis and the reader is referred to a specialist text on the subject for further information.

Bibliography

Chayes H. (1917) System of movable, removable bridgework in conformity with the principle that teeth move in function. *Dent. Rev.* **31**, 87.

Preiskel H. W. (1966) The use of internal attachments. *Br. Dent. J.* **121**, 564.

Preiskel H. W. (1971) Screw-retained telescopic prostheses. *Br. Dent. J.* **130**, 107.

Preiskel H. W. (1973) *Precision Attachments in Dentistry,* 2nd ed. London, Kimpton.

Rajezak E. J. (1971) Trouble shooting with pins. *Dent. Clin. North Am.* **15**, 711.

Schuyler C. H. (1953) An analysis of the use and relative value of precision attachment and the clasp in partial denture planning. *J. Prosthet. Dent.* **3**, 711.

Steiger A. and Boitel R. (1959) *Precision Work for Partial Dentures.* Zürich, Stebo.

13

ADHESIVE BRIDGES

The Acid-etch Technique
Selection of Pontic
The Rochette Bridge . Bonding Failures

W. M. TAY

In 1955, Buonocore's observation that acrylic resins could bond to an acid treated enamel surface opened up new possibilities in restorative dentistry. Since then the development of much harder and stronger composite resins with their low coefficient of thermal expansion and polymerization shrinkage has brought about a method of quickly and simply providing an inexpensive and aesthetic bridge with practically no need for the preparation of abutment teeth.

Replacement of missing teeth in the child or young adult, whether it be by fixed or removable prostheses, very often presents problems in technique and design. Conventional fixed bridgework requires the removal of tooth structure which, if sound, may seem quite radical in a young patient. Furthermore, such young teeth often have relatively short clinical crowns with large pulp chambers which make tooth preparation rather hazardous. It may be argued that conservative procedures such as partial veneer or pin-retained crowns can be carried out, but these often present aesthetic problems especially in the anterior region and frequently lack retention. Adhesive bridges largely overcome these problems and from the psychological aspect are ideally suited to the young patient because the procedure is relatively atraumatic. The reduced chairside time and the simplicity of the technique ensures that costs are relatively low, and in addition the teeth remain sound should the need arise for conventional bridgework. Indeed, Ibsen and Neville (1974) believe adhesive bridges are 'the single most important advance in bridgework in the last three decades'.

However, until more is known regarding the nature of the bond between composite and tooth the cautious practitioner should regard adhesive bridges as provisional prostheses. In fact, the self-limiting nature of the bond may itself not be a disadvantage because any potentially traumatic occlusal interference would cause the bond to fail long before any damage can be caused to the abutment teeth or periodontium.

THE ACID-ETCH TECHNIQUE

The key to the success of the adhesive bridge technique is the care taken in acid etching the enamel surface.

The application of a 30–50 per cent concentration of phosphoric acid to the enamel surface for 60–90 sec results in selective decalcification of the enamel rods and the formation of microscopic pores up to 25 μm deep. Acid etching also raises the surface energy of the enamel and this enables the applied resin to 'wet' the surface and penetrate the micropores.

The retention of the resin when set is mainly through mechanical interlocking with intermolecular (physicochemical) forces of attraction contributing a small part of the total bond strength.

The abutment teeth are cleaned with a bristle brush or rubber cup and a slurry of pumice or fluoride-free prophylaxis paste. All traces of pumice are then washed away and the teeth isolated with cotton-wool rolls or, preferably rubber dam. After blowing dry the surfaces, a 30–50 per cent aqueous solution of phosphoric acid is applied to the areas to be bonded only, care being taken to ensure that the surfaces are kept moist with acid. The acid may be applied with a pledget of cotton wool, synthetic sponge, or a fine artist's paint brush. It is not necessary, and in fact inadvisable to 'rub in' the acid lest any smearing of the micropores occurs. Etching time is between 60 and 90 sec. The acid must then be washed away with copious water directed at the etched surface for a minimum of 20 sec to ensure every trace of acid is removed. The surface is now blow-dried, whereupon it will appear frosty-white, indicating a successful etch. Extreme care must be taken at this stage not to contaminate the surface, and the resin should be applied straightaway.

The choice of composite resin is not critical, although the operator may find it easier to work with a system that enables him to modify the working time and viscosity of the resin than one that does not. With light-cured resins such as Nuvafil* and Alpha-Fil† which use ultraviolet light, and Fotofil‡ which employs blue light (440–480 nm) to activate the polymerization, the working time is fully under the control of the operator. Self-curing resins such as Concise Enamel Bond,§ Powderlite,|| and Restodent¶ enable the requisite viscosity of the final mix to be achieved by diluting the paste or powder with varying amounts of the liquid catalyst resin.

* L. D. Caulk Co., Div. of Dentists' Supply Co. of NY, Milford, Del. Toronto, Ontario, Canada.
† De Trey, A. D. International Ltd, PO Box 2AD, 26/40 Broadwick Street, London W1.
‡ Johnson & Johnson Co., Dental Div., Compare House, Brunell Way, Slough, Berks.
§ 3M Co., 3M House, PO Box 1, Bracknell, Berks.
|| S. S. White Co. of GB Ltd, 51 St Anne's Road, Harrow, Middlesex.

SELECTION OF PONTIC

■ A. Natural Tooth Pontic

The patient's own tooth, if it needs to be extracted, may be used as a pontic. Prior to extraction, and provided the tooth crown is relatively intact and in proper relationship with the abutment and opposing teeth, an impression of the lingual surfaces of the intended pontic and abutment teeth may be made in a silicone putty such as Optosil Plus** which can be moulded with ease without the need of a tray. The impression provides an accurate method of relocating the tooth pontic in its original position later. After extraction, and whilst haemostasis is taking place the root of the extracted tooth is sectioned about 1 mm below the amelocemental junction to allow for initial tissue shrinkage when the blood clot organizes. The pulp remnants are removed through the open canal which is then filled with a composite resin to avoid discolouring the crown. The amputated end is smoothed with abrasive discs, and the tooth cleaned and dried. When bleeding has stopped in the extraction socket the operation area may be isolated with cotton-wool rolls, and a trial location carried out with the pontic placed in the impression. Minor adjustments may be necessary at the amputated end. If the pontic fits satisfactorily it may be removed with the impression key and its abutment surfaces etched. Etching is also carried out at the same time on the corresponding surfaces of the abutment teeth. Resin is applied to the etched surfaces of pontic and abutments, and the pontic relocated with the aid of the impression key. After the resin has set, any excess may be trimmed away and the bridge polished.

¶ Lee Pharmaceutical, 1444 St. Anita Avenue, South El Monte, California 11733, USA.
** Bayer Leverkusen, Germany.

With an avulsed tooth, it is difficult to determine precisely the original arrangement of the teeth, and in this respect the impression key is not essential; however, the pontic preparation and acid etching of the tooth surfaces is as described above. The pontic is attached to the contacts of the abutment teeth with a small amount of resin. This initial attachment allows a certain degree of adjustment to be made until the correct position is judged to have been achieved. When this first layer of resin has set wood points may be inserted on either side of the pontic in order to maintain the interdental spaces whilst further increments of resin are applied. After 5–8 min when the resin has set the wood points may be removed and the composite finished in the usual manner, care being taken to ensure that the embrasures are free of excess resin (*Figs*. 13.1, 13.2). If necessary, the surfaces may be glazed with unfilled resin to acquire a smooth surface, albeit for a short period. The occlusion is then checked, and where indicated minor adjustments may be made.

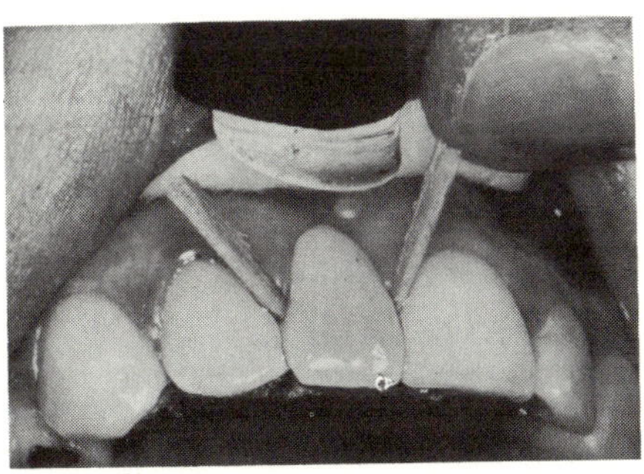

Fig. 13.1. *Resin tooth replacing 1|. Composition impression key on palatal surfaces to aid location of pontic. Interdental wood sticks maintain spaces for cleaning.*

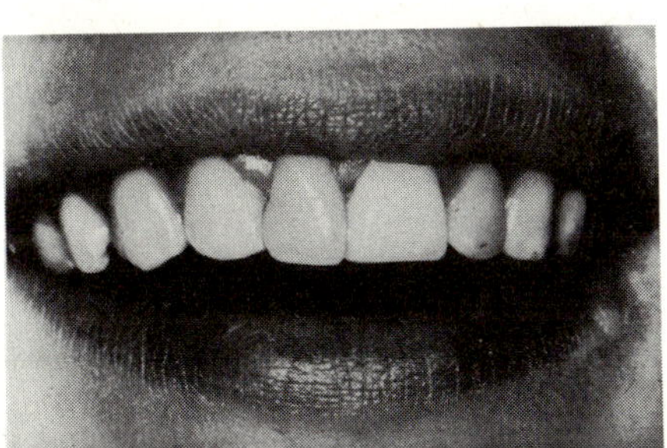

Fig. 13.2. *Finished pontic 1|.*

■ B. Resin Tooth Pontic (*Figs.* 13.3, 13.4)

A pontic may be fabricated in acrylic or composite resin in a cellulose acetate or polycarbonate crown form, or preferably selected from stock acrylic denture teeth because of the better colour stability of this material. The pontic is then trimmed at the chairside or in the laboratory on a plaster cast of the arch. If the latter technique is employed an impression key can be made to aid relocation of the pontic in the mouth. When an acrylic tooth is used additional mechanical retention in the form of grooves or undercut cavities need to be made in the lingual surface. These are filled with composite resin and attached to the abutment teeth as described for the

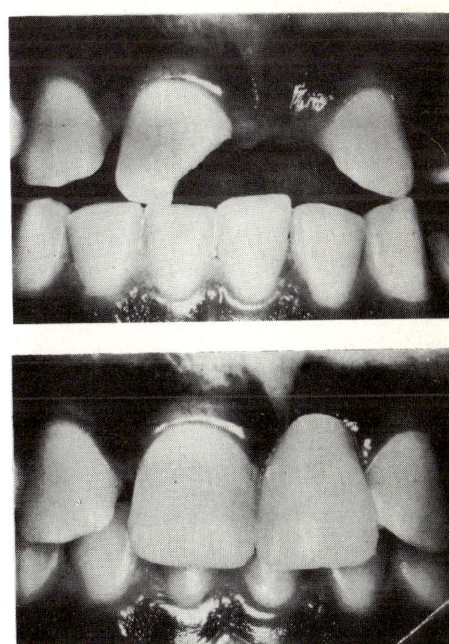

Fig. 13.3. *Acrylic resin pontic |1 bonded to 1|2. 1| form restored with the same etched-retained composite resin.* (By courtesy of Mr D. Rule.)

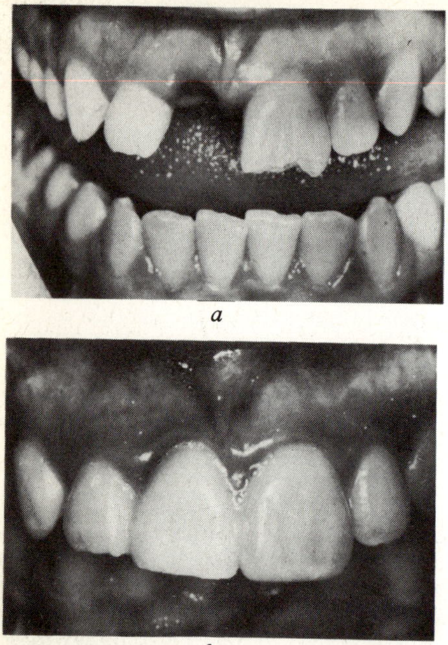

Fig. 13.4. *Immediate post-extraction replacement of* $\underline{1|}$ *with etch-retained acrylic pontic. Incisal edge of* $\underline{|1}$ *restored with composite resin.* (By courtesy of Mr D. Rule.)

natural tooth pontic. The bond between acrylic tooth and composite, or composite and composite is strong. However, polycarbonate crowns may not bond well to composite resins unless their surfaces are primed with acrylic resin.

So far it has been assumed that the surfaces of the abutment teeth are sound. If fillings are present they should be removed and the cavity margins bevelled and etched before placing and finishing a new composite filling. The pontic may then be attached with the same brand of composite in order to achieve a good bond.

Simonsen (1978) has described a technique using stainless-steel wire 0·8 mm in diameter incorporated in the pontic with the free ends embedded in the mesial and distal preparations of abutment teeth with composite resin. He recommends this technique in cases where more than one acrylic pontic is envisaged. The wire probably aids retention by stiffening the junction between composite resin and acrylic tooth.

THE ROCHETTE BRIDGE

Rochette (1973) in describing cast metal splints etch-bonded to periodontally involved teeth suggested that these splints could also incorporate an artificial pontic to bridge a gap. In 1977, Howe and Denehy reported the use of such a bridge in two patients, and gave clinical and laboratory details of its construction. Tay and Shaw (1979) described 3 cases from a series of 16 patients they had treated, a total of 17 Rochette bridges being successfully retained over a period of 19 months.

■ A. Clinical and Laboratory Procedures

Usually, only two appointments are required. At the first visit the abutment teeth are thoroughly cleaned, the shade of the pontic determined, and an impression of the teeth and tissues involved taken in an elastic impression material. The framework is outlined on the working model. The flanges should cover as much of the lingual surface of the teeth as possible without encroaching on the gingivae (*Fig.* 13.5). If the abutment teeth have translucent edges then the metal should not extend too far incisally lest a greyish discoloration be perceptible when the bridge is fitted.

Semi-precious alloys such as Victory,* Wiron S,† or Degucast U‡ are eminently suitable for the framework and will keep down the overall cost. The thickness of

* Uniteck Corporation, 2724 South Peck Road, Monrovia, California 91016, USA.

† Bego Ltd, Emil-Sommer Strasse 7, Bremen, W. Germany.

‡ Degussa Dental, Postfach 2644, D-6000, Frankfurt 1, W. Germany.

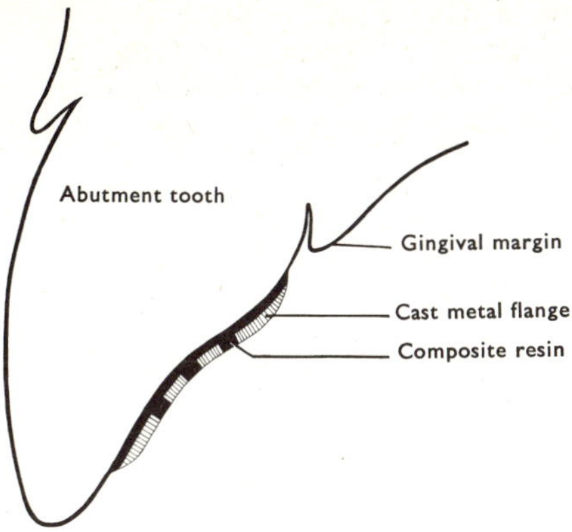

Fig. 13.5. *Rochette bridge: profile of flange to show retaining holes for composite resin. Note relationship of flange margins to incisal edge and gingival margin. (Diagram not to scale.)*

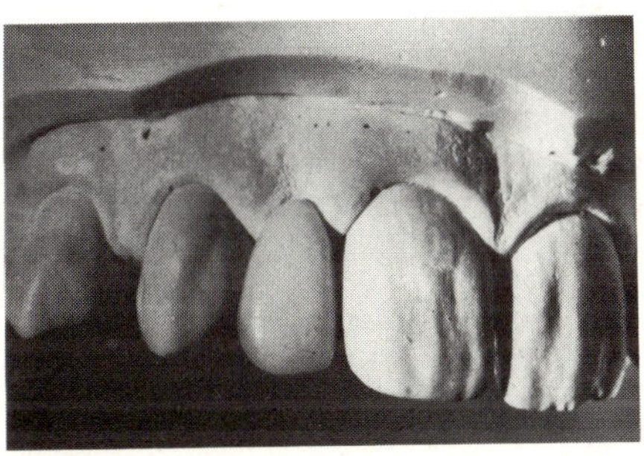

Fig. 13.6. *Rochette bridge. Master model showing labial aspect of baked-on porcelain pontic.*

each flange is approximately 0·5–1 mm and the margins are feathered. Several holes are drilled with a small rose head tungsten carbide bur such as Alston No. 2* which produces holes approximately 0·7–0·8 mm in diameter. The holes provide mechanical locking of the composite resin which is used to bond the framework to the teeth (*Fig*. 13.5). Porcelain is baked on to the framework, and the finished bridge is polished on the external surface only (*Figs.* 13.6, 13.7).

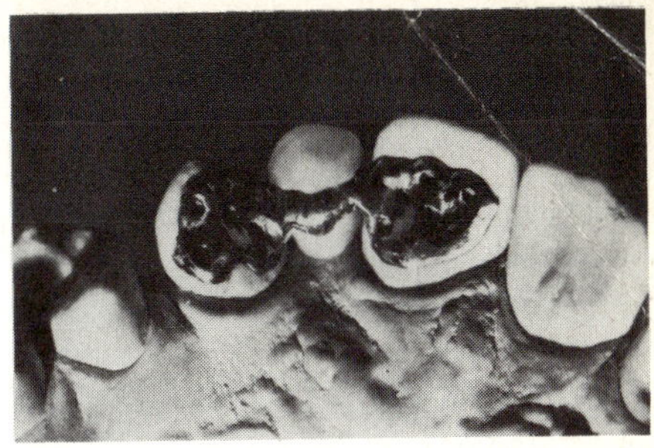

Fig. 13.7. *Rochette bridge. Master model showing polished (palatal) aspect of bridge with perforations in flanges. The flange margins are well clear of the incisal edge of* 1| *and gingival margins of* 3 1|.

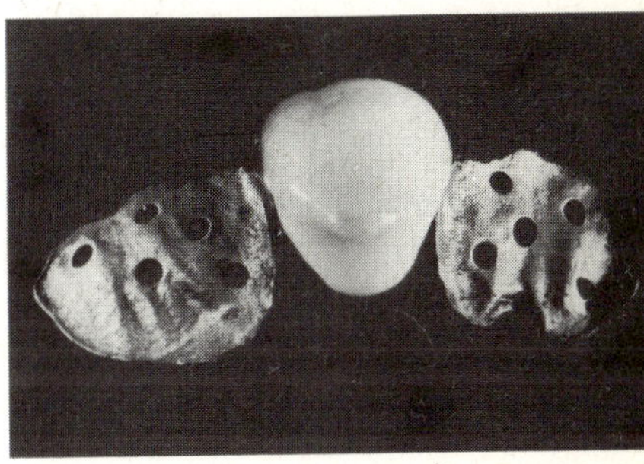

Fig. 13.8. *Fit surface of flanges which are sandblasted to assist mechanical retention.*

The fit surface should be sandblasted to increase roughness and aid mechanical retention of the bonding resin (*Fig*. 13.8).

At the second appointment the bridge is tried-in, and provided proper care has been taken at the earlier stages no adjustments should be necessary. The abutment teeth are isolated, etched, washed and dried, and a suitable direct bonding composite resin is mixed and applied to the fit surface of the flanges. The bridge is seated and held firmly in place, and any excess resin should be removed immediately with a probe. Three to five minutes later final finishing may be carried out with composite finishing instruments. The occlusion can then be checked and any adjustments made.

* D. M. Co., Preston New Road, Blackpool, Lancs.

■ B. Case Reports

Patient A. B. was a girl aged 18 who had undergone treatment of dental anomalies affecting the maxillary arch. The mal-erupted 3| had been extracted leaving a peg-shaped 2| in good position in the arch. There was congenital absence of |2, and |3 was surgically reimplanted in |2 space having been found previously in an unerupted horizontal position in the palate. Unfortunately, after reimplantation it did not proceed to erupt with the rest of the neighbouring teeth and was soon left in a 'submerged' and buccal position (*Fig.* 13.9). It was concluded that ankylosis had occurred, after unsuccessful orthodontic traction. The plan was now to extract |3 and fit immediately a Rochette bridge.

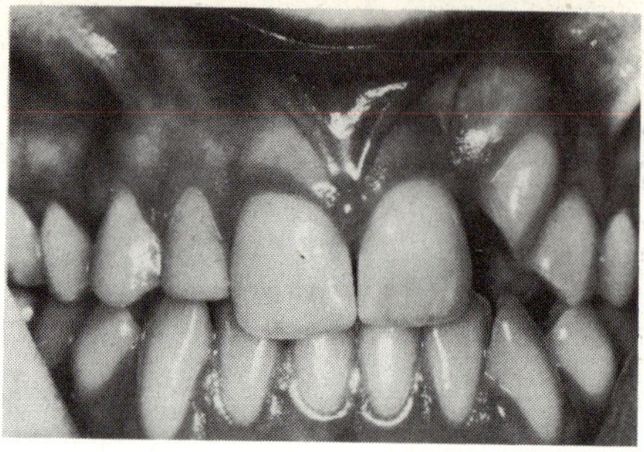

Fig. 13.9. *Patient A. B. Preoperative. |3 ankylosed in superior and buccal position. Peg-shaped 2| has been restored with etched-retained composite resin.*

In the laboratory, |3 was removed with a plaster knife and the ridge contoured to simulate the predicted post-extraction state. The bridge was fabricated, the flanges being placed on the lingual surfaces of |1 and |4. At the second visit, |3 was extracted and the bridge bonded in place (*Figs.* 13.10, 13.11).

Patient A. H. was a talented lad of 14 who had difficulty in playing the oboe because of air escaping through gaps in the upper lateral incisor region where 2|2 were congenitally absent (*Fig.* 13.12). His skeletal pattern was Class III with a reverse incisal overbite/overjet relationship. Also, the 3| had over-erupted reducing the interocclusal space in 2| region.

A pair of Rochette bridges were made to replace the missing lateral incisors, and were successful in enabling the patient to play his oboe without any problems. Only minor occlusal adjustments were necessary (*Figs.* 13.13, 13.14).

The Rochette bridge represents the intermediate stage between the exacting, precise and expensive nature of conventional bridgework and the economical, though less satisfactory etch-retained resin bridge. Because porcelain is baked on to the metal framework in the same manner as a conventional bonded porcelain bridge, proper pontic design with respect to aesthetics, physiological form and hygiene can be more easily achieved than with prefabricated acrylic pontics. In the latter, the embrasure form is often difficult to create without loss of strength of the bonding resin (*Fig.* 13.15) especially in the lower anterior quadrant (Jenkins, 1974).

To ensure success, it is necessary to select patients carefully. Obviously, it is unsuitable for patients with a heavy occlusion, and also should not be used in the posterior quadrants. Nor should more than two pontic spans be replaced, for it is doubtful whether adequate retention can be achieved. In the absence of any tooth reduction there should be sufficient interocclusal clearance to allow for the thickness of the cast metal flanges. Care must be taken to ensure that anterior guidance, if it is present, should be preserved. In this respect, it is much less of a problem to replace mandibular anterior teeth with Rochette bridges.

It may be possible to electroplate the fit surface of the flanges with a coating of tin (McLean, 1977), and then bond the bridge with a glass ionomer luting cement such as Chem Bond* which has an affinity for both the tin coating and etched enamel. This procedure, as yet untried, may go some way towards removing the need for drilling holes in the hard, miniscule flanges.

---

* De Trey, A. D. International Ltd., PO Box 2AD, 26/40 Broadwick Street, London W1.

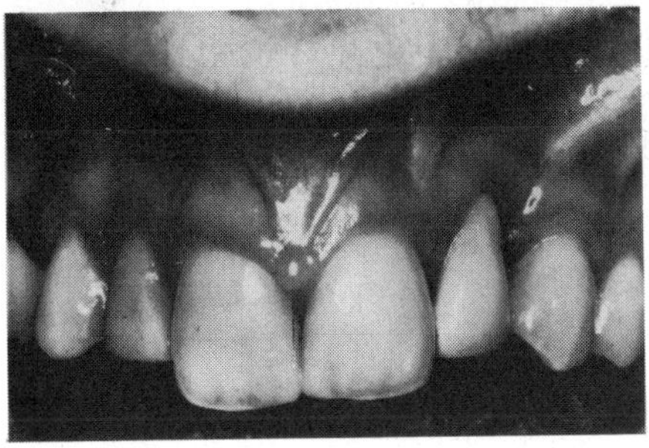

Fig. 13.10. *Patient A. B. Postoperative. |3 extracted and replaced by Rochette Bridge. Pontic is shaped as a |2 to balance aesthetically with 2|.*

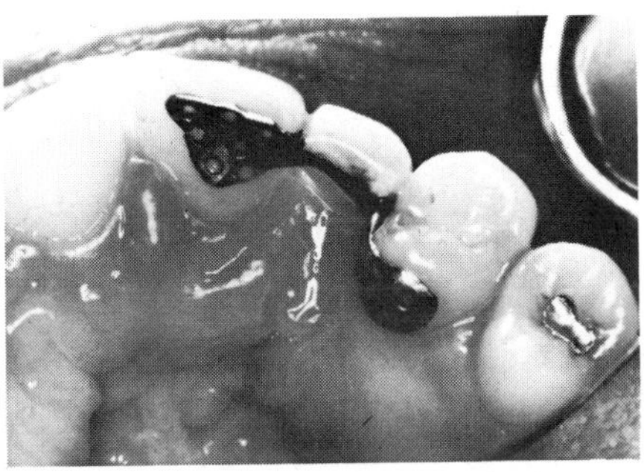

Fig. 13.11. *Patient A. B. Palatal aspect of Rochette bridge.*

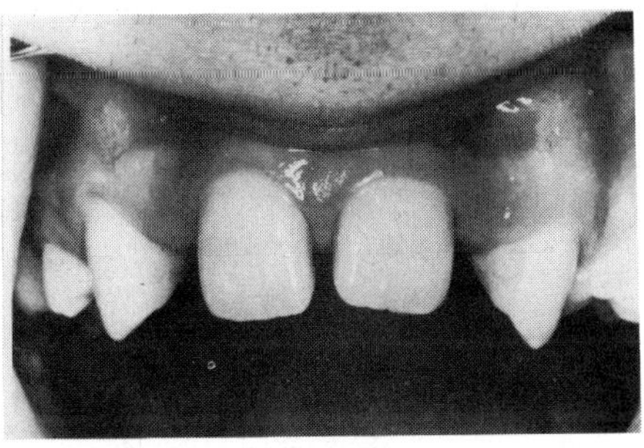

Fig. 13.12. *Patient A. H. Preoperative. Labial aspect.*

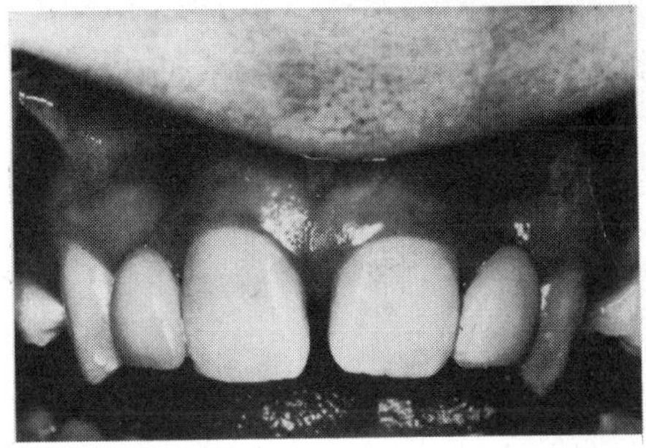

Fig. 13.13. *Patient A. H. Postoperative. Rochette bridges replacing 2|2 in position.*

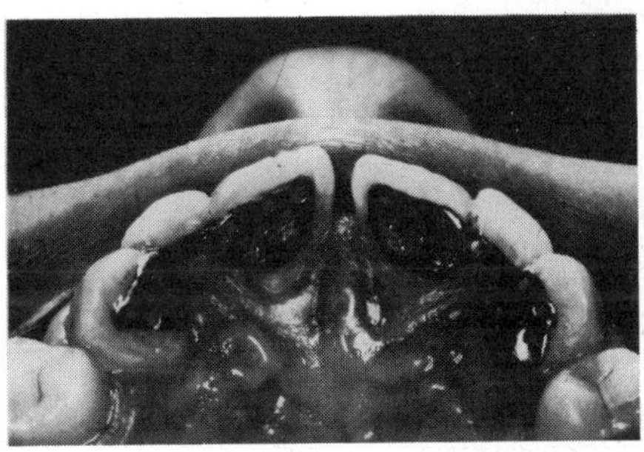

Fig. 13.14. *Patient A. H. Palatal aspect of Rochette bridges.*

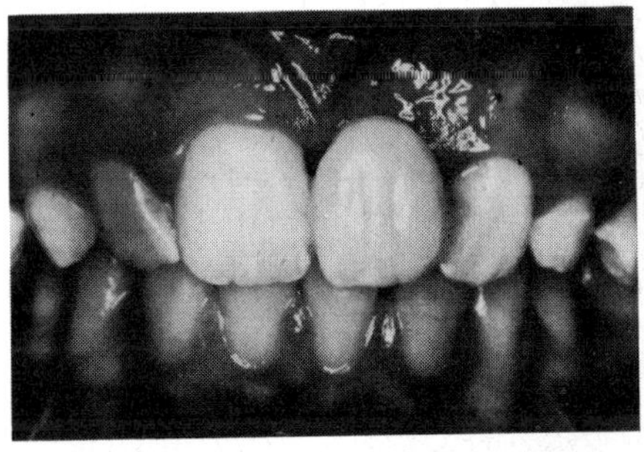

Fig. 13.15. *Etch-retained resin pontic showing difficulty in creating proper embrasures without weakening the bonding composite resin.*

BONDING FAILURES

Jenkins (1978), in his clinical survey of etch-retained acrylic bridges showed that the main mode of failure was in the cohesive strength of the composite resin. The technique is therefore limited only by the strength of the resin, and it is important to select the right cases for treatment. For instance, a high failure rate could be expected in patients with bruxism. It is also obvious that until stronger resins are discovered etch-retained posterior bridges are inadvisable.

If a bridge should become detached at one or both abutments it is quite feasible to rebond the bridge. The abutment tooth surfaces and pontic are polished with abrasive discs, e.g. Soflex,* until they appear smooth and shiny. In the case of Rochette bridges, the old composite resin should be removed from the flanges, and the fit surfaces cleaned by sandblasting. The tooth surfaces are then re-etched and the resin applied as before.

* 3M Co., 3M House, PO Box 1, Bracknell, Berks.

Bibliography

Buonocore M. G. (1955) *The Use of Adhesives in Dentistry*. Springfield, Ill., Thomas. p. 334.

Howe D. F. and Denehy G. E. (1977) Anterior fixed partial dentures utilising the acid-etch technique and a cast metal framework. *J. Prosthet. Dent.* **37**, 28.

Ibsen R. L. and Neville K. (1974) *Adhesive Restorative Dentistry*. Philadelphia, Saunders. p. 139.

Jenkins C. B. G. (1974) An adhesive bridge technique. *Dent. Update* **1**, 503.

Jenkins C. B. G. (1978) Etch-retained anterior pontics. *Br. Dent. J.* **144**, 206.

McLean J. W. (1977) A new method of bonding dental cements and porcelain to metal surfaces. *Oper. Dent.* **2**, 130.

Rochette A. L. (1973) Attachment of a splint to enamel of lower anterior teeth. *J. Prosthet. Dent.* **30**, 418.

Scheer B. and Silverstone L. M. (1975) Replacement of missing anterior teeth by etch retained bridges. *J. Int. Assoc. Dent. Child.* **6**, 17.

Simonsen R. J. (1978) *Clinical Application of the Acid Etch Technique*. Chicago, Quintessence Publishing Co., Inc. p. 71.

Tay W. M. and Shaw M. J. (1979) The Rochette adhesive bridge. *Dent. Update* **6**, 153.

14

PERIODONTAL PREPARATION OF THE MOUTH

Clinical Features of Chronic Inflammatory Periodontal Disease
Achieving Optimum Periodontal Health
Pocket Elimination Procedures Prior to Fixed Prostheses
Treatment of Edentulous Ridge Areas
Multirooted Teeth . The Attached Gingiva
The Place of Periodontics in the Sequence of Therapy

PROFESSOR IAN DAVIS

It must be taken as axiomatic that optimal health of the supporting tissues is achieved before any fixed prosthesis is inserted into the oral cavity, since clinical procedures involved in its construction must affect the status of the periodontium. It is equally important that a comprehensive examination of the supporting structures be carried out before the final restorative treatment plan is drawn up.

CLINICAL FEATURES OF CHRONIC INFLAMMATORY PERIODONTAL DISEASE

Chronic inflammatory periodontal disease is plaque induced. Initially it presents as a marginal gingival inflammation, the tissues exhibiting characteristic changes of colour, contour and consistency. Pink, firm, stippled tissues become red, soft, oedematous and glazed in appearance, and in turn become rolled and fibrotic as the inflammatory response becomes more chronic in nature (*Fig*. 14.1). As the disease affects the deeper tissues of the periodontium overt marginal signs may not be as apparent. Nevertheless, the effect of the expansion of a gingivitis into a periodontitis is the progressive loss of supporting tissues. The rate of loss differs from individual to individual and is the resultant of the pathogenicity of plaque and the nature of the host response.

Clinically, progressive loss of periodontal attachment may manifest itself as recession and loss of the attached gingiva. More commonly, however, the clinical result will be the formation of periodontal pockets (*Fig*. 14.2). Since these are normally painless, and the initial marginal gingivitis may well be no longer apparent, the only clinical means of detecting such pockets is through careful probing of the gingival sulcus area around all standing teeth. The use of the periodontal probe must therefore form an

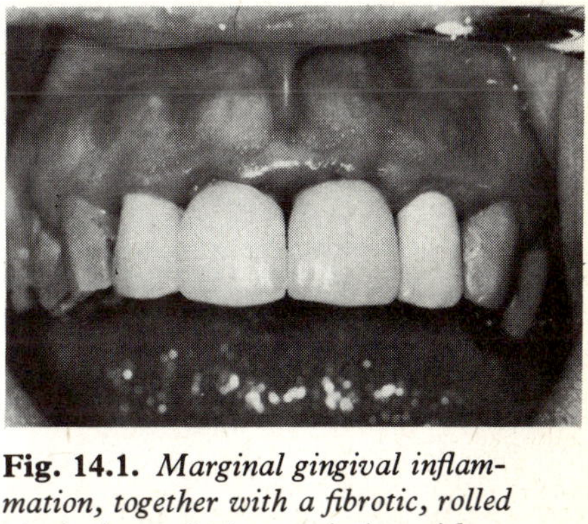

Fig. 14.1. *Marginal gingival inflammation, together with a fibrotic, rolled gingival margin in association with porcelain jacket crowns* 21|12.

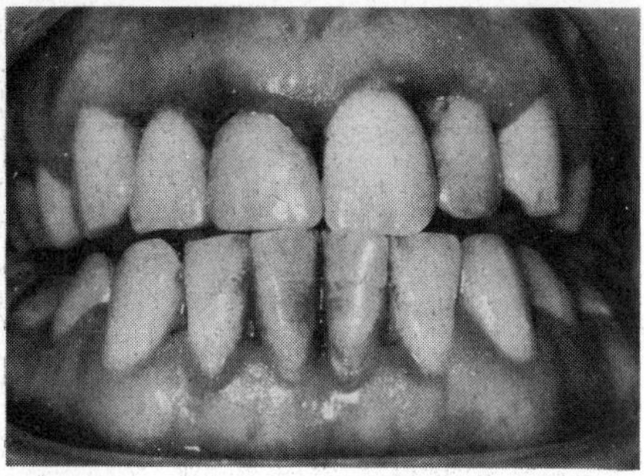

Fig. 14.2. *Chronic marginal periodontitis with increased probing depths, loss of interdental tissue and gingival recession, exposing the margins of a crown* |1*, which was once subgingivally placed.*

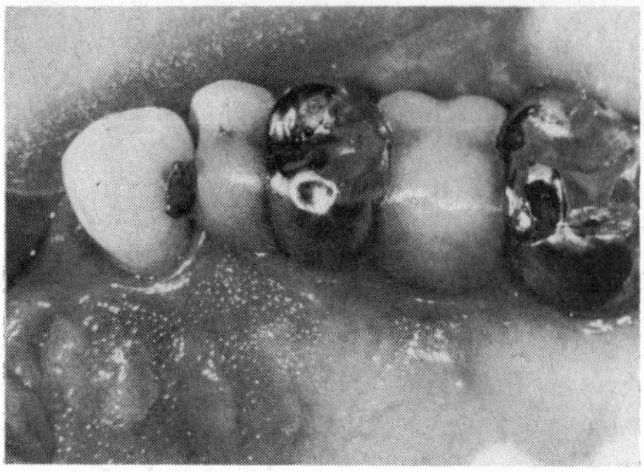

Fig. 14.3. *Total obliteration of embrasure spaces in a fixed prosthesis, together with ridge-lapped pontics* |4 *and* |6*, all rendering effective plaque control impossible.*

integral part of the clinical examination of a mouth about to be restored.

The actual numerical value of the probing depth is of significance in itself and should be carefully noted as it will give an indication of the rate of loss of attachment as time progresses. The clinical reaction of the gingival sulcus area during probing affords even greater evidence of the state of the deeper tissues of the periodontium. The presence of blood or exudate from the pockets during probing is a clear indication of progressive chronic marginal periodontitis. Inserting restorations into teeth with untreated periodontal disease of this nature is to court disaster.

Since the rate of periodontal destruction is related to the nature of plaque and to the nature of the tissue responses, factors affecting the pathogenic potential of plaque must be of primary importance in treating and preventing loss of attachment. Anything present in the oral cavity which contributes to the pathogenicity of plaque by rendering it inaccessible to normal cleansing procedures or allows it to age and mature adjacent to the marginal tissues is effectively a plaque-retentive factor. Often these factors are related to fixed or removable prostheses. Any prosthesis which diminishes the patient's ability to remove plaque or enhances plaque build-up near the gingivae, compromises the chances of successful maintenance of periodontal health. Poor pontic design and inadequate embrasure space in fixed prostheses are all plaque-retentive factors and can contribute to chronic inflammatory disease (*Fig.* 14.3).

Marginal gingival inflammation should respond to the removal of plaque, and plaque-retentive factors. Periodontal pockets, however, may continue to show signs of progressive breakdown after the marginal lesions have been controlled. It is imperative that progressive periodontal disease be adequately treated before fixed bridge prostheses are constructed. The only exception to this general rule is following orthodontic tooth movement in the adult, when temporary fixed prostheses may be used to retain and stabilize teeth in their new positions prior to definitive periodontal treatment.

ACHIEVING OPTIMAL PERIODONTAL HEALTH

Inasmuch as successful periodontal therapy is predicated entirely upon the patient's plaque control, so also must successful restorative dentistry be dependent upon the patient's ability to prevent the formation of plaque and to remove plaque once it has formed. This concern with 'cleansability' in the oral cavity should be reflected in the practice of all clinical dentistry.

The first stage of disease control consists of subgingival scaling and root planing while concurrently the patient is instructed in the control of dental plaque. The miniscrub toothbrushing technique using a flat-trim, relatively short-headed toothbrush with nylon bristles of a soft to medium texture has been widely advocated in periodontics. It has the advantage of efficiently removing plaque from the critical area of the gingival sulcus. Interproximal cleaning is of especial importance with fixed prostheses. The cleaning instrument advised for any individual patient should be selected on the basis of the anatomy of the embrasure spaces. Tight interproximal contacts will necessitate the use of dental floss or tape, often, in the case of fixed prostheses, in conjunction with some form of floss threader (*Fig*. 14.4). Larger spaces may accommodate wood sticks, while yet larger spaces, pontic areas or radicular surfaces exposed in multirooted teeth can best be rendered free of plaque by some kind of interproximal brush (*Fig*. 14.5).

Clearly, then, fixed prostheses must be designed with plaque cleansability in mind. This can be checked even before an appliance is inserted into the oral cavity (*Fig*. 14.6), while the position of solder joints and the area of contact between a pontic and the underlying edentulous ridge are all pertinent to this problem. Contour of restorations should also be considered, remembering that over-contouring protects plaque accumulating at the gingival margin, acting as another plaque-retentive factor. Under-contouring, on the other hand, rarely has any periodontal implications as is well exemplified by the 'natural' under-contouring of the peg-shaped lateral incisor.

The well-motivated patient may be recognized by the resolution of marginal gingival inflammation following the removal of plaque, calculus, plaque-retentive factors and necrotic cementum.

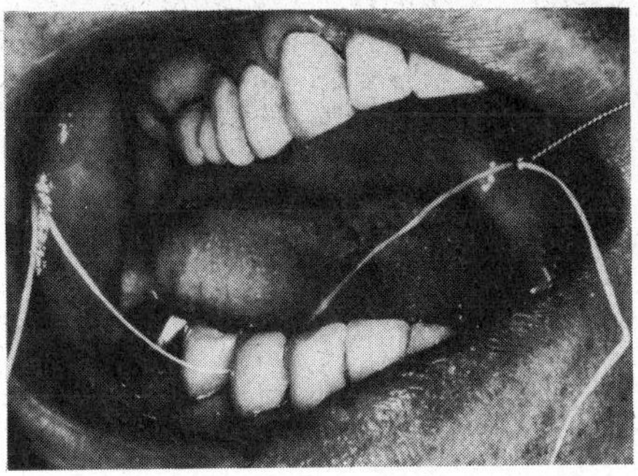

Fig. 14.4. *Use of dental floss and floss threader to remove plaque interproximally and beneath pontics in a patient with fixed bridgework.*

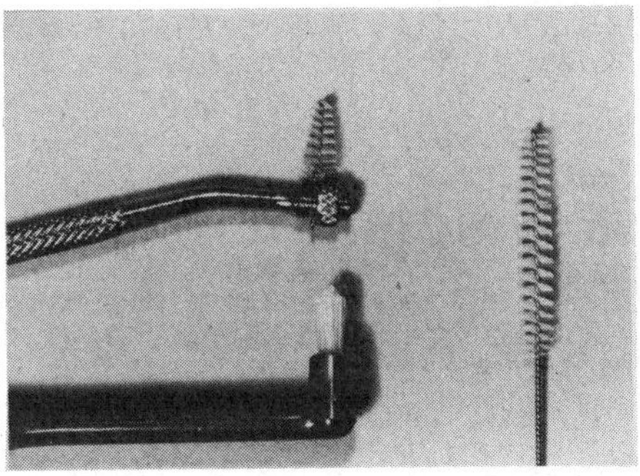

Fig. 14.5. *Types of interproximal brushes particularly useful for plaque control in patients with bridges.*

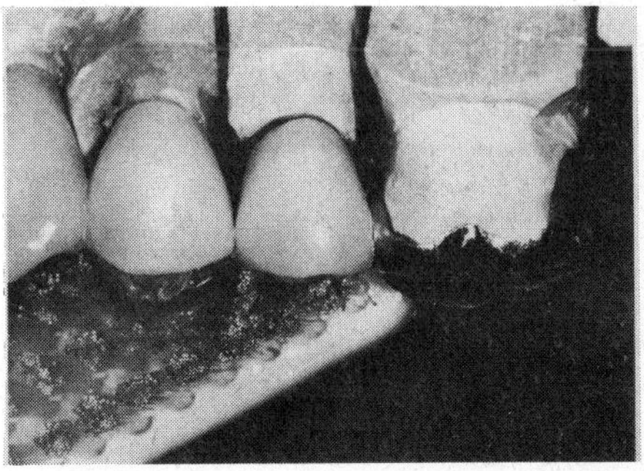

Fig. 14.6. *Good pontic and embrasure space design, allowing the passage of toothbrush bristles for plaque control.*

Persistent chronic inflammation within periodontal pockets, characterized by bleeding or exudate on probing, should be assessed prior to the final preparations for fixed bridgework, and areas of progressive disease must be treated by elimination of these pockets.

POCKET ELIMINATION PROCEDURES PRIOR TO FIXED PROSTHESES

Since optimal health of the periodontium is a prerequisite for successful fixed prostheses, it can be argued that total elimination of all pockets should precede the restorative phase of treatment. Teeth on which pocket elimination proves to be impossible should be regarded as of questionable prognosis as abutments, and appropriate design modifications made when planning the prosthesis.

A range of sophisticated surgical techniques has been developed as a means of eliminating periodontal pockets. Any one of these techniques may have a place in the choice of surgical therapy for any single patient. Essentially, however, all the techniques must concern themselves with gaining access to the root surfaces of the involved teeth in order to render them biologically acceptable to their investing soft tissues. At the same time the chronically inflamed lining of the pocket is removed, and, for teeth about to be utilized in fixed prostheses, a cleansable tissue anatomy must be created which results in minimal gingival sulcus depth postoperatively.

The use of the inverse bevel incision as an initial approach to surgical elimination of pockets has much to commend itself for the patient requiring restorative procedures. This incision, made at an angle of approximately 30° to the crown of the tooth at a point about 1 mm apical to the gingival margin successfully splits the chronically inflamed pocket lining from the remainder of the pocket wall and a mucoperiosteal flap may then be raised to expose the deeper portions of the periodontium.

Other advantages of the inverse bevel approach include:

i. Conservation of the maximum amount of the zone of keratinized attached gingiva.

ii. Good access to root surfaces thereby enabling them to be rendered free of all deposits and necrotic cementum.

iii. Routine access to the alveolar bone renders osseous problems visible for complete assessment and treatment.

iv. An ability to deal with bifurcation and trifurcation involvements in multi-rooted teeth.

After the initial incision, the flap is raised and the pocket lining removed by thorough curettage. The exposed root surface must then be planed free of necrotic cementum. As is usually the case there may be bony involvement and this is then accessible for analysis and osseous therapy. Optimal physiological osseous architecture is the goal in surgery prior to bridgework, and this hard-tissue architecture is achieved by ostectomy and osteoplasty procedures. Although a far from ideal tissue architecture might be well tolerated by the patient requiring solely periodontal treatment for dental health, in those requiring, in addition, complex restorative dentistry, every effort should be made to create an 'ideal' dentogingival relationship (*Fig*. 14.7).

Achieving such an 'ideal' architecture of the marginal tissues is dependent upon a knowledge of the functional anatomy of the gingival sulcus area. There are two types of epithelium lining the inner aspect of the gingival sulcus (*Fig*. 14.8)—the junctional epithelium, which is physically bonded to the enamel via hemi-desmosomes, and the oral-sulcular epithelium which is a transitional epithelium lining the gingival sulcus proper. Even when completely healthy, the junctional epithelium is a permeable 'barrier' at the dentogingival junction, allowing substances to pass from the gingival sulcus into the underlying connective tissue, and also the egress of gingival fluid into the gingival sulcus. Damage to the junctional epithelium will compromise the soft-tissue to hard-tissue seal yet further, and thereby initiate or

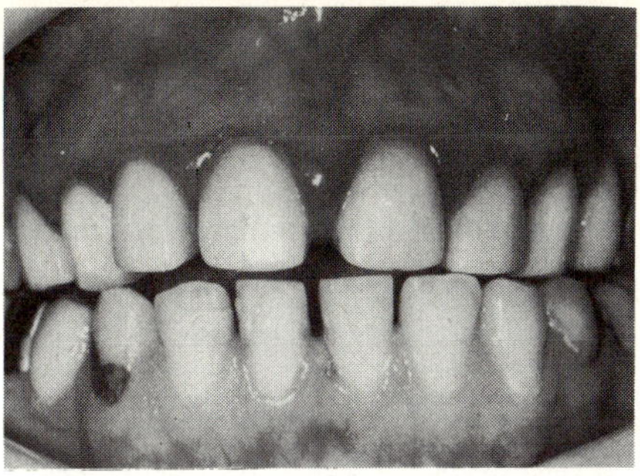

a

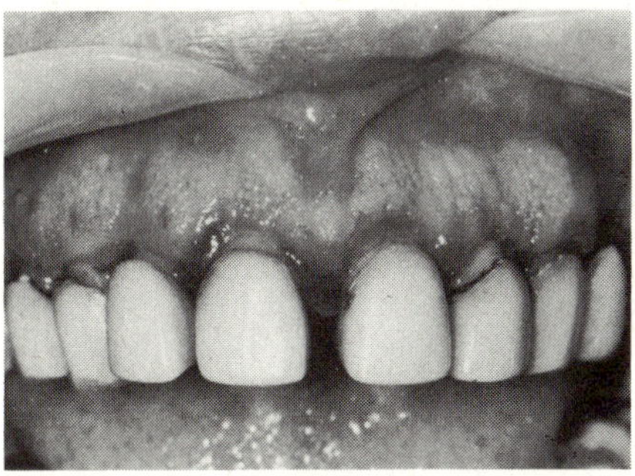

b

Fig. 14.7. *a, Extensive marginal gingival inflammation associated with poor subgingival crown margins in the maxilla. b, Periodontal pockets eliminated, the crown margins exposed and a satisfactory dentogingival junction forming ten days after apically repositioned flap surgery in the maxilla.*

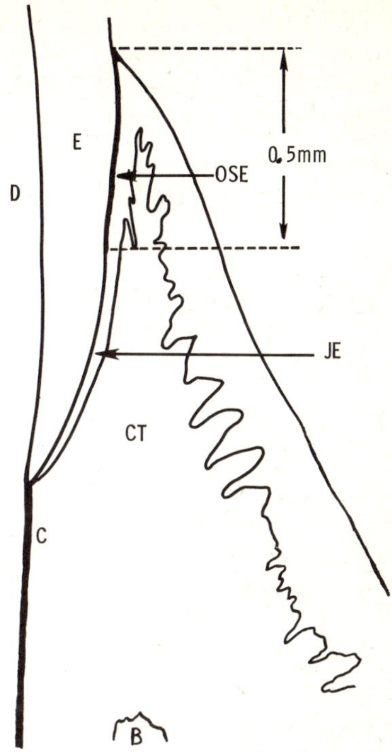

Fig. 14.8. *Diagrammatic representation of the normal gingival sulcus.* **E**, *Enamel;* **D**, *Dentine;* **C**, *Cementum;* **B**, *Bone;* **OSE**, *Oral sulcular epithelium;* **JE**, *Junctional epithelium;* **CT**, *Connective tissue of the gingival apparatus. The distance between the cement-enamel junction and the crest of the alveolar bone is 1–2 mm.*

compound inflammatory changes in the underlying connective tissue.

The dimensions of the gingival apparatus of the tooth are pertinent to the practice of restorative dentistry (*Fig.* 14.8). The depth of the true gingival sulcus, that portion bonded by oral-sulcular epithelium, is no more than 0·5 mm in health. It may thus be appreciated that, should subgingival margins be deemed necessary for aesthetic reasons, these margins should be no more than 0·5 mm below the gingival crest. To place them deeper would place them into junctional epithelium with all the consequent periodontal implications. Clearly, then, margins of restorations should be coronal to the gingival sulcus wherever possible. When there is no alternative to a subgingival margin, the sulcus area should be treated with respect. Burs and diamonds employed in this area must be used with the greatest care; gingival retraction must be performed very gently, and débridement of the gingival sulcus thereafter must be thorough.

In carrying out osteoplasty or ostectomy procedures, too, the normal anatomy of the healthy gingival apparatus is the yardstick. There is normally a physiological distance between the base of the junctional epithelium and the crest of the alveolar bone, of between 1 and 2 mm. This allows of the attachment of the supracrestal group of periodontal fibres into cementum. Even when subgingival margins are required by the restorative dentist, it is very important that no procedure involved in the preparation of the teeth should encroach upon this physiological width of connective tissue attachment. Equally, when periodontal surgery precedes the restorative treatment, flaps are carefully positioned on the correct height of alveolar crest to enable the normal dimensions of the dentogingival junction to re-establish themselves.

The routine access to the alveolar crest gained through the use of the inverse bevel approach to periodontal flap surgery has other possible advantages prior to fixed bridgework:

i. Extra supra-alveolar root length may be created for more retentive abutment preparations.

ii. Caries which has extended subgingivally is exposed and a gingival margin recreated on sound root structure.

iii. The fracture line in the roots of teeth which have been traumatized may be exposed.

TREATMENT OF EDENTULOUS RIDGE AREAS

The presence of pockets adjacent to edentulous ridge areas is relevant to the restorative dentist. Abutment teeth to be used in fixed prostheses must be periodontally sound, and pockets involving the pontic areas will have to be treated successfully before the bridge preparations are completed.

Once again, the inverse bevel approach may be easily adapted to cope with pockets mesial and distal to an edentulous area. In addition to giving access to the pockets, it will give access to the soft and hard tissues of the edentulous ridge and thereby allow these tissues to be recontoured to change the dimensions of the pontic space in an appropriate fashion for an individual patient.

The inverse bevel incisions are extended from the mesial and distal aspects of the abutment teeth along the crest of the edentulous area. The soft-tissue component of the ridge is then raised as part of the process of elevation of the buccal and lingual mucoperiosteal flaps. Any osseous problems related to the abutment teeth may be treated. The soft-tissue component of the pocket wall next to the ridge may be eliminated by excising a wedge of connective tissue from the undersurface of the flap when the flap is retracted away from the osseous crest. This creates a thin, knife-edged flap margin over the ridge consistent with the dimensions of the flap margins produced by the inverse bevel incisions elsewhere. On collapsing the flaps on to the underlying bony ridge, any excess of flap tissue may be taken up by moving one of the flaps apically. Alternatively, any redundant tissue may be excised to leave a butt joint of the flap tissues which can be sutured. This gives rise to rapid healing in the area, as no bone is left exposed, and there is an additional benefit for the restorative dentist in that increased tooth length is available for the preparation of the abutment teeth.

MULTIROOTED TEETH

Pockets which extend into the bifurcation and trifurcation areas pose difficult diagnostic, prognostic and surgical problems. Although techniques have been developed to help deal with these problems, one should be circumspect about utilizing severely involved multirooted teeth as critical abutments in a fixed prosthesis. Only when it is ensured that all progressive chronic periodontal disease has been eliminated may these teeth support bridges. In all other circumstances it would be sound practice to consider extracting these teeth before restorative treatment commences, or at the very least, contingency plans should be made during the design of the prosthesis to allow of the potential loss of a tooth with questionable prognosis.

Treatment of these involved furcation areas revolves entirely about rendering such areas cleansable of plaque. Early, or incipient, involvements may require only slight osteoplasty together with a suitable degree of apical repositioning of the flaps to achieve this. Severe involvement often necessitates the removal of one root as a root-resection or hemisection procedure, obviously after completion of the appropriate endodontic treatment.

The patient's plaque control has to be extremely good to ensure successful maintenance of these furcation areas and oral hygiene techniques may require the use of special instruments such as the interdental brushes (*see Fig.* 14.5). Even these have to be manœuvred with considerable manual dexterity. However, considerable evidence has accumulated in recent years that even isolated roots of multirooted teeth can serve as satisfactory abutments provided there is effective plaque control, sound remaining periodontal tissues and that the prostheses themselves do not act as plaque-retentive factors.

THE ATTACHED GINGIVA

The width of the zone of attached gingiva has for long been a matter of concern to the restorative dentist. It was recognized that narrow zones of keratinized, attached gingiva posed as hazards when clinical procedures used in the construction of a bridge compromised the physiology of the gingival sulcus area. Inflammation ensued and narrow bands of attached gingiva, especially when related to thin investing tissues, often suffered from progressive gingival recession.

An obvious solution to this problem is to keep the margins of abutment preparations well away from the gingival sulcus. This is particularly so when the tissues are thin and 'fragile' in clinical appearance or where there are already signs of gingival recession. There is then no risk of trauma during tooth preparation and impression-taking. The absence of subgingival margins will prevent any consequent reaction within the marginal gingival tissues, provided there is adequate plaque control by the patient.

On periodontal grounds alone there are very few reasons for extending the zone of attached gingiva. It is recognized that there is a great variation in the widths of the zone of attached gingiva and that it is perfectly possible for even minimal widths of keratinized tissue to function satisfactorily as attached gingiva as long as the marginal tissues are kept healthy through plaque control.

When such circumstances do not appertain, or when subgingival margins are considered essential adjacent to a narrow zone of attached gingiva, it is possible to increase the width of the zone surgically. Several techniques have been devised, including the denudation procedure, the periosteal fenestration technique together with flap procedures such as the laterally repositioned, the pedicle and the double-papilla flaps.

As techniques for predictably extending the zone of attached gingiva, prior to fixed prostheses, however, most of these procedures have been superseded by the free gingival graft. In this grafting technique a piece of keratinized tissue is removed from a donor site in the oral cavity, normally the palate. It is then placed on a recipient periosteal bed which has been prepared adjacent to the abutment tooth by a sharp, split-thickness dissection at the level of the mucogingival junction. After suitable dressing the healing is usually uneventful and within two weeks it should be clinically apparent that there is an increased width of attached gingiva at the abutment tooth. This should enhance the protective functions of the attached gingiva at the dentogingival junction after the insertion of the final restorations.

THE PLACE OF PERIODONTICS IN THE SEQUENCE OF THERAPY

A logical sequence of treatment can be constructed only after the nature of the patient's problem has been fully elucidated. This depends entirely upon a thorough history and a complete examination of the oral cavity and the whole masticatory system. The nature of the dental disease present should be noted and the causative factors for these clinical changes must be sought.

Examination of the periodontium will obviously be a component part of any comprehensive oral examination. It will involve:

i. The presence or absence of marginal inflammation.

ii. The degree of tissue recession or hyperplasia.

iii. The depth and distribution of periodontal pocketing.

iv. The involvement of bifurcation and trifurcation areas.

v. The mobility patterns of the teeth.

vi. The distribution of plaque and plaque-retentive factors.

The clinical findings should be related to any radiographic changes of chronic marginal periodontitis. Accurate full-mouth radiographs will reveal the extent and nature of bone loss, the thickness of the periodontal ligament space, the degree of furcation involvement and presence of any radio-opaque plaque-retentive factors such as overhanging margins of restorations or subgingival calculus. Data from the periodontal examination will be combined with that obtained from the remainder of the whole mouth examination of the patient requiring fixed prostheses. The status of the teeth themselves, together with their position and the quality of the pre-existing restorations can then be linked with the periodontal findings. An occlusal analysis, as described in Chapter 17, will help clarify the causes of any increased tooth mobility patterns and will be fundamental to an understanding of the masticatory system for an individual patient. The information so acquired will enable the clinician to arrive at a prognosis for individual teeth and for the dentition as a whole, and then to establish a logical sequence of treatment.

The usual temporal sequence of therapy for a patient who is to receive bridgework is as follows:

■ 1. Treatment of Acute Lesions

These lesions may be within the tooth, such as active caries or an acute pulpitis, or an acute lateral periodontal abscess in the supporting tissues. Acute symptoms must be alleviated and a stable clinical state produced which will allow the remainder of the treatment to proceed in a logical fashion.

■ 2. Removal of the Causative Factors of Disease

For both caries and periodontal disease, the cause is plaque. The first step in the treatment plan is therefore to reduce the level of plaque to that which does not cause disease. This requires sufficient time to produce a motivated patient in whom all the plaque-retentive factors, such as calculus and inadequate restorations, have received attention.

Such a process can be time-consuming, but it must be recognized that disease control is impossible without elimination of the causative factors of disease. Proceeding with complex periodontal or restorative treatment without adequate plaque control should only be contemplated in the knowledge that repair therapy will not in itself prevent that patient from suffering from further tissue breakdown, be it tooth or periodontium, in the future.

■ 3. Extraction of Teeth with a Hopeless Prognosis

It is as well to remove badly involved teeth, in the restorative case, as early as possible in treatment. This will allow sockets to heal, it may minimize adjacent periodontal defects and it will also enable the restorative dentist to decide on the distribution of key abutment teeth early on in treatment planning.

■ 4. Dealing with Problems of Increasing Hypermobility and of Drifting Teeth

Mobility patterns may prove a problem for patients who have lost a considerable amount of periodontal support through progressive disease and who also have a deranged occlusion. If this be the case, the occlusal factors incriminated should receive attention during the plaque control phase. If the patient is suitably motivated and the restorative commitment to fixed prostheses becomes certain, any minor orthodontic tooth movement considered necessary for restorative, aesthetic or functional reasons should take place concurrently.

In patients who have a clinical problem of progressive mobility after minor tooth movement has been carried out, it will normally be found necessary to stabilize the segments involved, while the remainder of the treatment plan is executed. Since the patient under consideration does indeed require fixed prostheses, the most logical way of stabilizing such teeth is by means of temporary bridges, carefully constructed so as not in any way to complicate the patient's efforts at plaque control.

■ 5. Monitoring of Patient and Tissue Responses

Effective plaque control means the resolution of marginal gingival inflammation. This is the clinical index to be used for the patient's level of achievement in oral hygiene procedures. Persistent inflammation from within periodontal pockets will require periodontal surgery before the continuation of restorative treatment.

■ 6. Periodontal Surgery

For the patient about to have bridges, surgery aims at total elimination of the pocket, together with the establishment of optimal dentogingival contour postoperatively. Thus, apical repositioning of the flaps raised via an inverse bevel incision is the usual practice, the tissues being placed upon the most favourable contour of the underlying bone. As has been described above, root caries or root fractures can be exposed by this means, or abutment teeth be given longer clinical crowns for retention.

Because it is an unpredictable way of totally eliminating periodontal pockets, techniques involving the reattachment of the pocket wall to the root surface of the tooth are rarely used preparatory to fixed prostheses. The only circumstances in which they might be employed is for aesthetic reasons in the anterior segments. Since the dentogingival junction so created is weaker than that supported by alveolar bone, the precautions already advised concerning the dangers of subgingival margins in such areas become all the more obvious.

It is at this stage, if there are any restorative reasons to do so, that the zone of attached gingiva would be increased at particular regions considered likely to be vulnerable to breakdown following the restorative instrumentation.

■ 7. Re-evaluation of the Status of the Supporting Tissues

A comprehensive periodontal examination is again carried out to ensure that pockets have been eliminated and the best possible tissue contour obtained. Should any additional orthodontics or occlusal therapy be required, this treatment may be provided during the period of evaluation. Further information may be gleaned about the patient's ability to control plaque with the new tissue contour. More advice will undoubtedly be necessary on the appropriate instruments to use for plaque control on the root surfaces exposed through periodontal surgery.

Teeth which continue to give rise to doubts concerning their long-term prognosis after such therapy should be considered for extraction. If they are not key abutment teeth, they may be left in situ to function for as long as possible, but it would be a great risk to include them in a fixed prosthesis.

Treatment planning in this sequence should deal with all the most commonly encountered periodontal problems in a logical manner in therapy. The point will then have been reached when the patient who requires the bridgework is well-motivated in plaque control, free of progressive periodontal disease and has an optimal tissue contour. These, it has already been stated, are the pre-requisites for successful restorative dentistry and the final preparations for the fixed prostheses may now be commenced.

Bibliography

App G. R. (1961) Effect of silicate, amalgam and cast gold on the gingiva. *J. Prosthet. Dent.* **11**, 522.

Cohen D. W. and Chacker F. M. (1964) Criteria for selection of one treatment plan over another. *Dent. Clin. North Am.* March 1964, 3.

Hazen S. and Osborne J. W. (1967) Relationship of operative dentistry to periodontal health. *Dent. Clin. North Am.* March 1967, 245.

Kieser J. B. (1974) An approach to periodontal pocket elimination. *Br. J. Oral Surg.* **12**, 177.

Larato D. C. (1969) The effect of full crown margin extension on gingival inflammation. *J. S. Cal. Dent. Assoc.* **37**, 476.

Leon A. R. (1977) The effect of approximal carious lesions on the periodontium. *Br. Dent. J.* **143**, 18.

Lindhe J. and Nyman S. (1977) The role of occlusion in periodontal disease and the biological rationale for splinting in treatment of periodontitis. *Oral Sci. Rev.* **10**, 11.

Nyman S. and Lindhe J. (1976) Considerations in the treatment of patients with furcation involvements. *J. Clin. Periodontol.* **3**, 4; Persistent tooth hypermobility following completion of periodontal treatment. *J. Clin. Periodontal.* **3**, 81.

Polson A. M. (1977) Periodontal considerations for functional utilisation of a retained root after furcation management. *J. Clin. Periodontol.* **4**, 223.

Ramfjord S. P. (1974) Periodontal aspects of restorative dentistry. *J. Oral Rehabil.* **2**, 107.

Silness J. (1970) Periodontal considerations in patients treated with dental bridges. *J. Periodontol. Res.* **5**, 225.

15

GENERAL AND CASE ASSESSMENT; TOOTH RESTORATION AND PREPARATION

Periodontal Considerations . Correction of Occlusion . Routine Conservation
Selection and Treatment of Abutment Teeth
Detailed Design Considerations
Preparation of Abutment Teeth

The initial assessment of a patient is probably the most important aspect not only of fixed bridge prostheses but of dentistry in general.

To try and emphasize this, a case is illustrated of a lady who, some twenty years ago, when she was in her early twenties, was advised successively by three independent practitioners to have all her teeth extracted because of bone loss which averaged 70–75 per cent (*Fig.* 15.1). She then attended the practice of a colleague, who carried out periodontal treatment for her and, above all, explained very carefully why she had periodontal disease and how she could prevent its recurrence and progression.

It will be seen that this initial treatment was so successful that some seventeen years later (*Fig.* 15.2) there had been only a minimal increase in bone loss. However, the upper laterals in particular were now very unsightly and the patient was extremely conscious of this (*Fig.* 15.3). It was thus decided to extract the laterals and place a fixed prosthesis involving 3 1|1 3. Although some operators would be reluctant to carry out relatively complex procedures on teeth with such a large degree of bone loss, it must be remembered that remarkably little bone had been lost in the previous seventeen years and, provided that the patient continued her high standard of oral care, there is no reason why any appreciable deterioration should take place in the next seventeen years.

The teeth were roughly prepared, an

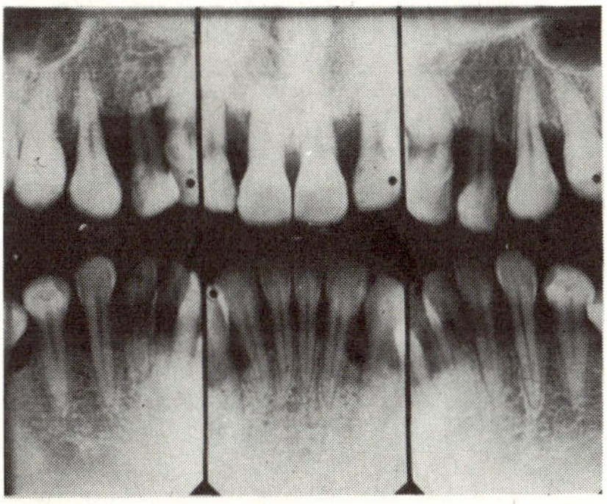

Fig. 15.1. *Patient at initial presentation when in her early twenties, with bone loss averaging 70–75 per cent.*

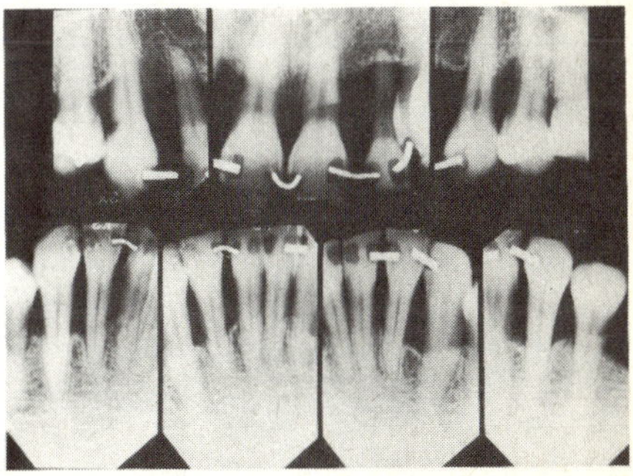

Fig. 15.2. *Patient some seventeen years later. Note negligible increase in bone loss compared with Fig. 15.1.*

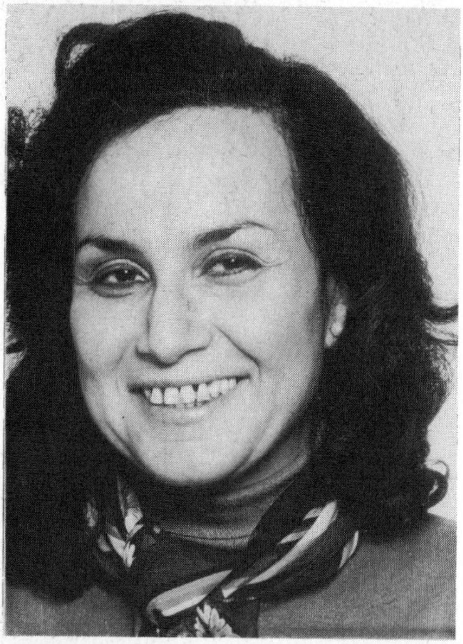

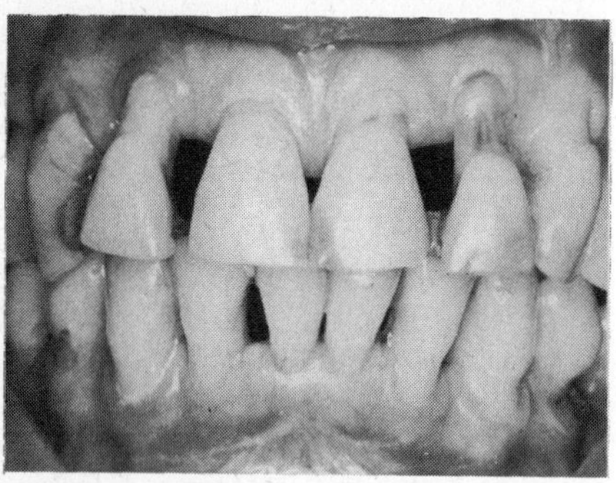

Fig. 15.3. *Clinical picture prior to bridgework, with unsightly* 2|2.

impression taken, and cast, the laterals removed from this (*Fig.* 15.4) and temporary bridges made in the laboratory prior to extracting the teeth. The temporary bridges were now modified at the chairside and in the mouth until the patient was fairly happy with the general morphology of the teeth. An impression was then taken of the temporary bridge in situ and a model made of this (*Fig.* 15.5) which, with detailed notes, gave the technician a guide to the final aesthetic result which the patient required.

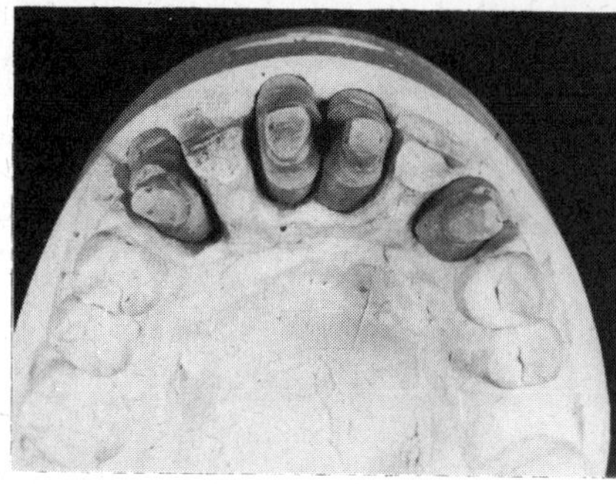

Fig. 15.4. *Rough preparations of* 3 1|1 3 *for temporary bridgework, prior to extracting* 2|2, *which have been removed from the model.*

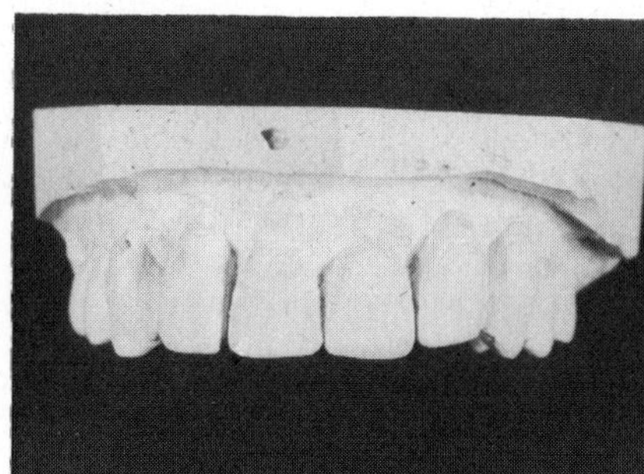

Fig. 15.5. *Model of temporary bridge in situ.*

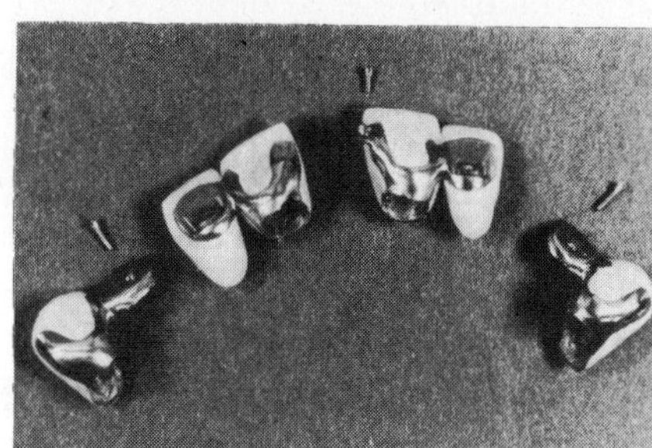

Fig. 15.6. *The prosthesis was fabricated in four separate units linked with dovetails.*

On final preparation of the teeth, it was found that the preparations on 3 1|1 3 could not be aligned without devitalization of at least two teeth. To avoid this and also to preserve as much tooth tissue

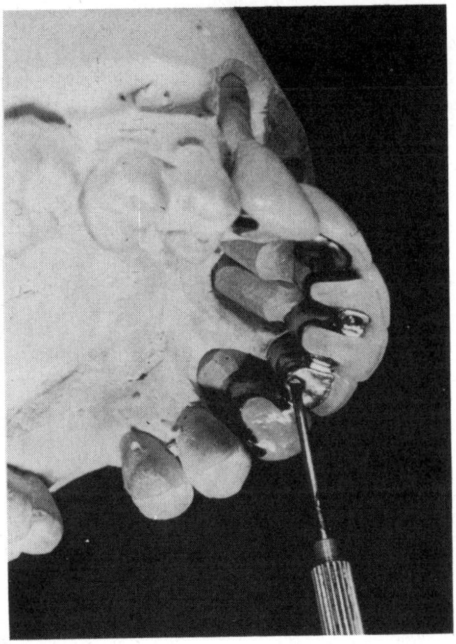

Fig. 15.7. *Screws used to provide final positive fixation of the various components of the bridge.*

as possible, each tooth was prepared without regard to the alignment of any of the others. The prosthesis was then made on a parallelometer in four different units (*Fig.* 15.6), each dovetailing into the other and being finally locked together with screws (*Fig.* 15.7).

When assembled in the mouth, the prosthesis had all the benefits of fixed-fixed bridgework. Dovetails were cut in the laboratory into the distal aspects of 3|3 and then filled with composite (*Fig.* 15.8), so that should posterior bridges or splinting be required at a later date, these could be linked to the anterior prosthesis without disturbing it in any way, by removing the composite and taking an impression of the slot at the same time as the posterior bridge abutments.

The patient was delighted with the aesthetic result, and to say that it transformed her life by removing her self-consciousness of her teeth is probably not too much of an exaggeration. Some three years after placement

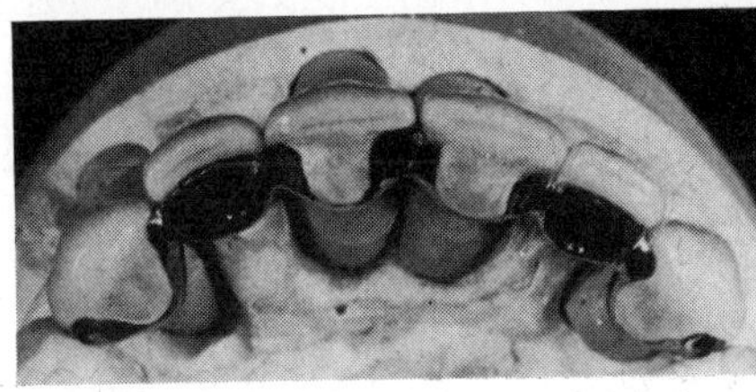

Fig. 15.8. *Occlusal view of prosthesis in place. Note screws and also the dovetails filled with composite in the distal aspects of* 3|3 *to permit linkage with posterior bridgework at a later stage, should it prove necessary.*

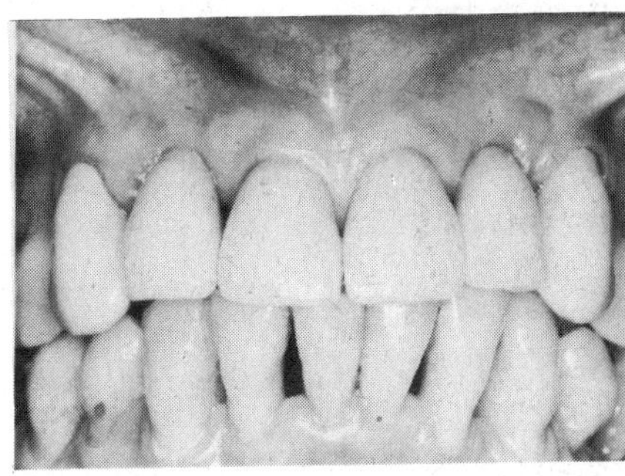

Fig. 15.9 *The completed prosthesis 3 years after cementation.*

of the bridge (*Fig.* 15.9), no deterioration could be detected.

It is necessary to know the outlook on life of patients and their attitude to dentistry. If they show little interest in their general welfare and health and, more specifically, in the condition of their mouth, there is little point in carrying out any prolonged or expensive operative procedures. Obviously considerable dental education will be needed and it should be seen that this has been effective before proceeding with anything other than simple treatment.

Having considered the foregoing, attention can be given to the general condition of the teeth and associated tissues. If oral hygiene is poor the patient must be taught how to take care of his mouth. There is little point in proceeding with a complex bridge if it is doomed to fail after 4–5 years because of cervical caries resulting from food stagnation.

The last general consideration is whether the patient will be able to withstand the prolonged operative procedures necessary for fixed bridge prostheses. This often depends on their temperament. Other factors such as age and general health have already been discussed in Chapter 3.

A careful case history, full mouth X-rays, electric pulp tests, and study models, possibly articulated, as well as a detailed intra-oral examination, are necessary to assess the general condition of the mouth. From this the treatment that will be required before bridge work is commenced can be considered. This may be conveniently divided into periodontal treatment, the correction of any occlusal irregularities, and routine conservation.

PERIODONTAL CONSIDERATIONS

These may be divided into two, those concerning the mouth in general and those relating specifically to the bridge abutments.

■ A. General

Obviously the general periodontal condition must be assessed and any relevant treatment carried out before fitting a prosthesis. Indeed, unless the long-term periodontal prognosis of the teeth is known it is impossible to select the most suitable type to use. Thus if it is considered likely that one or more teeth may be lost in a relatively short time, allowance must be made for this eventuality, and in the majority of cases a removable type of prosthesis supplied. Similarly the periodontal treatment plan may indicate the desirability of some form of splinting, in which case a fixed-fixed bridge is usually indicated.

It is important from the very first examination that continuity of treatment is planned and allowed for throughout the patient's life, and the doubtful prognosis of any teeth or restorations taken into account when assessing this.

■ B. Local

The periodontal and gingival condition of a patient should always be rendered as healthy as possible before constructing a bridge. This matter has already been dealt with in some detail in Chapter 14. At a strictly practical level it must be remembered that if the periodontal condition is poor there is a greater likelihood of bleeding occurring during the preparation and more particularly when taking impressions of the teeth. Similarly the gingivae may be enlarged and therefore their correct contour will not be known. The teeth must always be free of calculus so that there is absolutely no chance of finishing a preparation on to a false edge created by it.

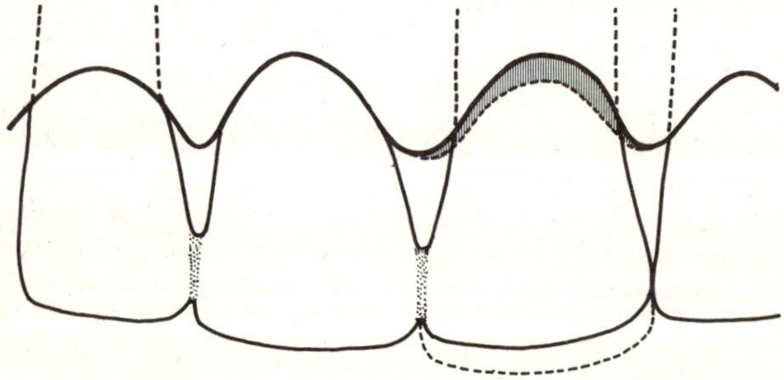

Fig. 15.10. *By carrying out a gingivectomy on* |1 *(shaded area represents tissue removed) an even gingival contour can be established for the bridge and thus a better appearance achieved.*

There are two occasions in which a gingivectomy or other periodontal surgery may assist in the construction of a bridge:

a. By increasing the effective length of the crowns of the teeth and thus enabling better retention to be obtained, i.e. removing 'false' pockets.

b. By adjusting the gingival contour so as to improve the aesthetics of the final restoration (*Fig*. 15.10).

c. By altering the gingival contour and thus simplifying the patient's maintenance after the prosthesis is fitted.

CORRECTION OF OCCLUSION

Before proceeding with a bridge it is desirable to assess any occlusal defects which may be present. Thus a premature contact may be causing a deviation of the mandible which, unless adjusted before the prosthesis is constructed, may result in incorrect occlusal records being taken. This will cause a bridge to be placed in a position and in a dentition out of harmony with the joints and muscles.

Similarly an over-erupted tooth may be locking the articulation (*see Fig*. 2.2, p. 8), rendering it inefficient and preventing any accurate records of the occlusion in lateral and protrusive excursions. In fact when the occlusal defects are corrected, masticatory efficiency may be so increased as to render a bridge unnecessary for that particular reason. An example of this is a colleague's patient who requested a bridge to replace |7 because he could not eat efficiently on that side of the mouth. Prior to construction of the prosthesis 8| was extracted as it was grossly over-erupted and locking the articulation. When the patient attended 3 weeks later to have the teeth prepared for a bridge he stated that he no longer required it as he could now eat perfectly well.

The foregoing are only a few examples of the reasons why occlusal equilibration is necessary before proceeding with fixed bridge prostheses. In a book of this nature it is impossible to go into this matter in any great detail and the reader is therefore referred to one of the specialist textbooks on this subject which are currently available.

ROUTINE CONSERVATION

Having completed any periodontal treatment required and corrected the occlusal irregularities the general condition of the teeth must be assessed and any necessary routine conservation carried out. Thus caries, overhanging margins, and faulty contacts should be eliminated and if any apical infection is present this must be treated. The prognosis of all the teeth needs to be ascertained before a bridge can be satisfactorily designed. If a tooth in the same arch is lost shortly after the prosthesis is fitted, the whole purpose of the treatment may be invalidated.

Should the condition of any of the teeth be at all doubtful it is often best to wait for at least 6 months until their prognosis is more certain before proceeding with the bridge (*Fig*. 15.11). However, this will obviously vary with the urgency of the restoration and the area involved. Thus, the replacement of a lower molar which has been missing for several years is far less urgent than the replacement of a central which has just been extracted.

SELECTION AND TREATMENT OF ABUTMENT TEETH

The choice of abutment teeth will depend on their apical and periodontal condition and also on such factors as the length of span, the occlusion and the type of bridge to be used, which has already been more fully discussed in Chapter 2.

Having selected the most suitable teeth, it may be necessary to carry out some initial treatment to make them

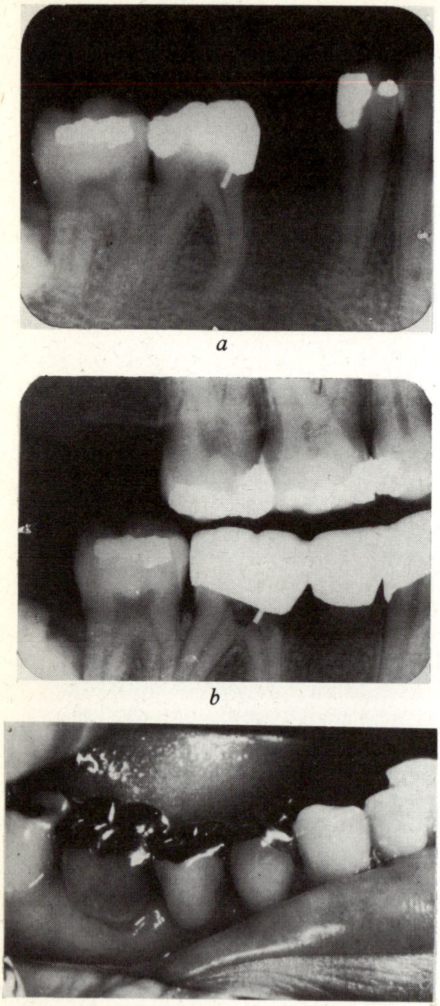

a

b

c

Fig. 15.11. a, *A very deep cavity in* 6⏋ *was restored with a pinned amalgam and then a bridge placed.* b, c, *One year after fitting the bridge. Extensive internal idiopathic resorption has rendered the abutment unsavable. Conclusion: Always wait until the prognosis of the abutment teeth is certain before proceeding with a bridge.*

satisfactory as bridge abutments. Thus if they have an apical area this must be dealt with and the treatment seen to be successful before proceeding. When placing the root filling it simplifies the subsequent placing of posts or screws in the canal if only the apical 3·00 mm is filled. However, this consideration should not be allowed to affect the operator's choice of what is felt to be the correct endodontic therapy.

It is important that the crown of a non-vital tooth be strengthened by such means as a post or screws to reduce any chance of its fracture after the bridge is placed.

■ Restoration of Crowns

One of the big advantages of the extra-coronal restoration is that any caries may first be treated, the crown restored, and the tooth then prepared for the relevant restoration (*Fig*. 15.12). This appreciably improves the prognosis of the tooth, particularly when it is already heavily restored.

It is important that any amalgam used for restoring an abutment be firmly fixed to tooth tissue. If the filling is of any size the most satisfactory method of doing is by using pins (*see Fig*. 6.49, p. 109). These obtain their retention either by being cemented in place, by friction or by being threaded into the dentine. They are usually positioned so that they are divergent from each other. Thus when the amalgam has been placed around them they cannot become dislodged unless either they, the dentine, or the amalgam breaks.

The threaded pins may be divided into two types, relatively large ones which are used in root canals (*Fig*. 15.13), particularly those of multirooted teeth, and smaller ones to be placed in dentine (*Fig*. 15.14). They are easy to use and give excellent retention. Examples of these are marketed by Courtin* under the name of Dolphin (*Fig*. 15.15) and Whaledent† under the trade name of TMS.

These latter pins are in four sizes: Minuta (0·013 in, 0·3 mm), Minikin (0·017 in, 0·4 mm), Minim (0·021 in,

* Courtin Ltd, Courtin House, Horsham Road, Capel, Surrey, England.

† Whaledent International, 236 5th Avenue, New York, NY 10001, USA.

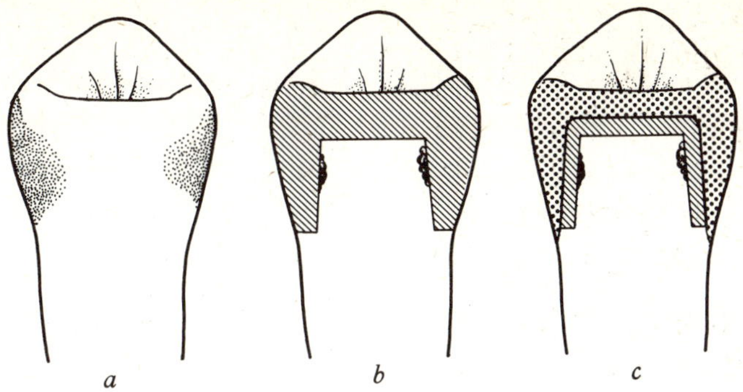

Fig. 15.12. *An advantage of extracoronal restorations is that the tooth may first be restored in amalgam (b) and then the three-quarter of full crown placed over this (c), thus providing two lines of protection from recurrent caries.*

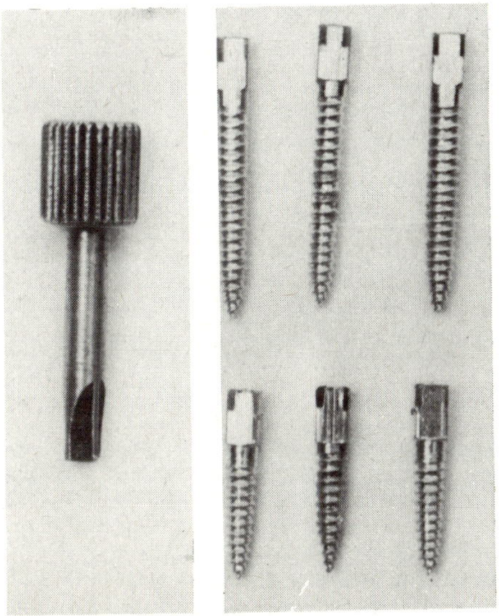

Fig. 15.13. *Dentatus screws, complete with key, for use in root canals.*

0·5 mm), and Regular (0·027 in, 0·7 mm) and are also available in the form of a 2-in-1 pin which incorporates a weak or 'sheer' point in it so that one half may be used as the first pin and the remaining half as the second pin.

Technique

The areas of the tooth at which additional retention is required are assessed and may be marked with a half-round

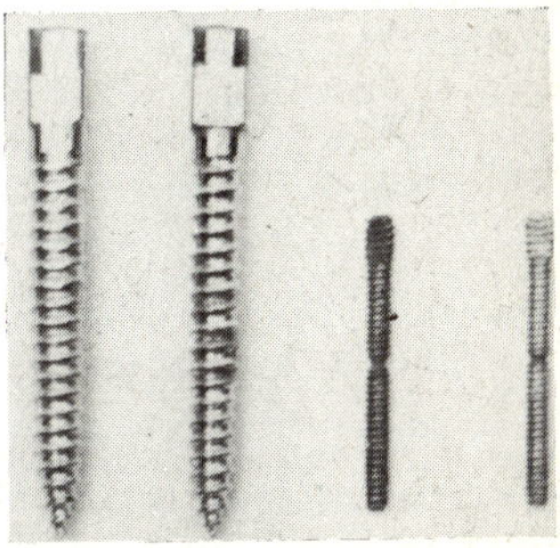

Fig. 15.14. *Comparative sizes of screws used in root canals and dentine.*

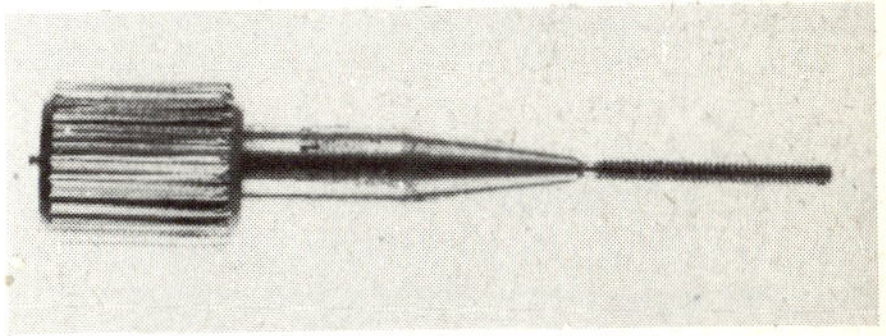

Fig. 15.15. *The Dolphin self-shearing threaded retention pin.*

bur, which is also used for starting the pin holes. X-rays must be available to make certain that the pulp will not be penetrated. The reduction of tooth tissue and amalgam which will be necessitated by the extracoronal preparation should also be taken into account and the pins placed where they will not subsequently be disturbed. However, they cannot be placed in enamel.

Having assessed the number, position and angulation of the pins required, the holes for these are drilled with a matched twist drill of slightly smaller diameter than the pins. A handpiece with a 10 : 1 reduction gear facilitates this procedure. It has been shown that a depth of 2 mm will give optimum retention and nothing will be gained by going beyond this point. Thus with the 4-mm pin 2 mm is buried in tooth tissue and 2 mm is available to provide anchorage for the amalgam.

The self-tapping pins may now be inserted either by hand using the tool illustrated or by using a limited slip chuck in a contra-angled handpiece. The latter, again with a 10 : 1 reduction, is usually to be preferred as it is easier to handle and to obtain the correct angulation for the pin, particularly in the posterior region. The limited slip chuck has the advantage that the pin cannot be overtightened and thus the thread cut in the dentine cannot be damaged or the pin broken.

The 2-in-1 pin will sheer when the first half is fully seated to its correct depth. The second half, which is still in the handpiece, can then be inserted into a second pin hole.

After insertion the pins can be bent to any desired angle with a suitable tool which is supplied with the kit.

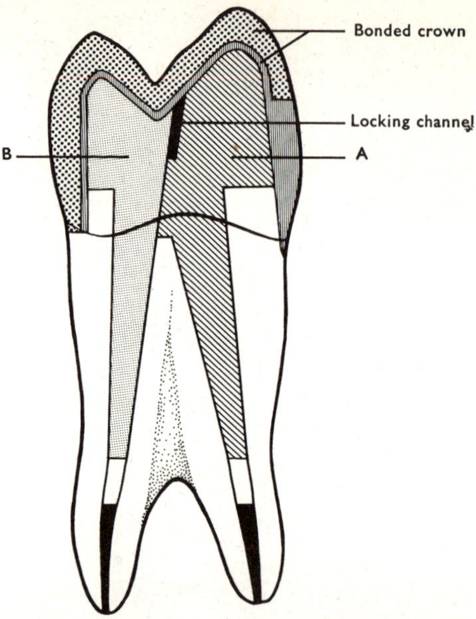

Fig. 15.16. *The split post technique. This may be used for a tooth with divergent roots. A post* A *with part of the core is inserted into one root canal and then a second post* B *is placed which carries the remainder of the core which 'keys' into that already placed. A bonded full crown is then usually fitted.*

■ Restoration of Non-vital Teeth

Where a non-vital tooth has to be restored in the anterior region a post crown will usually be required. The design of this has already been dealt with in Chapter 6; suffice it to say here that every effort must be made to obtain the maximum retention and as much tooth tissue as possible should be retained for this purpose (*see Figs*. 6.64 and 6.65, p. 117).

With the non-vital tooth in the posterior region, other than possibly the lower premolars, it is difficult to place an adequate post crown because of the multiplicity of roots and their divergent angulation. This may sometimes be overcome with a split post technique as shown in *Fig*. 15.16. An alternative to the technique illustrated is to cast one post and all the core as a single unit and then pass the second post down through the core and into the other root canal. More often it is better to restore the tooth first by placing suitable screws such as those marketed by Dentatus (*see Fig*. 15.13) into the root canal together with fine threaded pins in the dentine (*Fig*. 15.17) and then rebuilding the tooth with amalgam. This will give better retention than any other system (Lovdahl, 1977).

After this any type of full crown preparation can be carried out. Where possible it is best to extend the margins of this on to sound tooth tissue (*see Fig*. 6.50, p. 109) so as to provide an accurate fit cervically and to transfer as many of the stresses of occlusion from the amal-

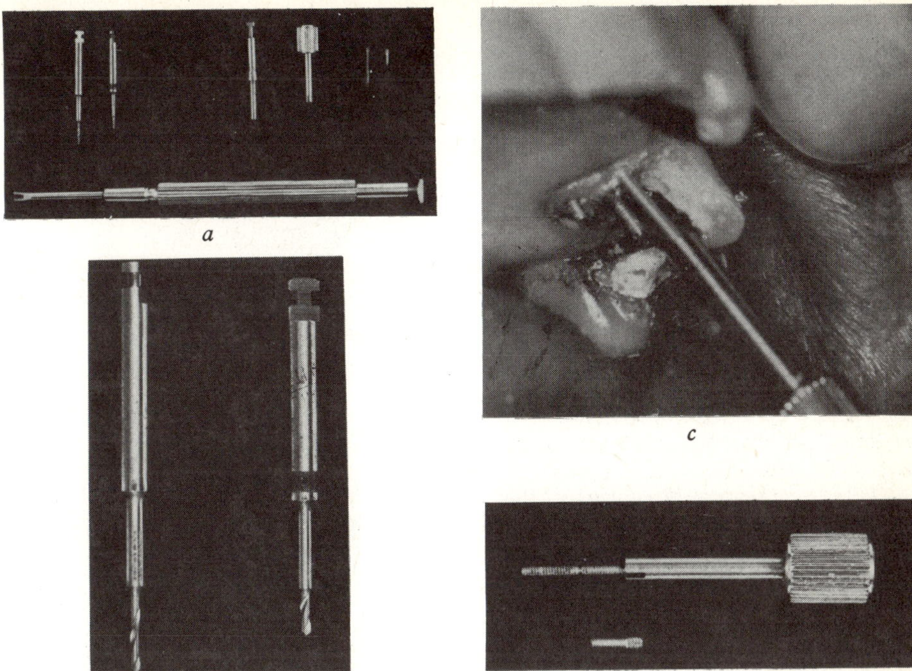

Fig. 15.17. *a, The TMS kit for using self-tapping pins, consisting of hand wrench, limited slip chuck, bending tool, drills, and pins. b, Shouldered drills for penetrating dentine to a predetermined depth. c, TMS threaded pins being inserted with a hand wrench. d, A 'two-in-one' self-shearing TMS pin in a hand chuck.*

gam core to tooth tissue at a point where it is stronger.

DETAILED DESIGN CONSIDERATIONS

There are many factors to be considered prior to actually preparing the teeth. Among these are:

The size and position of the pulp.

Any rotation or tilting of the teeth.

The provision of space for any connectors.

The possible use of any precision retainers.

The position of the correct finishing margins.

The degree of gold which may be displayed.

The treatment of any opposing teeth.

■ The Size and Position of the Pulp

This is one of the most important factors to be assessed before preparing a tooth and may well determine the correct choice of retainer. Where the pulp is large, particularly in the young patient, it may be impossible to obtain sufficient reduction of tooth tissue for an adequate retainer without devitalization. This is especially true of the bonded porcelain restorations, where quite drastic reduction of tooth tissue is essential if a good aesthetic result is to be obtained. However, devitalization should never be resorted to unless it is absolutely essential, as it destroys more tooth tissue, makes the tooth more liable to fracture and occasionally, even in the most skilled of hands, results in an apical area.

On occasions where devitalization is required it is far better if this is elective rather than haphazard, following an exposure. In the posterior region a bite-wing X-ray is the best method of assessing the correct position of the pulp. With anterior teeth an X-ray taken with the ray at right-angles to the crown of the tooth is to be preferred to the usual apical view. On occasions it will be necessary to take X-rays at two or three different angles mesiodistally to show the pulp clearly.

With pinlays the assessment of the position of the pulp is absolutely essential if an exposure is to be avoided.

■ Rotation or Tilting of Teeth

The position of the teeth is important on several counts. Thus if they are rotated it may be possible to correct this in the preparation so that a more aesthetic abutment tooth will result. Likewise there is often a greater liability for gold to be displayed and the preparation will need modifying accordingly (*Fig*. 15.18) if this is to be avoided.

Finally, where a fixed-fixed bridge is to be placed the preparations will have to have a common line of insertion. This must be obtained without pulpal exposure and also without producing retainers of poor retentive value on one or more of the abutment teeth. If this cannot be achieved the design must be modified, possibly by converting it to a fixed-movable type (*see Fig*. 6.4, p. 84) or by the incorporation of precision retainers. However, even with a fixed-movable design it is desirable to have fairly similar lines of insertion for the retainers, otherwise the housing of the dovetail in the minor retainer becomes difficult (*Fig*. 15.19).

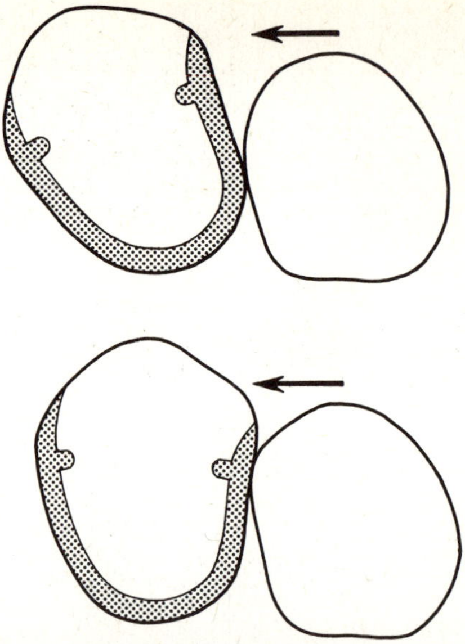

Fig. 15.18. *When a three-quarter crown is placed on a rotated tooth, then there is likely to be an increased display of gold labially, unless the preparation is modified.*

■ The Provision of Space for any Connectors

Where a connector such as the laboratory-made dovetail and slot is to be

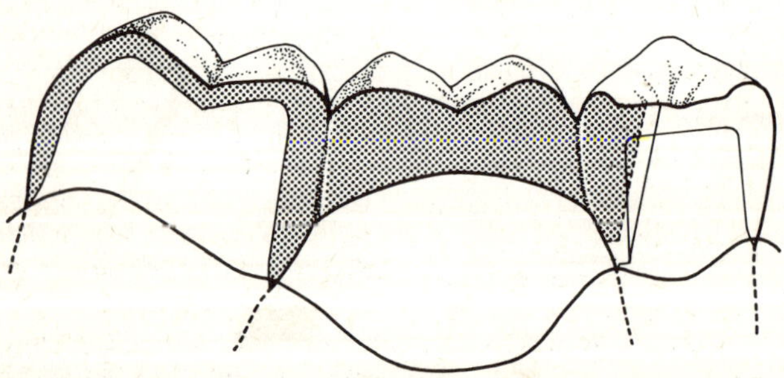

Fig. 15.19. *The box cut in the minor abutment should have approximately the same alignment as the preparation for the major retainer so as to house the dovetail. With severe tilting of the teeth this becomes difficult.*

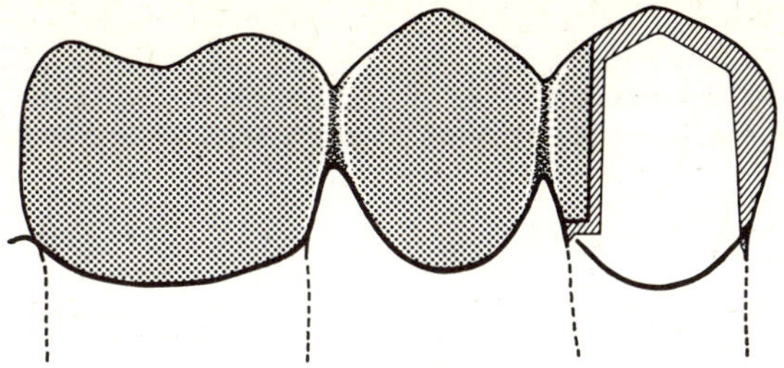

Fig. 15.20. *With a fixed-movable design a box must always be cut in the minor abutment to allow a strong dovetail to be provided which can be housed intracoronally and permit good interproximal embrasures.*

used it is essential that the tooth be prepared so that a dovetail can be housed intracoronally which will be of sufficient length, depth, and width to provide adequate strength and at the same time give good interproximal embrasures. This necessitates the provision of a box in any tooth which is to be used as a minor retainer in a fixed-movable bridge (*Fig.* 15.20).

■ The Use of Precision Retainers

If precision retainers are to be incorporated in a bridge this should be taken into account before commencing tooth preparation. The first consideration is to decide whether they can improve the design of the bridge in any way, possibly by providing for continuity of treatment should the prognosis of one of the abutments be suspect. Likewise it may be thought desirable to allow for a removable saddle area should there be considerable soft tissue loss.

Where precision retainers have to be incorporated in a bridge it is usually desirable to house them intracoronally. Thus it is essential to make certain that the tooth can be reduced sufficiently to permit this before proceeding with the bridge. In this context it is worth bearing in mind that precision retainers are nearly all larger than they appear and require teeth having longer clinical crowns than normal with well receded pulps before they can be accommodated satisfactorily.

The only accurate method of assessing this is by initially carrying out the preparations on a plaster model and then checking the particular retainers in situ. This will also prove of value when actually preparing the teeth.

■ The Finishing Margin

The correct position of the finishing margin requires careful consideration before tooth preparations are commenced. Several factors influence this. If the retainer is of the extracoronal type it is usually desirable to extend the margins beyond any existing restoration and on to sound tooth tissue. Similarly, if there is a tendency to cervical caries or if it is in a region where oral hygiene is difficult, such as the buccal aspect of the upper third molar, it should be extended to or just below the gingival margin.

Other factors which will affect the position of the finishing line are the length of the clinical crown, the retention required, and periodontal considerations. Thus if the crown is short and maximum retention is required the preparation will have to be extended as far subgingivally as possible. However, where the clinical crowns are reasonably long and other factors are favourable the preparation should always be terminated about 1·5–2 mm supragingivally. Providing the external contour of the crown is correct this situation is ideal from the periodontal aspect, as it will cause the minimum of gingival irritation. It will also enable the best possible marginal adaption to be obtained. This subject has already been discussed more fully in Chapter 6.

■ The Degree of Gold to be Displayed

The importance of this factor depends largely on the abutment tooth involved and the patient's own opinion on the matter. By careful design of the preparations any display of gold can be kept to a minimum. The curving of the slice on the mesial aspect of the three-quarter crown (*see Fig*. 6.41, p. 102) is an example of this. A further example is the use of the Selberg preparation in certain cases in preference to the three-quarter crown. On the occlusal aspect of the posterior teeth the method most commonly used to avoid any display of gold is the use of the bonded full crown. However, this requires a very drastic reduction of tooth tissue.

From all the foregoing it will be seen that a very careful assessment of the correct preparation in any particular case is essential before proceeding with any reduction of tooth tissue. Likewise, consideration has to be given not only to the abutment teeth but to the opposing teeth also.

■ The Treatment of any Opposing Teeth

Before proceeding with the preparation of the abutment teeth it is best to decide whether any adjustment of the occlusal surfaces of the opposing teeth is indicated. If this is of a relatively minor nature it is best to assess it and mark and correct the relative areas on the models prior to constructing the bridge in the laboratory. The necessary occlusal reductions are then carried out in the mouth immediately prior to fitting the bridge. This has the advantage that no over-eruption of the teeth is likely to occur while the bridge is being constructed.

Where a more drastic removal of tooth tissue is necessary it is best performed at the outset. It may even be necessary, because of the extent of the reduction required, to place a three-quarter or full crown on the opposing tooth. This should be done either immediately before the bridge is constructed or at the same time.

PREPARATION OF ABUTMENT TEETH

■ Occlusal Reduction

Having considered all the foregoing we are now in a position to commence tooth tissue reduction.

The general principles involved will be illustrated by describing the technique used for the posterior three-quarter crown. Those employed for other preparations are basically similar.

The exact methods of tooth reduction are not described in any detail as individual operator's techniques vary so much. However, in the majority of cases the preparations may be outlined with an airotor and then completed first with a precision low-speed handpiece and finally with hand instruments such as chisels, shoulder files, and hatchets. A set of high-speed diamonds principally for use in the air turbine and suitable for carrying out most abutment preparations has been developed by Mr Setchell of the Eastman Dental Hospital, London, in cooperation with Diamond Precision Tools Limited* (*Fig*. 15.21).

Study models and X-rays should always be to hand during tooth preparation and the first step is to decide the extent of occlusal reduction. This can generally be estimated best on the models. In some areas the tooth may need very little reduction and in others far more, but basically the contour of the existing occlusal surface should be followed. To make certain that the correct occlusal reduction is carried out

* Diamond Precision Tools Ltd, 263–269 City Rd, London EC1, England.

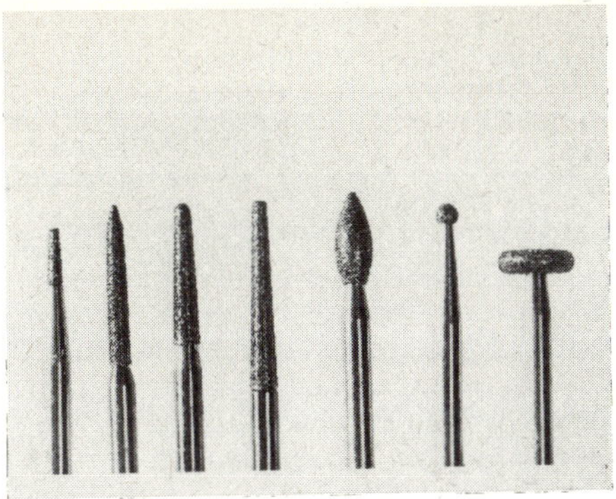

Fig. 15.21. *A selection of high-speed diamonds suitable for crown and bridge-work, developed by Mr D. Setchell.*

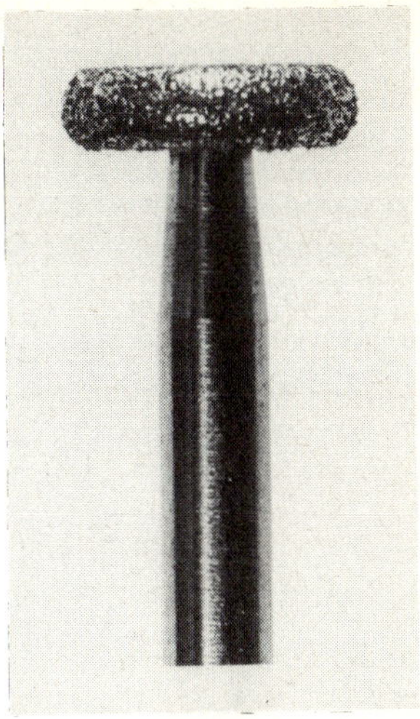

Fig. 15.23. *4-mm wheelstone, Hi-Di Ref. 513; suitable for occlusal reduction and concavities.*

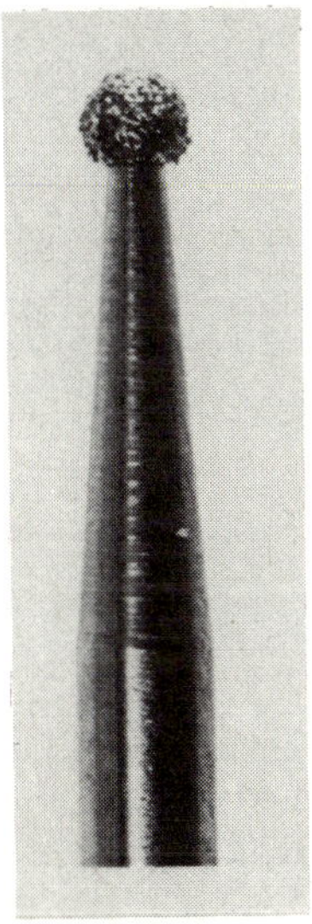

Fig. 15.22. *15-mm round diamond, Hi-Di Ref. 521; for cutting depth guides and endodontic access.*

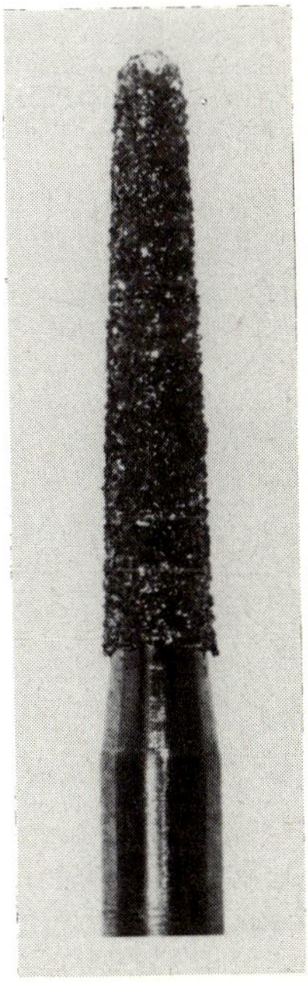

Fig. 15.24. *8-mm round-ended tapered diamond Hi-Di Ref. 501; suitable for occlusal or axial reductions and a chamfer finish.*

over the whole occlusal surface, depth limiting grooves may be cut in it, preferably with a round diamond (*Fig.* 15.22) before the main reduction is performed with a small wheelstone (*Fig.* 15.23) or a tapered round-ended cylinder (*Fig.* 15.24). On the lingual aspect of anterior teeth a biconvex diamond (*Fig.* 15.25) is often of use and this stone will also prove of value for some posterior occlusal reduction. A thickness of gold of at least 1 mm is usually required over the whole of the occlusal surface and this must be increased to 1·5–2·0 mm if bonded porcelain is to be employed. The correct clearance can be checked both visually and by periodically getting the patient to bite into a piece of soft red wax and holding this in front of the light. If necessary it can be sectioned with a scalpel to assess the thickness at any one point. It is important that an adequate clearance is provided to accommodate both lateral and protrusive as well as centric occlusion.

■ Preparation of Interproximal Areas

Before commencing the preparation of the mesial and distal aspects the position of the contact point must be assessed. This can usually be done with a probe. References to the patient's bite-wing X-rays may also be helpful.

In the majority of cases the contacts can be cleared by the use of a very fine taper diamond in an airotor, gradually working through from the lingual to the buccal or labial aspects (*Fig.* 15.26*a*). If a non-end cutting diamond such as shown in *Fig.* 15.31 is employed and the tip kept firmly against tooth tissue and the other end clear of the neighbouring tooth, then there is no way in which this can be damaged during the preparation.

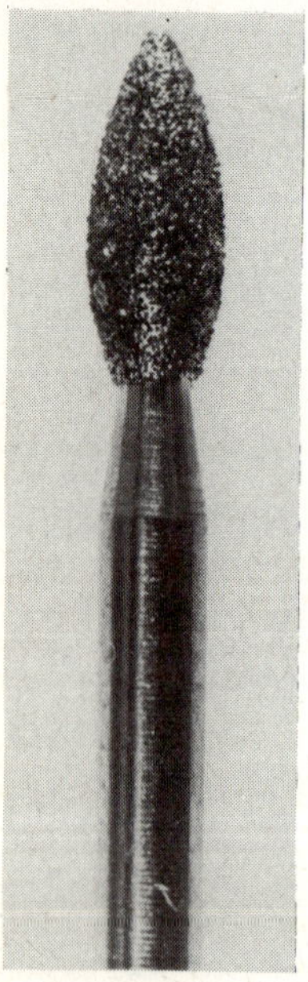

Fig. 15.25. *5-mm biconvex diamond, Hi-Di Ref. 564, which is particularly useful for lingual reduction on anterior teeth. It can also be used to produce a strong chamfer, but care must be taken or undercuts will result.*

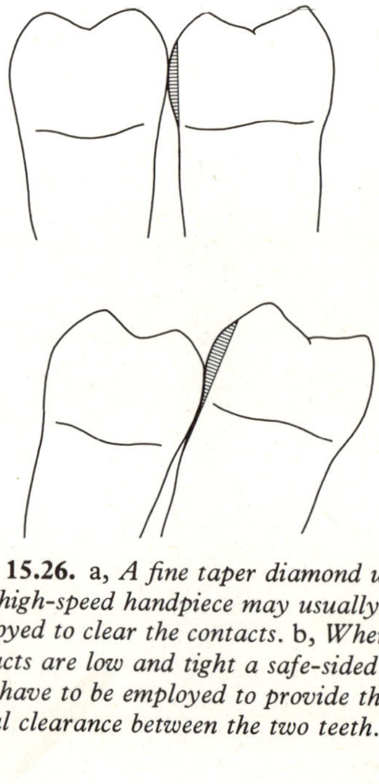

Fig. 15.26. a, *A fine taper diamond used in a high-speed handpiece may usually be employed to clear the contacts.* b, *Where the contacts are low and tight a safe-sided disc may have to be employed to provide the initial clearance between the two teeth.*

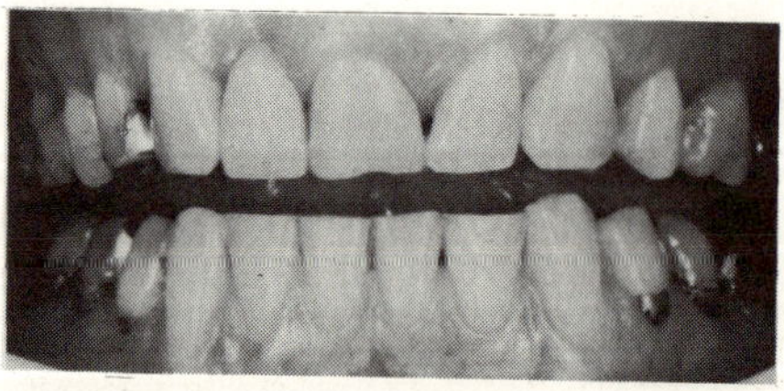

Fig. 15.27. *A slice preparation on* 4| *using a disc. Note the unnecessarily large amount of gold displayed which mars the otherwise good aesthetic result obtained by this spring bridge replacing* 2|.

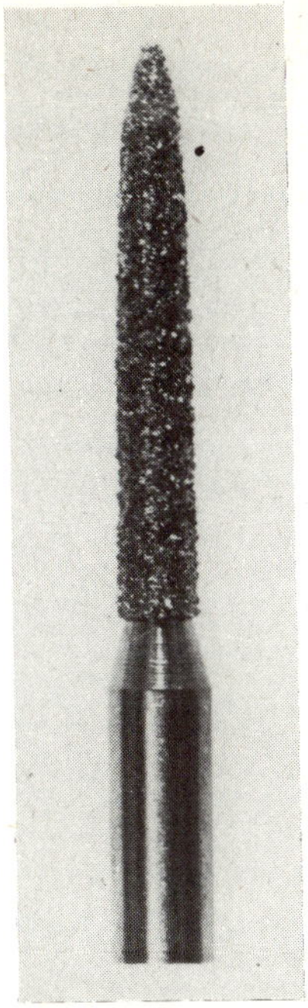

Fig. 15.28. *8-mm finely tipped thin flame diamond, Hi-Di Ref. 563, suitable for interproximal reduction, flares and bevels.*

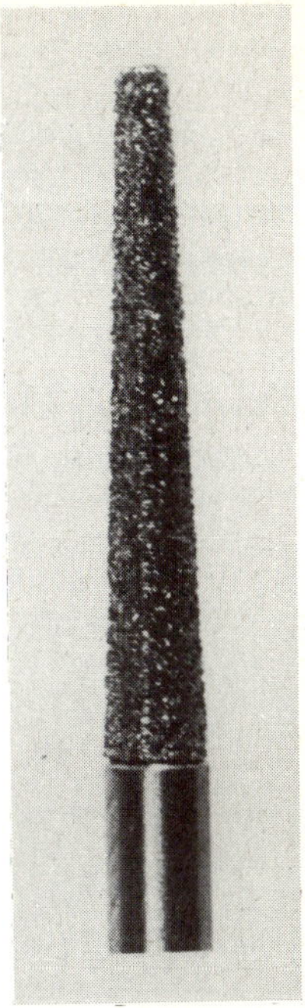

Fig. 15.29. *8-mm long tapered flat-ended diamond, Hi-Di Ref. 556, suitable for axial reduction to produce a shoulder finish.*

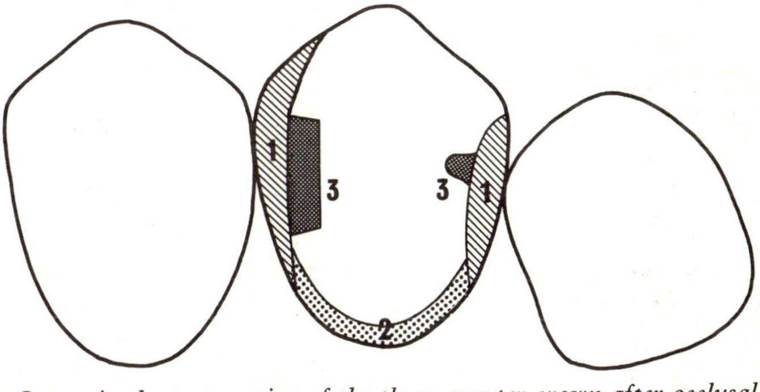

Fig. 15.30. *Stages in the preparation of the three-quarter crown after occlusal reduction has been carried out:* 1. *Mesial and distal slices;* 2. *Connection of slices;* 3. *Preparation of box distally, if three-quarter crown is to be used as a minor retainer, and slot mesially.*

An advantage of using a fine tapered diamond is that the slice need not be extended too far buccally and any display of gold may be kept to a minimum. This would be impossible if a disc were employed (*Fig.* 15.27), the use of which, however careful the operator, is always fraught with danger. If a guard is used visibility is reduced and in any case protection is only partial, but the risks involved in using a disc without a guard are too great to be acceptable.

However, where the contacts are low and tight (*Fig.* 15.26*b*) a disc has to be employed as however fine the taper diamond there will be the likelihood of some damage to the adjacent tooth. This may be mitigated by fitting a band to it. The only other alternative, provided the contact is sound, is to modify the preparation so as to avoid this area.

Having cleared the contact points either with a non-end cutting or a long narrow flame diamond (*Fig*. 15.28) the principal reduction of the mesial and distal aspects is completed. Both the mesial and distal slices will be curved (*Fig*. 15.30), the former to minimize any display of gold and the latter to provide increased retention. The margins will usually be extended to completely cover any existing restoration and to finish on sound tooth tissue. A round ended tapered cylinder (*Fig*. 15.24) is used, sinking the tip in to approximately half its depth so as to produce a chamfer finish as shown in *Fig*. 15.32.

The tooth must be reduced sufficiently mesially and distally to permit a casting of sufficient thickness and strength. In this context it should be borne in mind that the longer the span the greater the stresses which will be imposed on the retainers, pontics, and solder joints of the bridge and therefore the stronger they must be.

To increase the strength of the gold in the region of the solder joint further tooth reduction, either in the form of a box or a curve, may be indicated (*see Fig*. 6.46, p. 106).

■ Connection of the Mesial and Distal Slices

Having completed the preparation of the mesial and distal aspects of the tooth these can now be joined using a fine taper diamond in a high-speed handpiece. If the preparation is to be subgingival a stone may be used with a smooth tip to avoid any damage to the gingival tissues (*Fig*. 15.31).

In the majority of cases a diamond with a curved tip is indicated so as to produce a chamfer finish which will give a rather more positive finishing line and increase the thickness and thus the rigidity of the casting at this point (*Fig*. 15.32).

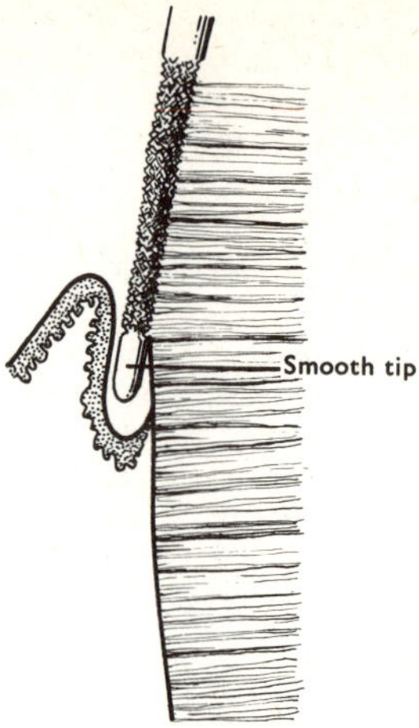

Fig. 15.31. *The use of a smooth-tipped diamond reduces gingival trauma.*

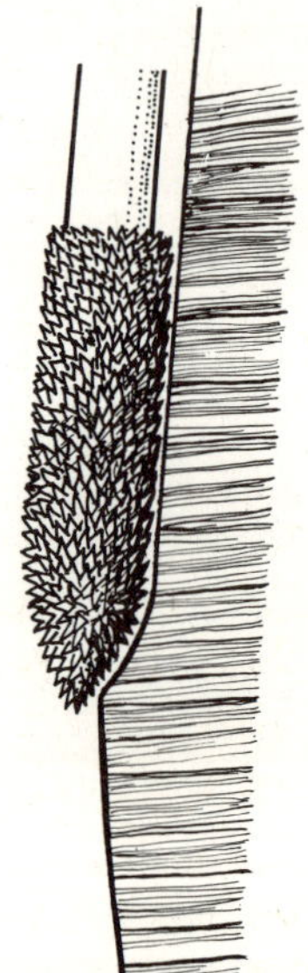

Fig. 15.32. *A diamond with a curved tip will provide a more positive finishing margin than a straight taper diamond.*

At this stage the preparation should be checked to see that there are no undercut areas and that it has been extended to the correct depth throughout.

■ Accommodation of Dovetail

If the abutment is to carry the minor retainer of a fixed-movable bridge the relevant aspect of the tooth must be modified to allow for the slot which will have to be cut in the gold to house the dovetail. This is usually achieved by a box preparation which may be done either before or after the preparation of the remainder of the tooth. The advantage of the former is that it is possible to see exactly how deep the box has been cut into the tooth, as its outer aspect is still intact. This is particularly important when preparing the teeth for precision retainers.

■ Finishing of Preparation

At this stage the whole of the preparation, except the rails, should have been outlined and it may now be finished with low-speed and hand instruments. First, diamonds of a fairly fine grit size are used to smooth the preparation and eliminate any minor irregularities. After this a still smoother surface may be obtained, if required either with multi-bladed high-speed tungsten-carbide finishing burs which may be obtained in various profiles or by using carborundum stones or sandpaper discs. The axial wall of any box is best finished with chisels, hatchets and gingival margin trimmers.

■ Cutting of Slots

The final stage of tooth preparation is the cutting of the mesial and distal slots. These should be placed well buccally to provide maximum retention and if possible cut into sound tooth tissue. If this is not possible then they may safely be placed in amalgam provided that this is adequately retained, usually by means of pins.

The size of the rails will vary with the size of the tooth but normally a 700 or 701 taper fissure bur will provide one of adequate thickness. It should be made as long as possible but should stop a little before the gingival margin of the preparation. Where the crown is short and retention lacking two rails may be provided on both the mesial and distal surfaces. If a box has already been prepared on one aspect of the tooth a slot will not also be needed there.

Finally any sharp margins, other than those at the edge of the preparation, should be lightly rounded. Little is gained by leaving them, as they are always liable to be damaged on the model in the laboratory.

■ The Bonded Full Crown

This preparation has already been considered in Chapter 6. However, there are a few practical points to take into account. The first of these is the assessment of the degree of labial reduction required. This will depend to some extent on the position of the tooth. If this is normal then it will be merely a matter of making certain that the whole of the labial or buccal aspect is reduced by at least 1·5 mm. This can be achieved most accurately by cutting three grooves with a cylinder diamond of the correct thickness to the depth required and then joining these together (*Fig*. 15.33) with a long tapered flat-ended cylinder diamond (*see Fig*. 15.29). On anterior teeth it is usually desirable to have a shoulder finish labially, so that the porcelain may be extended down to the finishing margin. However, on posterior teeth a strong chamfer is often to be preferred with a 1–2 mm gold finishing margin. This may

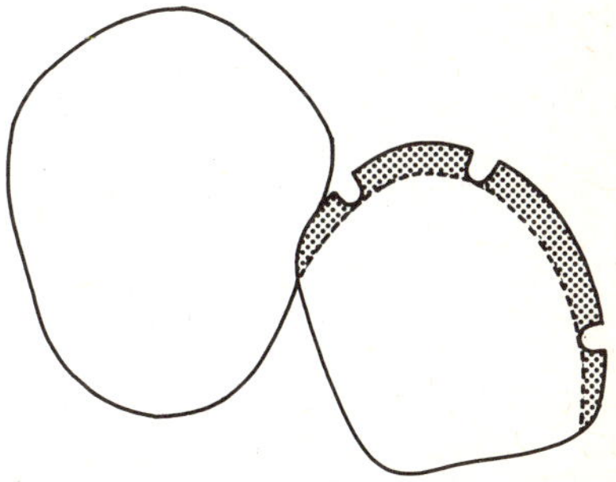

Fig. 15.33. *The degree of labial reduction may be predetermined by first cutting grooves in the tooth to the final depth required.*

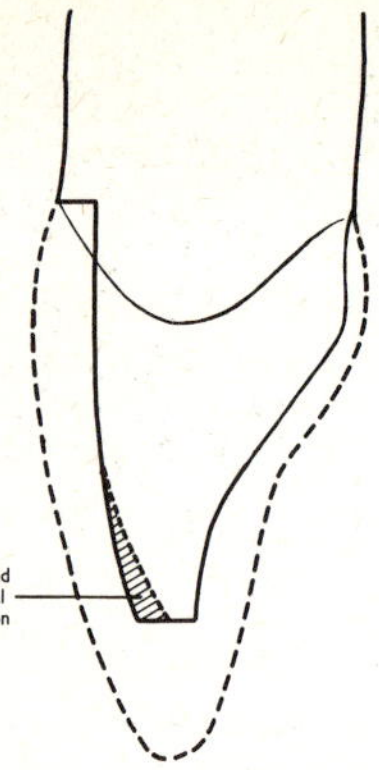

Fig. 15.34. *Labial reduction should be increased a little at the incisal edge to provide the best aesthetic result.*

be achieved with a relatively thick flame-shaped diamond.

The second problem which may arise is where it is impossible to establish an adequate shoulder on the labial or buccal aspect without undue destruction of tooth tissue. This applies in particular to the upper premolar, where it is relatively common for the buccal cusp to be the only standing sound tooth tissue. It is particularly undesirable to weaken this further by cutting into it to provide a shoulder. The problem may be overcome by using a chamfer finish and establishing the correct shoulder width for the porcelain in the gold a little above the finishing line (*see Fig.* 6.49, p. 109). The only disadvantage of this technique is that a small amount of gold will be displayed cervically and that the final contour of the tooth in this area may sometimes have to be a little wider than normal to preserve tooth tissue.

It may be mentioned here that some authorities prefer to use a chamfer finish for the buccal aspects of all posterior teeth and this has much to commend it, particularly if a gold finishing margin is employed, which will usually provide a better fit than porcelain. If it is necessary to have porcelain to tissue contact then a strong chamfer must be employed otherwise insufficient space will be created for the porcelain and either a poor aesthetic result, or, worse still, over contouring will result.

The other factors to be remembered when preparing an anterior tooth for a faced full crown are that the outer aspect should usually finish just subgingivally and that the incisal part of the labial surface of the preparation should be curved and rounded a little. This will provide the maximum thickness of porcelain at this point, which will make the provision of an aesthetically pleasing facing far easier for the technician (*Fig.* 15.34).

■ Paralleling of Preparations

Having completed the preparations it is necessary to make certain that they have a common line of withdrawal if the bridge is to be of fixed-fixed design. If it is to be fixed-movable the box cut in the minor abutment to house the dovetail will need to be roughly parallel with the line of withdrawal of the major retainer (*see Fig.* 15.19, p. 200).

Both these factors should have been borne in mind during the preparation of the teeth, but a final check will be necessary. In the case of a simple bridge this may be assessed by eye using a larger dental mirror than normal. A further aid is the use of a special front-surfaced steel mirror which has parallel lines machined on it (*Fig.* 15.35). This may be inserted in the buccal sulcus, one of the lines paralleled with a particular aspect of the preparation and then the other aspects compared to this.

With multiple preparations it is usually best to prepare all the teeth almost completely and then take an impression of these and assess the case on a model in the laboratory, marking any places where further reduction may be required.

There are several paralleling devices, such as the P.P. and Prec-in-Dent, which may be used to assist in the alignment of multiple preparations, particularly pinledges. The use of one of these has already been described in Chapter 6.

At this stage it may be helpful to summarize the various stages required in

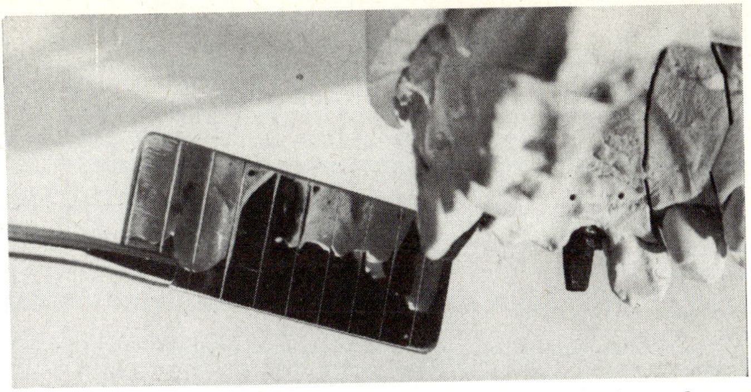

Fig. 15.35. *A front-surfaced mirror with vertical lines which may be used as a guide for paralleling preparations.*

the preparation of a bridge. Obviously all of these will not be necessary in every case but it does help to remind us of each of the factors involved:

1. *Patient assessment.* Attitude to and tolerance of patient to dentistry. Patient's requirements.

2. *Medical and dental case histories,* to eliminate any contraindications or complications.

3. *Initial investigations.* Examination; X-rays; vitality tests; study models.

4. *Restoration of the rest of the mouth.* Routine conservation and endodontics; periodontal treatment; correction of occlusal irregularities, premature contacts, deviations, etc.

5. *Bridge assessment and design,* including patient consultation.

6. *Restoration and treatment of abutment teeth.*

7. *Detailed design considerations.*

8. *Trial assessment of case on models,* including preparations in the stone teeth to consider such problems as the housing of any precision retainers and the paralleling of the preparations.

9. *The construction of a special tray,* and where indicated a *mock-up* of the final result to assess aesthetics.

10. *Almost complete preparation* of the teeth and impressions to assess the alignment and adequacy of these on models.

11. *The placing of a temporary bridge.*

12. *Detailed impressions.* Occlusal records; selection of shade; refit of temporary bridge.

13. *Try-in of bridge.* Check fit and finish of margins; check and adjust occlusion; check and adjust contacts; check tissue contact, adjust and, if porcelain, reglaze; check aesthetics.

14. *Cement bridge.* Recheck margins; recheck occlusion; make certain no cement is left subgingivally.

15. *Review* 1 *month after cementation.* Check: margins, articulation, gingival condition, colour, and tissue contact, and again check for any cement left subgingivally; note all details of bridge construction; instruct patient in care of bridge; arrange regular recalls.

Bibliography

Blair H. A. (1971) The role of endodontics in restorative dentistry. *Dent. Clin. North. Am.* **15**, 619.

Brecker S. C. (1964) How to prevent failures in crowns and bridges. *Dent. Practnr Dent. Rec.* **14**, 261.

Dawson P. E. (1970) Pin-retained amalgam. *Dent. Clin. North Am.* **14**, 63.

Guyer S. E. (1970) Multiple preparations for fixed prosthodontics. *J. Prosthet. Dent.* **23**, 529.

Harty F. J. (1977) Filling the root canal. *Dent. Update* **4**, 211.

Lovdahl P. E. (1977) Pin-retained amalgam cores *vs* cast-gold dowel cores. *J. Prosthet. Dent.* **38**, 507.

Miller F. I. and Feinberg E. (1962) Electronic surgery. *N.Y. J. Dent.* **32**, 172.

Nicholls E. (1963) The restoration of root filled teeth. *Dent. Practnr Dent. Rec.* **13**, 459.

Winstanley R. B. (1971) Pin retained amalgam restorations. *Br. Dent. J.* **130**, 327.

16

IMPRESSION TECHNIQUES, SHADE TAKING AND TEMPORARY BRIDGES

Gingival Retraction . Mixing of the Impression Material
Construction of Special Tray
Injection Technique . Testing for Set
Modified Techniques . Checking of Impression
Transfer Copings
Recording Tooth Colour and Shade
Temporary Bridges

The use of only one material, polysulphide, will be described in this chapter. Most of the other materials are used in a similar fashion for bridge work but where differences do occur these will have already been mentioned in the section on impression materials in Chapter 4. The technique described here is the one which is most universally applicable to bridge work and is likely to produce the best results.

All periodontal treatment should be completed prior to bridge work and the gingivae brought into as healthy a state as possible. Inflamed and swollen gingivae bleed easily and make the taking of an accurate impression difficult, if not impossible. The position of the gingival margin may also alter appreciably. It is particularly important that the teeth are carefully scaled before taking the impression. It is pointless to finish a gold margin to a piece of calculus.

Where the preparations are supragingival which they should be whenever possible, or just subgingival, the impression can be taken immediately after completion of the preparations. However, if these are well subgingival it may be best to allow the gingivae to settle and delay impression-taking until the next visit. Even a small subgingival haemorrhage will ruin a complex impression.

GINGIVAL RETRACTION

Electrosurgery may often be of value in preparing the gingival crevice or adjusting the gingival contour before the impression is taken and is particularly helpful if bleeding is likely to occur. There would seem to be little difference in the adverse effects of the gingival retraction whether it is performed with an electrosurgical unit or a retraction cord.

In order to aid the flow of the impression material into the gingival crevice, retraction may be employed. This is basically the tucking of a thin cord (*Fig.* 16.1) into the gingival crevice,

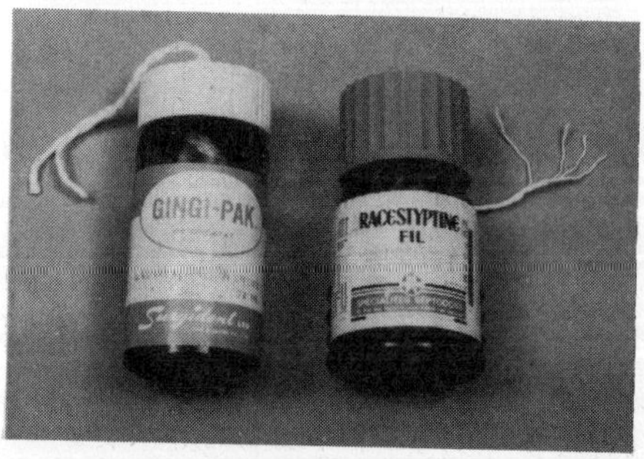

Fig. 16.1. *Gingival retraction cords with 2 and 4 strands. The thicker variety is best used where the gingival crevice is deep.*

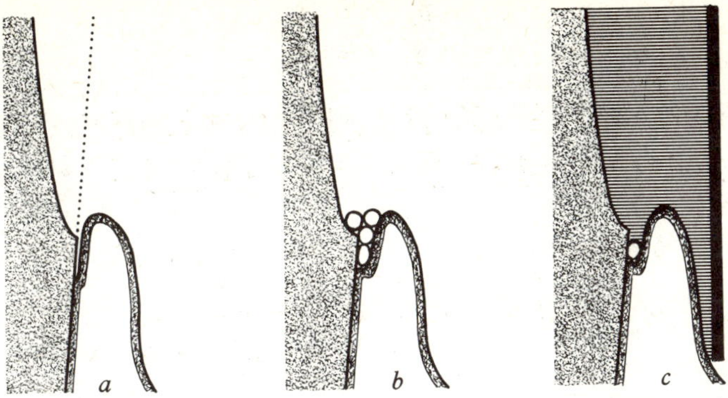

Fig. 16.2. *Gingival retraction. a, Gingival tissues close to margin of preparation. b, Lateral displacement of tissues by retraction cord. c, Impression being taken with one strand of cord being left in position below margin of preparation to reduce the liability of a recurrent haemorrhage.*

thus displacing the gingivae laterally sufficiently to allow the easy passage of the polysulphide around the margin of the preparation (*Fig.* 16.2).

The cord used is impregnated with a material which aids haemostasis and reduces the crevicular exudate. Adrenaline and aluminum trichloride are employed for this purpose, a suitable solution being adrenaline 8 : 100 with 1 per cent benzyl alcohol as a preservative. Ten per cent zinc chloride has also been recommended. However, this is an escharotic and literally burns the tissues, although normally to only a limited extent. Unfortunately a severe reaction, possibly allergic, occasionally takes place with sloughing of the adjoining gingivae and even generalized oedema of that side of the face. For this reason its use is best avoided.

An alternative to the incorporation of the medicaments in the retraction cord is to bathe the gingival tissues with a suitable solution for 2 minutes (Wilson and Tay, 1977) prior to inserting plain retraction cord. An advantage of this technique is that it appreciably reduces the period for which the tissues are subjected to any chemical irritation. A suitable solution would be 0·4 ml of a saturated solution of potash alum containing 1 per cent adrenalin acid tartrate and 0·1 per cent sodium metabisulphate.

The cords employed are usually made of several strands. Where there is a deep crevice which, of course, should normally have been treated beforehand, the cord may be used as it stands, but where there is only a small gingival sulcus one strand of the cord may be inserted first (*Fig.* 16.3*a–d*) and frequently this alone will be sufficient; however, it may be followed up with the other two or three strands (*Fig.* 16.3 *e–h*). If bleeding is likely to occur the best technique is to make certain that the strand placed first is entirely below the margin of the preparation and an exact collar fit. This is then left in place whilst the impression is being taken.

The cord may be gently eased into the gingival crevice with a flat plastic instrument (*Fig.* 16.3*c*) and is usually left in place for 5–15 min, the time varying with the gingival condition, the likelihood of haemorrhage, and the type of medicament incorporated in the cord.

MIXING OF THE IMPRESSION MATERIAL

Many techniques have been advocated for mixing the polysulphides, but only one will be described here. The material is required in two consistencies, thin or medium for use in the syringe and thick

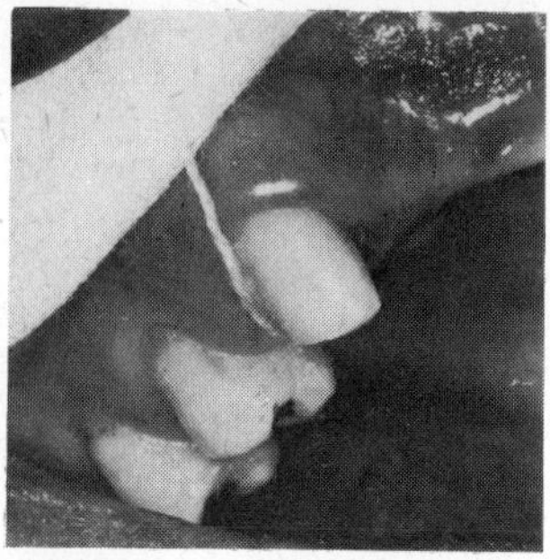

a

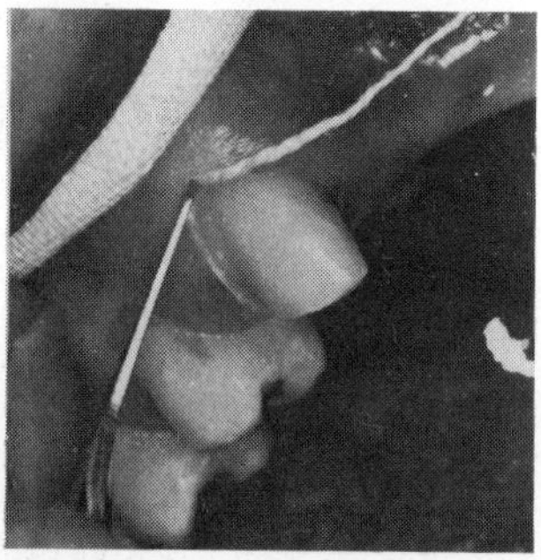

b

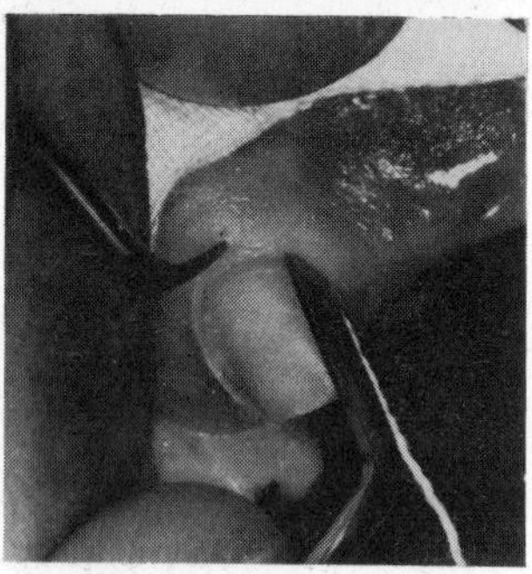

c

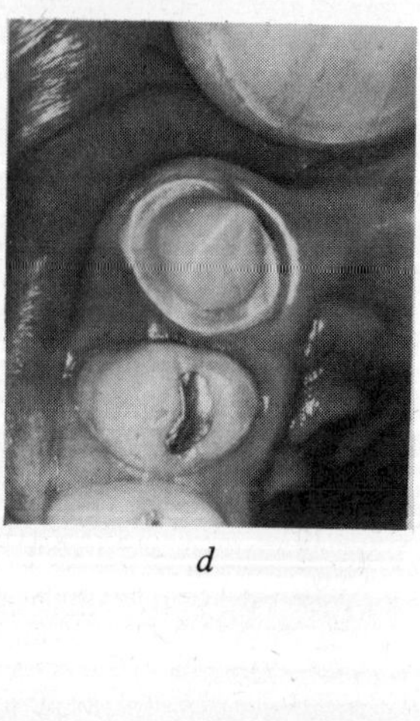

d

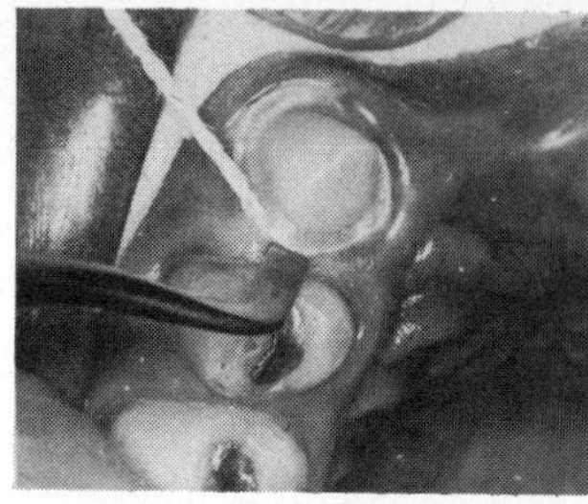

e

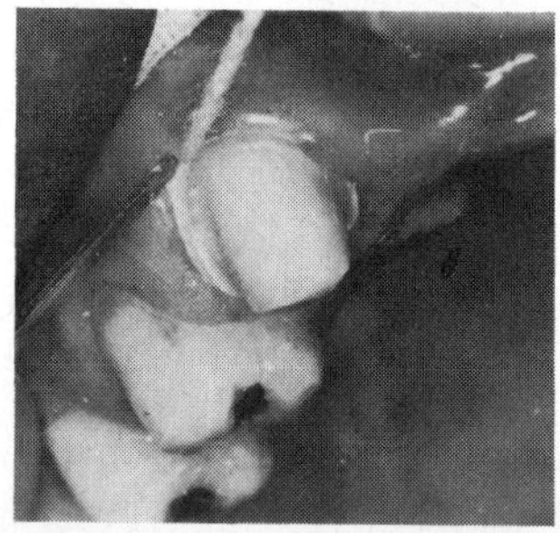

f

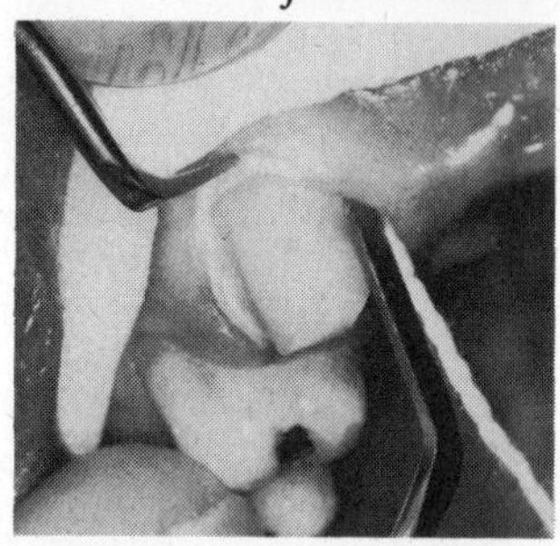

g

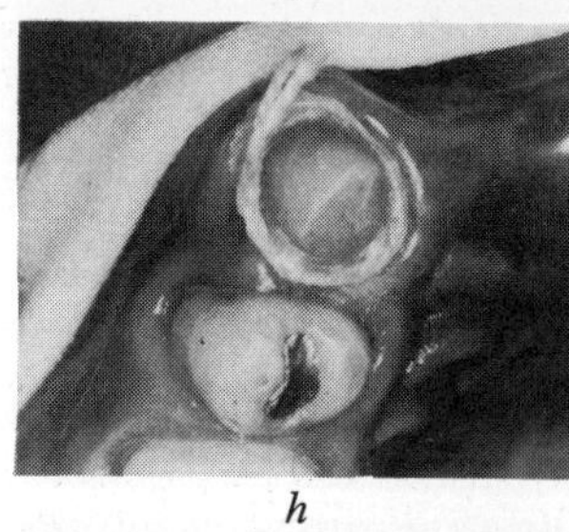

h

Fig. 16.3. *a, The initial insertion of the cord is made interstitially. b, The cord is placed in a clockwise direction to prevent unravelling. c, Flat plastics may be used for inserting the cord. d, Completion of insertion of the single strand. e–g, Two further strands of cord being positioned. h, The completion of gingival retraction.*

for use in the tray (*Fig.* 16.4*a*). Some manufacturers sell it in these viscosities, whereas others only supply it in the heavy form, a lighter bodied material being obtained from this by thinning it. Alternatively, one of medium consistency may be used for both syringe and tray, but this is usually only satisfactory for the simpler case.

■ Mixing and Loading of Light-bodied Material

This material is usually supplied in two tubes, catalyst and polysulphide rubber, and equal lengths of these are dispensed on to a disposable paper slab. As they are relatively thin they mix fairly readily, the best action being to hold the spatula vertically and mix the material with the tip of the instrument, using a circular motion (*Fig.* 16.4*d*). Care must be taken to see that no unmixed constituents remain on the slab, as these may then become incorporated in the impression and result in a defect. When the material is a completely even colour throughout it is fully mixed. However, it is important to adhere to the mixing times and schedules recommended by the manufacturers.

■ Syringe

The purpose of injecting the impression material is to make certain that all the prepared surfaces of the teeth are covered with polysulphide and no air is trapped beneath the impression. A photograph of a typical syringe is shown in *Fig.* 16.4*b, c*—and is self-explanatory. Various angles and thicknesses of nozzle are available to ensure access to even the most difficult cavities, including pinholes. It is possible to alter the shape of plastic nozzles to suit an individual case by immersing them in hot water for a few seconds, after which they can be easily bent.

To load the syringe both nozzle and plunger are removed. The impression material is then driven up into the body of the syringe by scraping it across the slab (*Fig.* 16.4*e*). The nozzle and plunger are then replaced and the latter depressed, one finger being kept over the end of the nozzle as this is done, to drive any air out of the syringe. This is now ready for use and is put to one side until

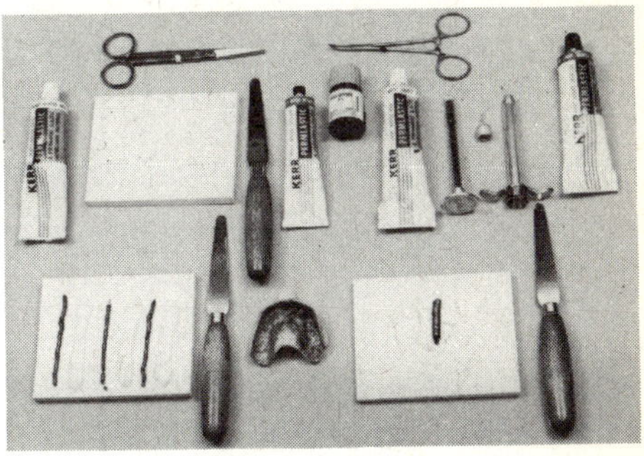

a

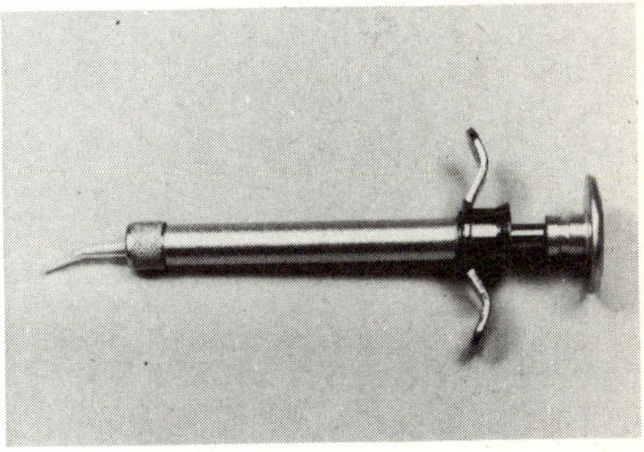

b

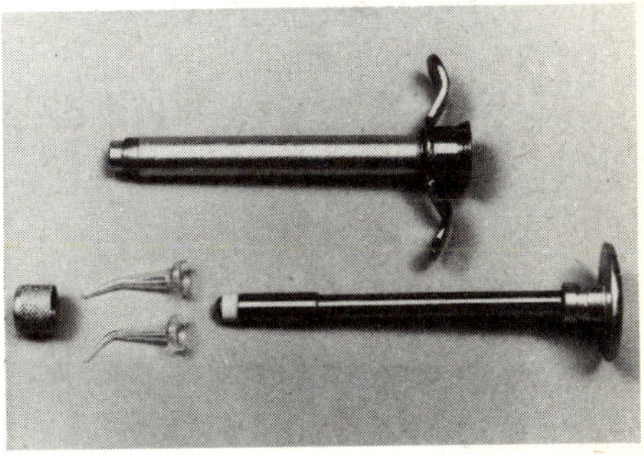

c

Fig. 16.4. *a*, *Trolley laid up for a polysulphide impression including light- and heavy-bodied materials, special tray, syringe and retraction cord. b, c, Syringe used for injecting impression material. Note the fine nozzle for use with pinlays.* (*Continued on page 214*)

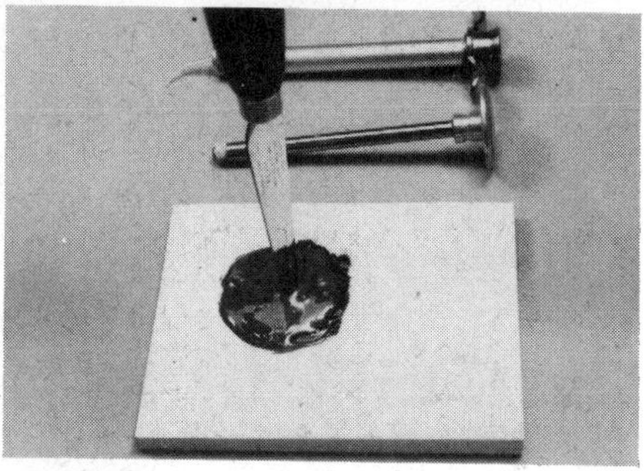

d

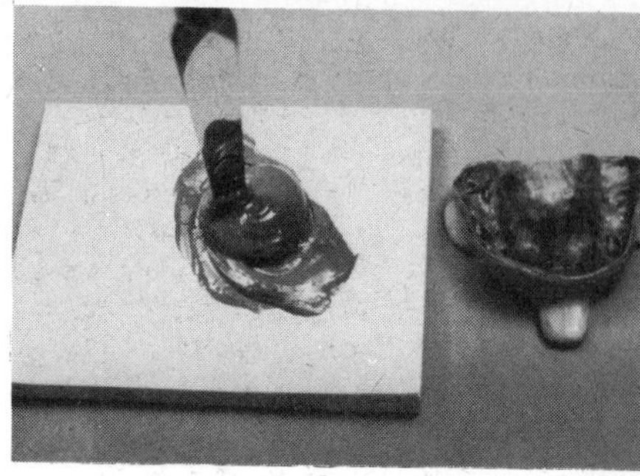

h

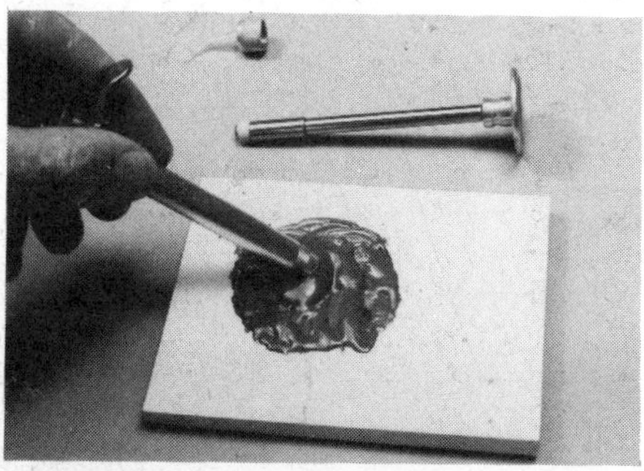

e

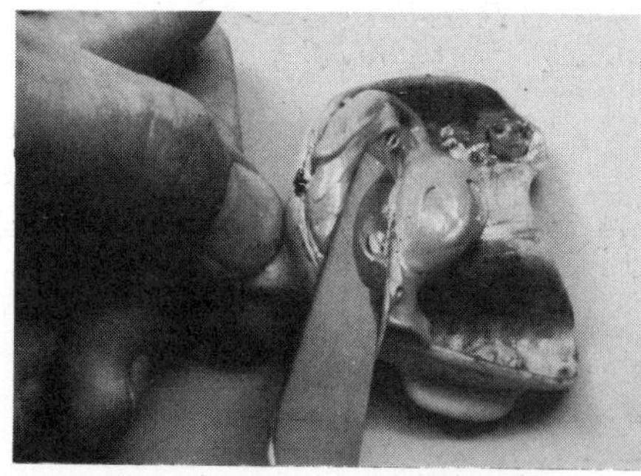

i

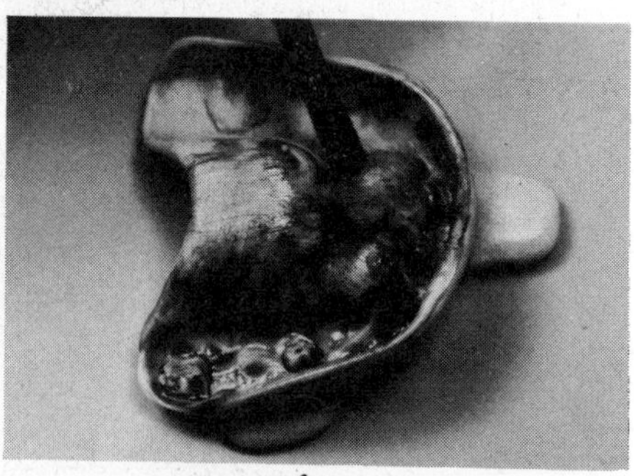

f

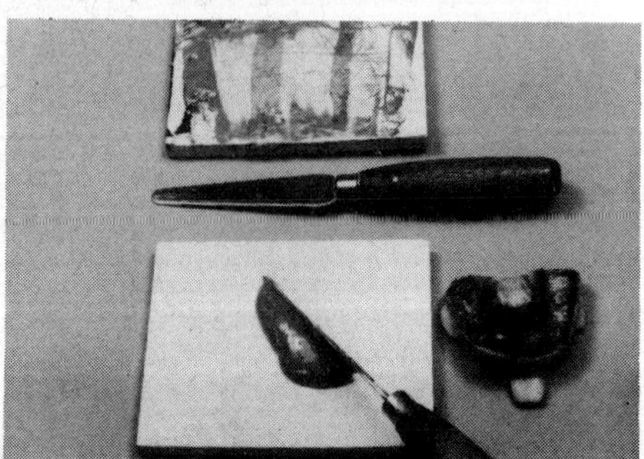

g

Fig. 16.4. *d, The light-bodied polysulphide being mixed, with the spatula held vertically to avoid the incorporation of any air. e, Syringe being loaded by scraping it across the slab with the nozzle removed. f, The special tray being coated with adhesive. g, The heavy-bodied material being transferred to a clean slab for completion of the mix, using a fresh spatula. h, i, Completion of mix of heavy-bodied material (note vertical spatulation) and the loading of the tray.*

the heavy-bodied material is almost mixed as the setting time is adjusted to allow for this procedure.

■ Mixing of Heavy-bodied Material

This is far more difficult to mix completely than the light-bodied type. One of the main problems is the adhesion of the thick unmixed polysulphide rubber to the spatula and to a lesser degree the slab which can result in unmixed material being transferred to the tray. This can be prevented either by coating them prior to mixing with the catalyst which is thinner and less adherent, or by using a two-slab technique which will now be described.

The actual method of mixing is similar to that already discussed for the light-bodied type (*Fig.* 16.4*h*). However, after the mix has been almost completed the material is transferred to another slab and a new spatula used to complete the procedure (*Fig.* 16.4*g*). In this way the unmixed material, which tends to stick to both the first spatula and slab, is eliminated. The material is now ready for loading into the tray (*Fig.* 16.4*i*).

CONSTRUCTION OF SPECIAL TRAY

The special tray is made in such a way that only those records required for the construction of the bridge will be obtained. Thus all the articulating surfaces will be required, the entire surface of all teeth which may be necessary to assess the correct morphology of the bridge, and, finally, in great detail, all the prepared teeth and the adjoining tissues. Most compression will be required in this latter region to force the light-bodied material firmly up around the prepared teeth and thus the tray is taken to maximum depth in this area. Where it is only necessary to record the occlusal surfaces the tray is taken just a little below this level (*Fig.* 16.5).

The tray is relieved by two thicknesses of wax or asbestos in the region of the prepared teeth and by one thickness elsewhere. This is then covered with tin-foil prior to laying down the acrylic. Three or four stops are provided by cutting through the wax to the occlusal surfaces of the unprepared teeth to make certain that the tray will seat correctly in the mouth.

The tray is best constructed of a quick-setting acrylic and must be made sufficiently thick to avoid all chance of fracture or distortion during removal. It should be completed at least 24 hours before use to allow for complete polymerization. The incorporation of flanges in the posterior region is advisable to assist in the removal of the impression.

It is best to try the tray in the mouth to check its extension, make certain it does not hurt the patient and to get used to its exact position when fully seated before taking the actual impression. At this stage any marked undercuts such as

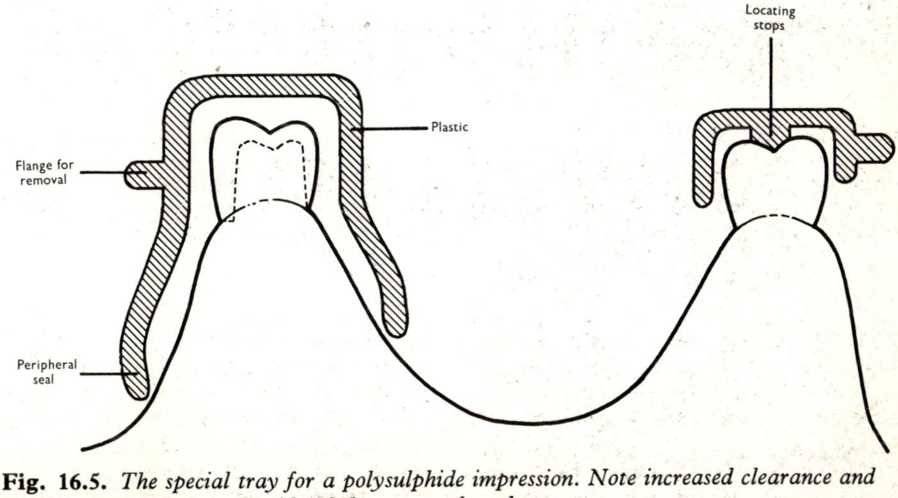

Fig. 16.5. *The special tray for a polysulphide impression. Note increased clearance and maximum extension on the side of the prepared teeth.*

those caused by a sanitary pontic or large interproximal embrasures can be eliminated with soft wax.

The fit surface of the tray is painted with adhesive at least 10 minutes before it is loaded (*Fig.* 16.4*f*). Unless this adhesive is completely dry before it comes into contact with the polysulphide the strength of the bond will be seriously reduced.

INJECTION TECHNIQUE

When all is ready the gingival packs are removed with the possible exception of one fine strand lying below the margins of the preparation which is left in place if it is felt that there is a chance of bleeding occurring whilst the impression is setting, and any excess moisture is blown away. The abutment teeth should be free of blood or any other contamination and their surfaces should be very slightly moist. If they are too dry, which may easily happen in the upper anterior region if the patient's mouth has been open for a long time, the material may adhere to them. If they are too wet, moisture will be trapped beneath the impression, which could cause a discrepancy.

The tip of the syringe is placed in the most difficult point of access and injection is then commenced (*Fig.* 16.6*a*). The nozzle is gradually moved around the margins of the preparation, constantly keeping it in contact with tooth tissue so as to avoid incorporating any air (*Fig.* 16.6*b*, *c*). When the prepared surfaces of the teeth have been coated the other surfaces of these teeth are also covered and finally the pontic area is dealt with. Care must be taken to avoid using too much of the light-bodied material otherwise it will tend to run off the teeth and can produce folds (*Fig.* 16.6*d*) and blow holes as well as inadequate compression from the heavy bodied material in vital areas when the tray is seated.

Immediately injection is completed, the tray, loaded with heavy-bodied material, should be inserted and firmly seated in position, using a rocking motion (*Fig.* 16.6*e*).

TESTING FOR SET

The material will usually set within 6–8 min of insertion. However, the only way in which one can be certain that the impression is ready for removal is by pushing a flat plastic instrument into both the light- and heavy-bodied materials at periodic intervals. When no permanent deformation can be achieved, the impression is left for a further 2 minutes before removal (*Fig.* 16.6*f*). If at the time of injecting the light-bodied material some of it is deposited on to a tooth in the opposing arch, it is easy to check the set without disturbing the tray.

When it is suspected that the impression has been spoilt by bleeding, it is best to leave the impression in the mouth for at least 5 min longer than normal. This will often provide complete haemostasis and a second impression can then be taken immediately after the first is removed. Fresh packing will rarely be necessary.

If appreciable bleeding has occurred it is usually best to abandon the attempt until another visit. A well-fitting temporary bridge will greatly assist in this matter.

MODIFIED TECHNIQUES

There are three occasions when the technique may need modification:

a. Where the control of saliva is very difficult.

b. For pinlays.

c. For post crowns.

■ A. Where Saliva Control is Difficult

This applies in particular to the lower third molars and in these instances it may

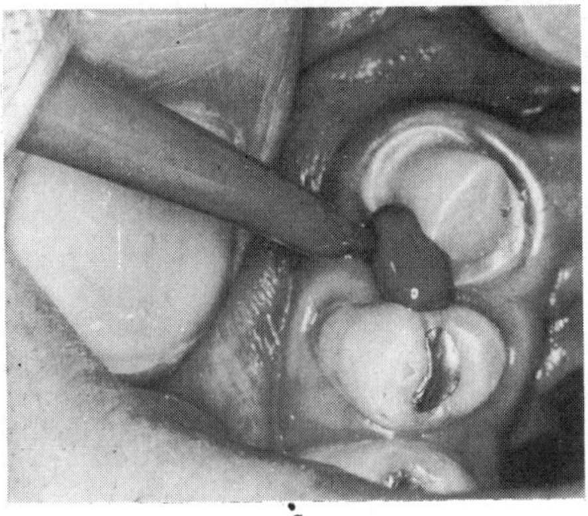

a

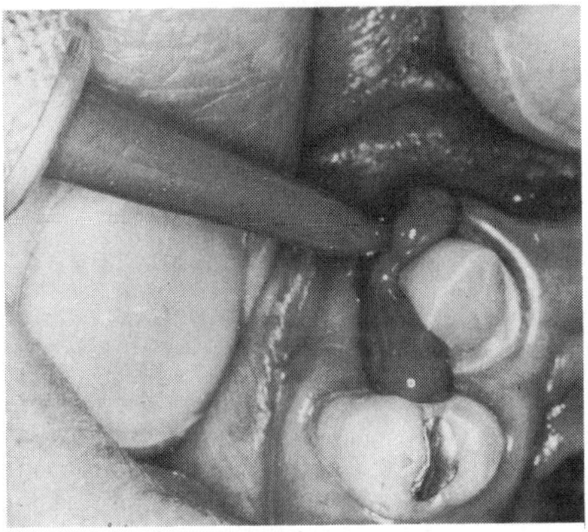

b

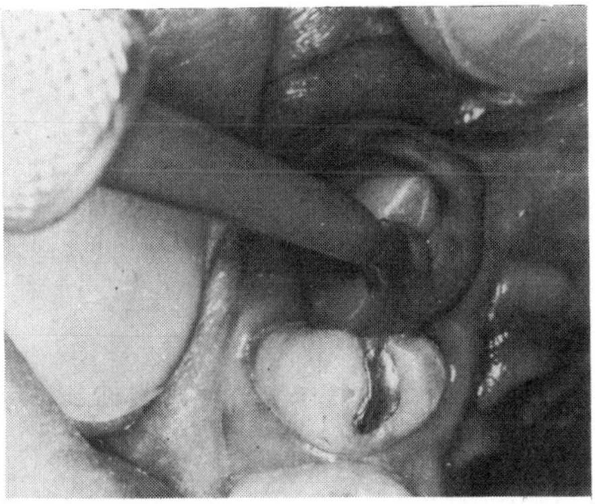

c

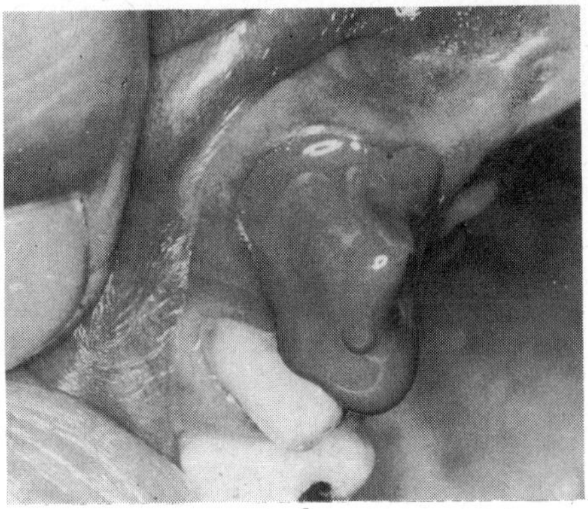

d

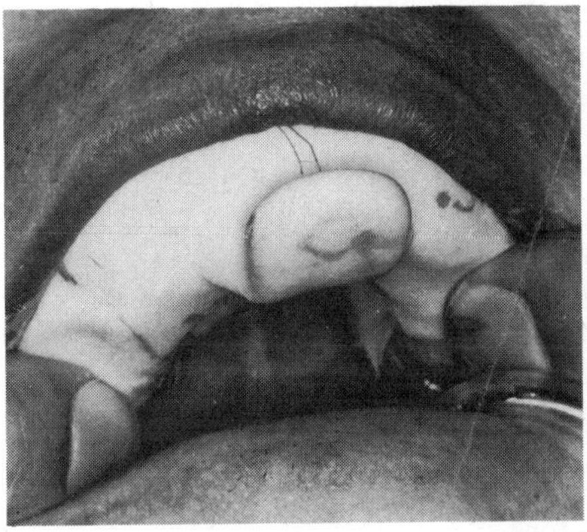

e

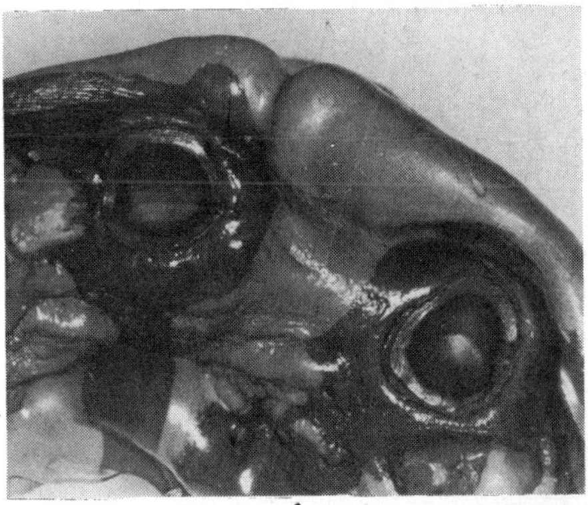

f

Fig. 16.6. *a, Commencement of injection of light-bodied material into gingival crevice. b, c, The injection is continued around the whole margin of the preparation, keeping the syringe in contact with the tooth to prevent air being trapped. d, If too much light-bodied material is injected folds may occur. e, Impression in situ. f, Final impression.*

prove desirable to take an individual impression in a copper ring. This must be rigid and a loose fit otherwise it may distort on removal. The top should be sealed with acrylic or any other suitable material.

The inner aspect and edges of the ring are painted with adhesive and this is allowed to dry. It is then loaded with heavy-bodied polysulphide and seated on to the tooth. Just before taking the impression it is best to get the patient to rinse out thoroughly to try and eliminate any thick saliva and then to quickly isolate the tooth. Antisialogogues may also be of help.

From the copper ring impression a die can be made which may then be seated in an overall impression before it is cast.

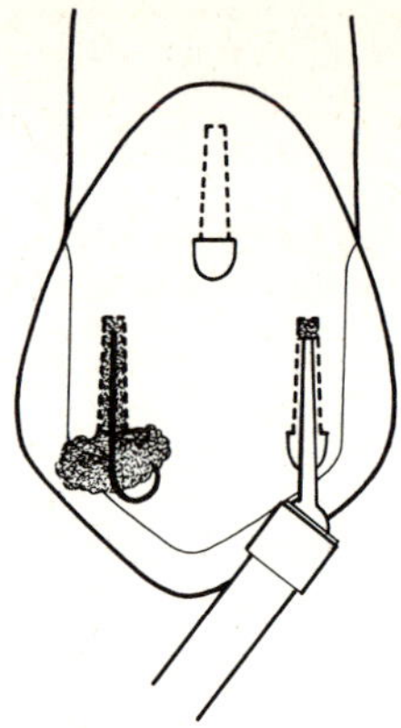

Fig. 16.7. *Rubber base impression material being injected down pinholes, after which stainless-steel wire is inserted.*

■ B. Pinlays

When an impression is being taken of pinlay preparations suitable pins, normally either plastic (perlon), stainless steel or iridioplatinum, will have to be seated in the pin holes beforehand. It is important to make certain that sufficient of the pin protrudes from the tooth for the impression material to grip it firmly. In the case of metal pins they may be bent over to provide more positive retention.

After removal of the impression and before casting, the pins are sleeved. These sleeves will then be incorporated in the model and allow an accurate replacement of the pins to be incorporated in the casting.

Alternatively, where the pin holes are larger, rubber base may be injected down these holes with a very fine nozzle and a spiral root-canal filler used to ensure adequate filling of the holes. This is followed up with a piece of fine stainless-steel wire, coated with adhesive and incorporating a retentive loop at the free end (*Fig*. 16.7).

After this the injection of the rest of the cavity is completed and the overall impression taken.

To achieve the best results a system such as that marketed by Svenska (*see* p. 93) which employs matched drills, impression and retention pins should always be used.

■ C. Post Crowns

There are numerous ways of making post crowns and thus the impression techniques must vary also. Where a prefabricated type of post is to be used, this is seated prior to the impression, unless it is of the screw type. A sufficient amount of the post must protrude from the tooth to make certain that it is withdrawn with the rest of the impression without any displacement.

Where a cast post is to be used the light-bodied rubber base is injected down the root canal and this is then followed up with a stainless-steel post coated with adhesive prior to taking the rest of the impression in the heavy-bodied polysulphide. However, the best results will probably be obtained, as with the pinlays, by using matched drill, impression and pattern pins for instance, that marketed by P.D. (p. 119). Alternatively, a system such as the Wiptam technique described on p. 118 may be employed.

CHECKING OF IMPRESSION

After removal of the impression it should be carefully washed, dried, and checked. Particular points to watch out for are that the impression material is still firmly attached to the tray and that there are no tears in the material which would allow it to distort on casting. Also that the tray is not showing through the impression material, particularly around the margins of the preparation. The trapping of air or blood will be indicated by a smooth round area somewhat shinier than the surrounding material and needs to be looked for very carefully.

After checking, the impression should be cleaned with a detergent, washed, and then poured up (or electroplated) between $\frac{1}{2}$ and 1 hour after removal from the mouth.

It is extremely important that whatever impression material is used it is correctly handled and its assets and limitations are fully understood if a good result is to be obtained (Bell and von Fraunhofer, 1975). This subject is more fully dealt with in the chapter on materials.

TRANSFER COPINGS

Where any doubt exists as to the accuracy of the impression then transfer copings may be used. These are of particular value in complex cases especially those incorporating precision retainers and obviate the need to obtain an accurate impression of every single abutment at the same time.

A model (or models) is made from the impression(s) and copings constructed either in a material such as Duralay or a soft metal, which has the correct peripheral extension and fits the margins accurately. They are also made so that they have positive retention in the overall impression. Each coping is now individually checked in the mouth and if all are satisfactory an impression is taken to record their correct relationship. Should any of the copings fail to fit then an individual impression may be taken of the relevant tooth and a new die and coping made, which may be tried in before the overall impression is taken. Alternatively, the detailed impression of any one tooth can be incorporated in the overall impression but then, of course, a slight risk is being run as the fit of the casting on this tooth will not have been checked prior to completing the bridge, unless a special appointment is made for this purpose.

RECORDING TOOTH COLOUR AND SHADE

This is one of the most difficult aspects of bridge work, as so many factors will affect the choice of the correct shade.

■ Ultraviolet Radiation and Fluorescence

Light may be described as radiation which is detectable by the human eye and fluorescence as the absorption of radiation of a particular wavelength and its re-emission as a radiation of longer wavelength. Ultraviolet light is in the frequency range 30–390 mμ, violet around 400 mμ and red 700 mμ.

Natural teeth fluoresce at the blue and ultraviolet end of the spectrum and also in sunlight and thus ideally dental materials used for aesthetic purposes should do the same.

Unfortunately acrylic does not fluoresce and this is one of the reasons for its variable appearance under different lighting conditions. It will, for instance, virtually disappear in a room lit only by ultraviolet light, however, porcelain can be made to produce a yellow-white fluorescence, similar to natural teeth, by the addition of sodium diuronate to the porcelain frit. This poses no danger to the patient as the level of radiation is very low, but it does mean that technicians should handle the powder with some caution and avoid, for instance, licking their brushes.

Facing Material

First the material which will be used for the construction of the facing must be considered. This will be either acrylic or porcelain.

Acrylic

Although acrylic may provide a good aesthetic result, initially at least, this is not always easy to achieve. The material is relatively translucent and thus the background, which may be either the cementing media or the gold of the box, tends to shadow through. The greater the thickness of the acrylic the less susceptible it will be to its background colour and similarly the darker the shade the less the colour will be altered. Thus it is usually better to err on the side of a darker rather than a lighter shade.

Porcelain

A porcelain facing may be of two types, a manufactured stock pontic such as the long pin and trupontic, which are seldom used nowadays, or it may be made in the laboratory. Examples of the latter are the jacket crowns and also those fabricated from porcelain bonded to gold.

Where a stock porcelain facing is being used the choice is limited to the shades made available by the manufacturer and ideally the actual pontic to be incorporated in the bridge should be tried in to assess if it is satisfactory.

The cementing media has far less effect on porcelain than acrylic. However, it can still influence the result and this is particularly true of the air-fired varieties. With the aluminous and vacuum-fired types the core mass will mask the effect of the cement, except at the cervical margin.

As with acrylic, the thickness of porçelain is important. If it is too thin the core material or cement will shadow through. This is most liable to occur with the lighter shades. The bonded porcelains are especially critical in this respect, a full 1·0 mm of porcelain being necessary if a good aesthetic result is to be achieved.

Light

The light in which the shade is recorded will have an appreciable effect on the correct choice. Although the majority of dental lights are colour-corrected it is still far better in most cases to use daylight, ideally with the patient close to a north-facing window. Direct sunlight is to be avoided as also is the evening and early morning light.

Should the patient be involved in theatrical or similar employment the lighting to which his teeth will be subjected must be considered. Thus the shade of a tooth will vary appreciably under daylight, fluorescent, spot, flood, and flashlights. It may therefore prove necessary to check the shade with several different light sources and consider which will be the most important for each individual case.

Shade Guides

The way in which individual manufacturers' shade guides are laid out varies. However, it is usually best to decide first which colour group is indicated, for instance whether the teeth are basically yellow, brown, or grey. After this it is possible to decide how dark or how light the shade should be.

With a manufactured pontic it is only possible to choose the overall hue and shade, but if the facing is being fabricated in the laboratory it can be made up exactly to requirements as in the case of a porcelain jacket crown. In these instances the best way is to draw a picture of the tooth and mark on this drawing the basic distribution of the various shades and then indicate any additional features required such as staining, check lines, and white spots. A typical shade record is shown in *Fig*. 16.8.

Ideally the technician should always see each case and record the shade himself so that he knows exactly what he is trying to achieve. Unfortunately, however, this is not always possible.

Whereas the shade guide will give a fairly accurate indication of the powders to be used when building up the porcelain it must be borne in mind that each

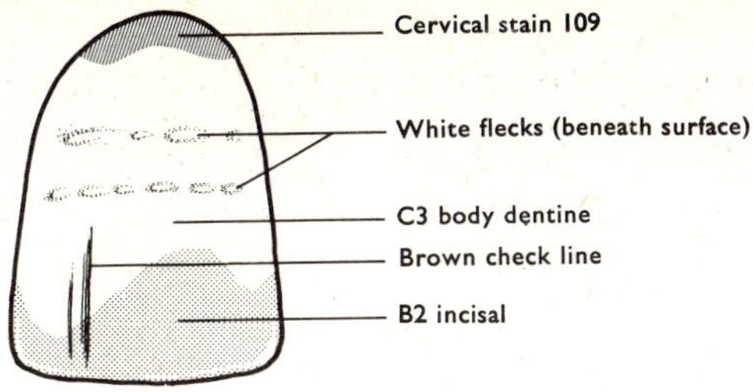

Fig. 16.8. *A typical shade record for a porcelain crown.*

batch of powder produced by the manufacturers varies a little in colour. Thus to achieve the best results small buttons of porcelain should be fired from each batch of powder and these buttons used to check finally the shade prior to build up. Preoperative photographs can be helpful in selecting the shade although both the colour fidelity and stability of most film is somewhat suspect.

■ Alterations of Shade at Fit Stage

Having recorded the shade and constructed the bridge pontic to this the colour may still be modified to some extent at the fit stage if necessary. In the case of the manufactured pontic, surface stains may be added and sometimes low fusing porcelain. With the laboratory-made porcelain facing, particularly the porcelain jacket type, far more extensive changes can be carried out provided that it is tried in with the platinized foil still in place or that it is bonded to metal. Thus, should the incisal shade be incorrect this area may be ground away and replaced. Surface stains may also be added. It is, therefore, sometimes considerably easier to obtain an aesthetically pleasing pontic if it is made in the laboratory.

In conclusion it must be stated that there are so many variables in the assessment of the correct shade for any particular case that it is only with considerable experience and in particular a close liaison with the laboratory that consistently good aesthetic results can be achieved.

For further consideration of shade taking the reader is referred to textbooks which deal with laboratory technique.

TEMPORARY BRIDGES

After completing the preparation of the teeth, obtaining a detailed impression, taking occlusal records, and deciding on the correct shade, it is desirable to fit a temporary bridge before dismissing the patient. This has many advantages:

1. It protects the teeth, avoiding any discomfort for the patient and preventing damage to the preparations.
2. It provides an aesthetically acceptable temporary prosthesis.
3. It stabilizes the abutment teeth and maintains their correct relationship to each other.
4. It prevents any over-eruption of the abutment and opposing teeth.

The main property required of a temporary bridge is that, at least in the anterior region, it will be aesthetically acceptable. It must also be comfortable for the patient, smooth to the tongue, strong enough to resist the forces of mastication, and capable of removal and reinsertion without damage.

It is important that it should cause the minimum of gingival irritation and in this respect care must always be taken to trim and polish the margins carefully. A slightly negative edge is to be preferred to a positive one, as any overhang is always likely to have an adverse effect (*Fig.* 16.9). This may lead to gingival recession and thus when the bridge is

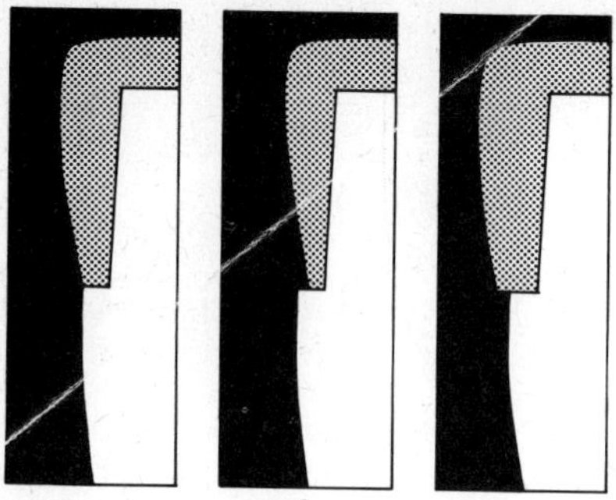

Fig. 16.9. *The margins of a temporary bridge. a An accurate fit at the gingival margin is obviously best. However, a negative edge b is to be preferred to a positive one c because less gingival irritation will result.*

fitted the margins of the retainers will be exposed.

The tissue contact of the temporary bridge in the pontic area needs to be fairly precise otherwise depression or proliferation of the tissues in this region may be stimulated.

■ Methods of Construction

There are several ways of making a temporary bridge and the selection of which type to use will depend on its size, the individual operator's preference and, above all, how long it has got to last. Thus if it has only to be in situ for 10–14 days, the time usually taken by a laboratory to construct the prosthesis, then it may usually be made entirely of acrylic or an epimine resin. However, if it has to remain in place for several months or possibly even up to a year, because it has been used as an immediate replacement or it is felt best to await the outcome of periodontal therapy before placing the permanent prosthesis, then gold and acrylic are usually best employed because of the greater strength obtained and the reduction in wear which may be achieved, thus preventing any movement of the teeth and alteration of the occlusion.

Thus the provision of temporary bridges will be divided into two types: (*a*) short-term and (*b*) long-term.

■ Short-term Temporary Bridges

If any existing fixed prosthesis is being remade it is usually best to modify this and use it as a temporary restoration. The fit will obviously be poor after the teeth have been re-prepared but this can be remedied by relining it with acrylic. This is best done in the mouth, the prepared teeth being greased and the bridge retainers filled with a self-curing acrylic and then replaced in the mouth. The bridge is removed before the acrylic is set hard and then taken in and out several times to make certain that it will not be too tight a fit. A possible disadvantage of this technique is the exothermia of the acrylic which could affect the pulp. After the acrylic has set completely the margins are trimmed and polished and it may then be replaced with a temporary cementing media such as a quick-setting zinc oxide and eugenol cement. If retention is good it may be best to grease the abutment teeth first and only put the temporary cement around the margins of the crowns.

If no previous bridge exists there are three common ways in which the temporary restoration may be constructed.

a. From the Original Study Models

This method has the advantage that the bridge is constructed, usually at the same time as the special tray, before the teeth are prepared.

The abutment teeth are shaped on the original study model so that they approximate to the final preparations. They are always under-prepared so that the temporary bridge will fit easily in the mouth. This is now waxed up, processed in acrylic, and polished. Final adjustments to the occlusion, contacts, etc., can be made in the mouth. The fit may be improved if necessary by relining it with a cold curing acrylic at the chairside.

b. From a Model of the Completed (or almost Completed) Preparations

In this case an impression is taken as soon as the preparation of the teeth has been almost completed. A model is then cast from this on which the temporary bridge is made. If there is a laboratory close to hand the bridge can usually be constructed, using self-curing acrylic, by the time the operator has finalized the preparations and taken detailed impressions and occlusal records.

Alternatively, if the final impressions are not to be taken at this visit, individual temporary crowns may be placed and the temporary bridge prepared for placement at the next visit. It is only after the taking of the impressions on which the bridge will be made that it is essential to prevent all tooth movement.

c. In the Mouth

i. Using an Impression 'Mould'

In many ways this is the simplest of all techniques and involves no laboratory time or expense. It has the advantages that the original morphology of the teeth is exactly reproduced in the temporary bridge and that the occlusion should always be correct.

An impression of the teeth in the region of the bridge is taken before they are prepared, preferably with one of the silicone impression materials. This will give extremely good reproduction of the fine detail of the labial surfaces of the teeth. It also stores far better than an alginate impression. If there is no tooth present where the future pontic will be this can be simulated in wax. Alternatively, if a prosthesis is already present the impression may be taken with this in place.

Instead of taking an impression in the mouth one can be taken of the model (*Fig.* 16.10*c*) after the pontics have been built up on this in wax (*Fig.* 16.10*a, b*). The advantage of this is that it is easier to build up the pontics out of the mouth and keep them in place while the impression is being taken. Another advantage is that the labial or palatal aspects of the abutment teeth may be thickened with wax on the model which will result in a stronger temporary bridge.

The impression is now laid on one side until the preparation of the teeth is completed. At this stage it is trimmed to remove any excess and to enable it to be taken in and out of the mouth easily. It need only extend a little way beyond the cervical margins of the teeth.

Relief channels are cut in the impression on its lingual aspect next to the abutments which are now isolated and greased. The area of the impression containing the preparations is filled with a suitable plastic such as Kerr's Tempspan,* which is a quick-curing acrylic, Scutan† which is an epimine plastic (*Fig.* 16.10*d*) or Trim‡ which is based on butyl methacrylate. The latter two materials have the advantage that they generate far less heat than a conventional acrylic and flow more easily. The materials may be injected into the impression (*Fig.* 16.10*e, f, g*) in the region of the abutments and pontic by means of the special syringe provided (*Fig.* 16.10*h*) or by using any of the plastic disposable medical syringes without a needle. This will avoid any air bubbles and thus porosity. The impression is now seated in the mouth, using firm, continuous pressure. The relief channels on the lingual aspects of the abutments will allow any excess to flow out. It is best to remove the impression initially before the material has completely set, to make certain that the temporary bridge will come away from the teeth easily (*Fig.* 16.10*i*). After this it can be reinserted until the material is hard. It is then removed, trimmed, polished and the occlusion and contacts adjusted before cementing it into place with a material such as a quick-setting zinc oxide (*Fig.* 16.10*j*). The strength of some temporary cementing media such as Tempbond* may be modified to suit the retention required in any specific instance.

---

* Kerr Mfg Co., Romulus, Michigan 48174, USA.
† Espe, GMbH, Seefeld/Oberbay, W. Germany.
‡ Harry J. Bosworth Co., Chicago, Illinois 60605, USA.

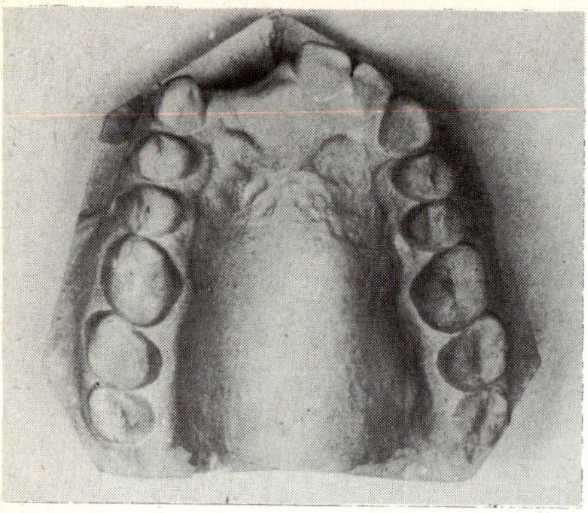

a

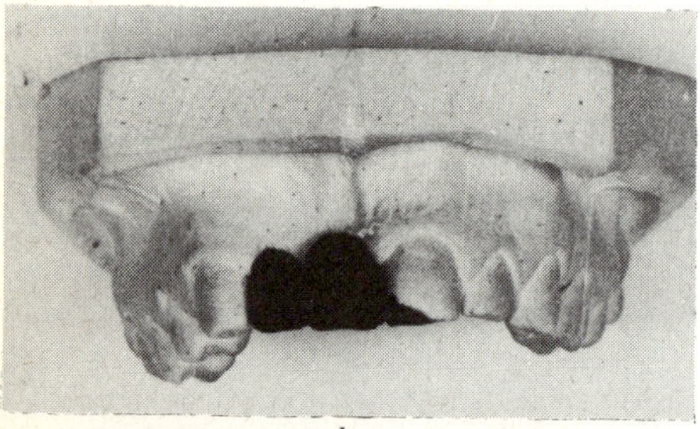

b

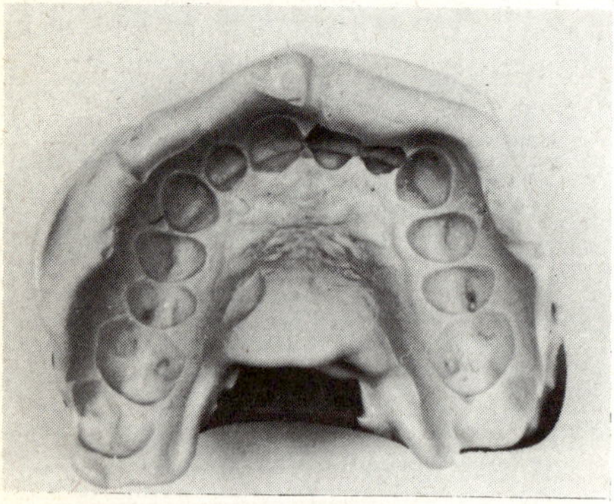

c

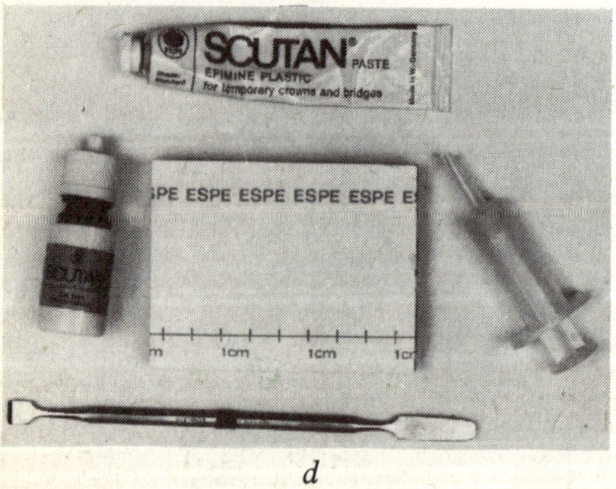
SCUTAN® PASTE
EPIMINE PLASTIC
for temporary crowns and bridges
ESPE ESPE ESPE ESPE ESPE
1cm 1cm

d

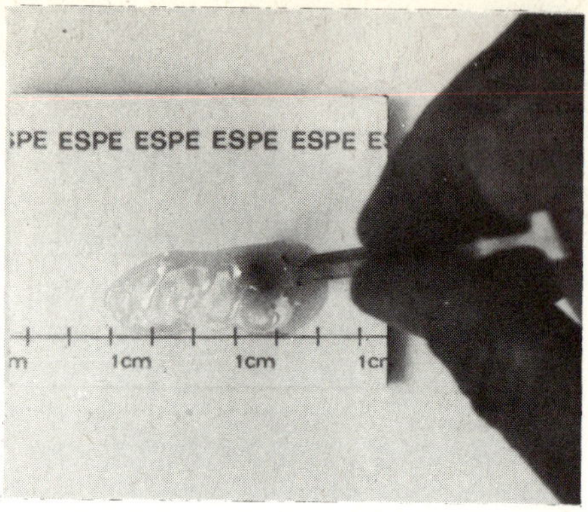
ESPE ESPE ESPE ESPE ESPE
1cm 1cm

e

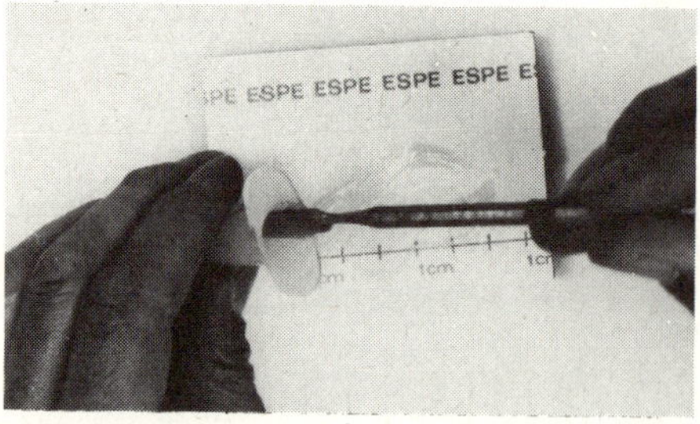
ESPE ESPE ESPE ESPE ESPE

f

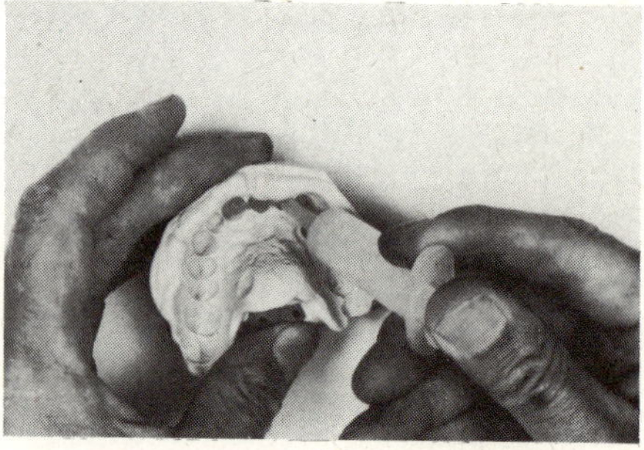

g

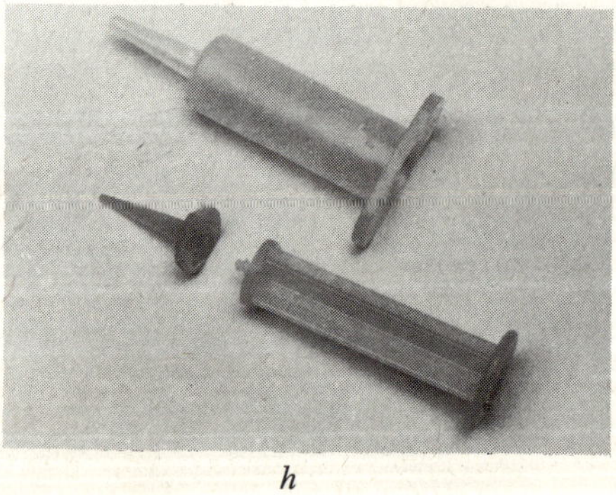

h

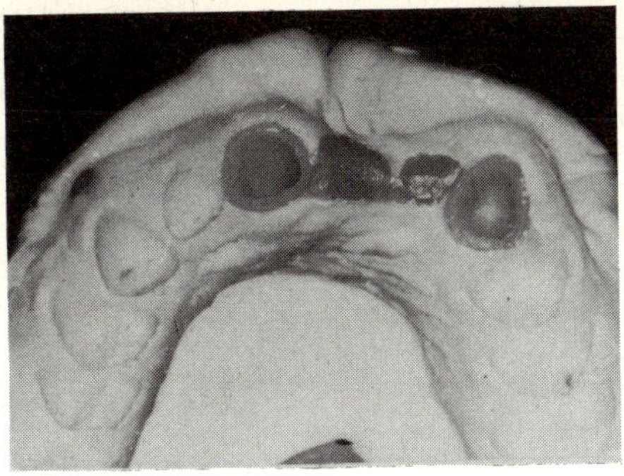

i

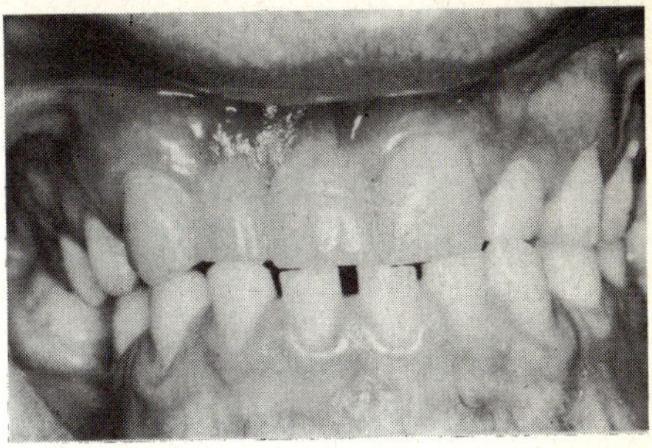

j

Fig. 16.10. *a, b, A model is made on which the missing teeth are waxed-up together with any defects of the teeth to be crowned. c, A silicone impression is taken of the model. d, The temporary bridge kit, consisting of epimine plastic, catalyst, mixing slab, and gun. e, Vertical spatulation is used to prevent the incorporation of air. f, Loading of the syringe. g, Injection of the plastic into the impression. h, Syringe for injecting temporary-bridge material. A thread is incorporated on the end of the barrel to engage any residual material and simplify its removal. i, The silicone impression containing the temporary bridge. j, The temporary bridge in situ.*

Finally it is important that the margins be carefully checked to make certain that no excess of the cementing medium is left subgingivally where it may result in irritation.

ii. Hand Moulded Quick-curing Acrylic
If only a relatively simple temporary bridge is required it may be constructed by moulding a mass of quick-curing acrylic to fit the abutment teeth and then getting the patient to bite on it. The pontic can be roughly shaped up at the same time. The whole is then removed from the mouth for trimming, shaping and polishing. Where necessary, additions may be made. The main disadvantages of this method are that the acrylic tends to be porous and that considerable heat is generated when it is setting. It must also be borne in mind that the self-curing methyl methacrylate resins will cause appreciably more soft-tissue irritation than the epimine plastics such as Scutan (Dahl et al., 1974).

Pinlays and Post Crowns
When placing a temporary bridge over a pinlay it is important to prevent the cement passing up into the pin holes where it will be difficult to remove. The easiest way of doing this is by inserting paper points, soaked in a material such as cavity varnish, into the pinholes before placing the temporary bridge. On no account should plain paper points be used as they will swell when moist and be very difficult to remove.

An alternative is to use plastic pins a little smaller in diameter than the drills used for the pinholes. The advantages of this technique are that the pins are easy to remove and that they provide a suitable anchorage point for the rest of the temporary restoration, which will usually be made of acrylic.

In the case of post crowns a pledget of cotton-wool, impregnated with grease, or a piece of gutta percha may be inserted into the root canal, leaving just enough space for a short post for the temporary bridge.

■ Long-term Temporary Bridges
These have many applications. Thus they may be used after the traumatic loss of a

tooth or when one has to be extracted for a variety of reasons. They are usually designed to last until a suitable time has come for the placing of a permanent prosthesis. This may be after complete healing has taken place following an extraction or when periodontal therapy has been completed, and the prognosis of the other teeth can be more accurately assessed. An asset is that the prosthesis may be removed as and when necessary to assist in any periodontal surgery.

A big advantage of using temporary bridges as opposed to dentures is that far less harm is likely to occur to the periodontium in general and that of the teeth adjoining the gap in particular. Moreover the degree of soft-tissue loss is likely to be less (*Fig*. 16.17). A further advantage is that whereas a temporary denture may be difficult to provide as in *Fig*. 16.12, because of lack of space between the lower incisors and the palate in which to accommodate the plate this creates no difficulty so far as a bridge is concerned. Indeed patients will usually be far happier with a temporary bridge than a denture however well this is constructed.

Several methods exist of constructing temporary bridges and some of these have already been mentioned by Mr Tay in Chapter 13. Another alternative is to screw threaded pins into the teeth on either side of the gap and then fix the pontic onto these with an auto-polymerizing acrylic resin.

Although it may be thought that temporary bridgework is much more expensive than a denture the difference in

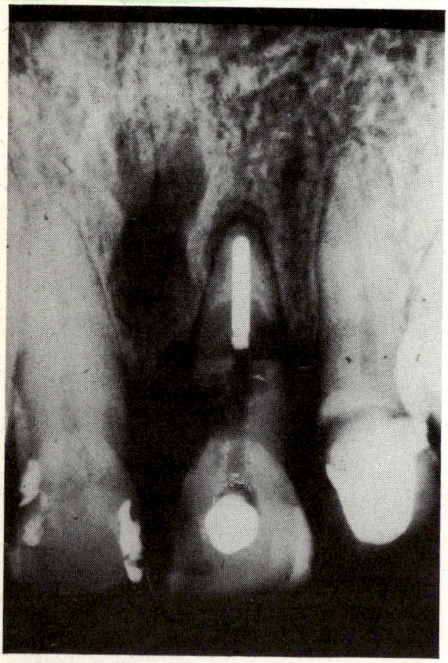

Fig. 16.11. *Root resorption making the loss of* |1 *inevitable.*

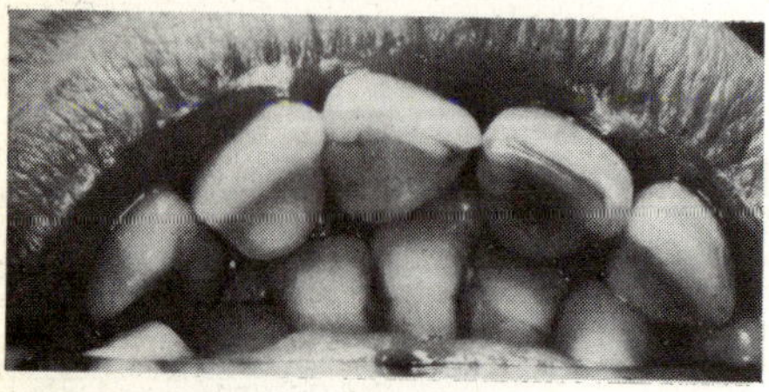

Fig. 16.12. *An extremely close bite leaving no space for a temporary partial denture* (see also Fig. 16.16).

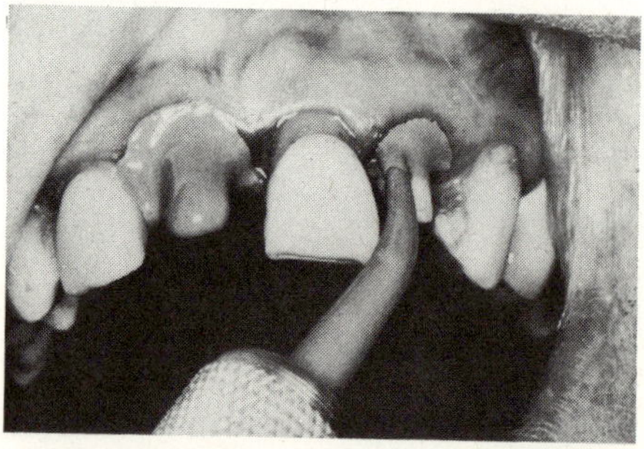

a

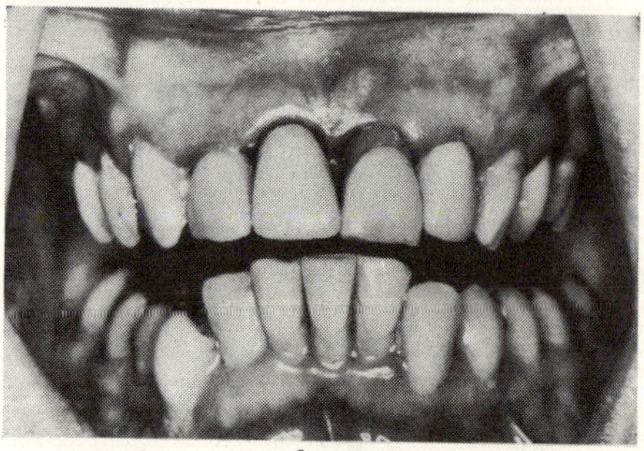

b

Fig. 16.13. *a, b Teeth on either side of the one to be extracted were prepared, impressions taken and temporary crowns placed.*

cost between the two is probably relatively small when one bears in mind that the abutment teeth will have to be prepared in any case when the permanent bridge is provided. When a tooth has to be extracted (*Fig*. 16.11) but is giving only minor symptoms, the teeth on either side may be prepared first, an accurate impression taken (*Fig*. 16.13), temporary crowns placed and a model made (*Fig*. 16.14) on which crowns may be constructed for the proposed abutment teeth. These are then tried in and if satisfactory the tooth to be extracted is then removed from the model and the temporary bridge made. In the particular case illustrated it was anticipated that it would be required for 1–2 years and thus, in view of the occlusion (*Fig*. 16.12), was constructed in gold and acrylic with gold on the occluding surfaces to make certain that no wear and consequent over-eruption of the opposing teeth, took place.

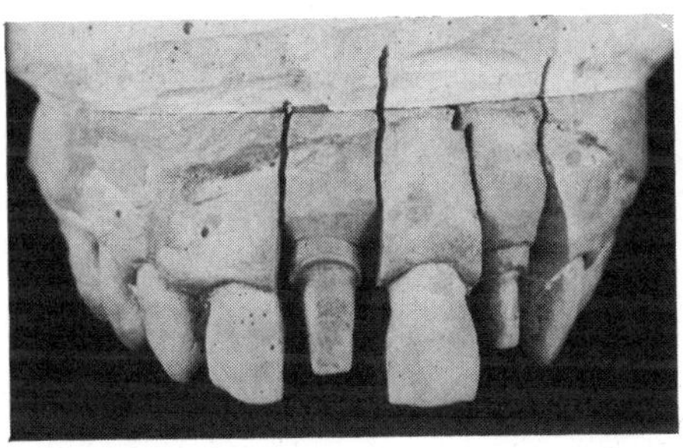

Fig. 16.14. *A model was made on which initially crowns were constructed for 1|2.*

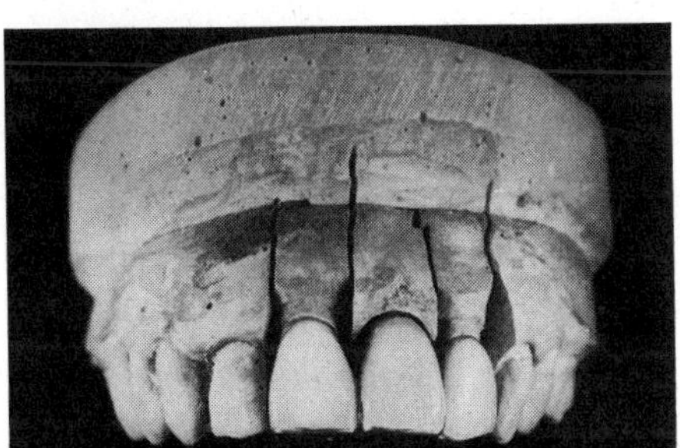

Fig. 16.15. *After the crowns had been checked |1 was removed from the model and a pontic fabricated which was soldered to the retainers.*

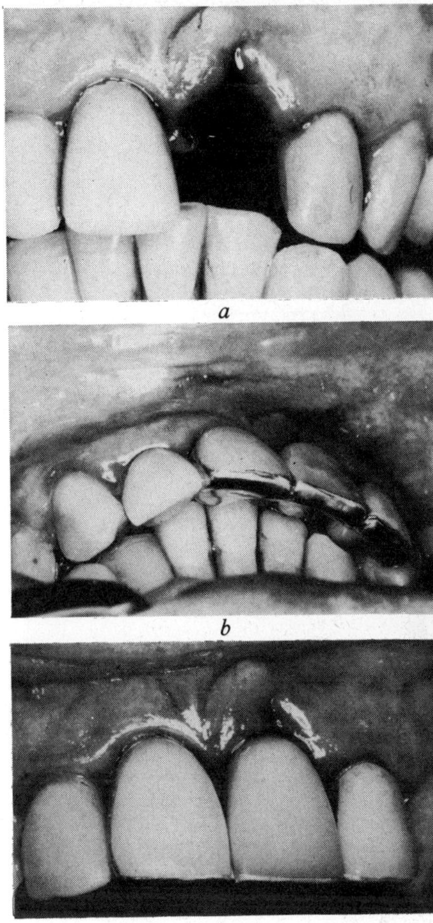

Fig. 16.16. *a, b, c. The |1 was extracted and the bridge placed. Note difficult occlusion contraindicating a removable prosthesis.*

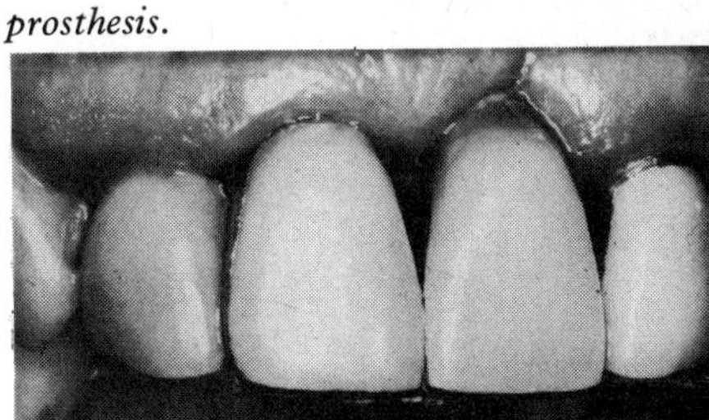

Fig. 16.17. *The temporary bridge 4 months after placement. Note how little recession has occurred around the abutments and the relatively small loss of soft tissue beneath the pontic.*

The tooth is now extracted (*Fig.* 16.16*a*) and the temporary bridge placed. (*Fig.* 16.16*b, c*). It is interesting to see how little soft-tissue loss has taken place around the abutments or beneath the pontic after some 4 months (*Fig.* 16.17).

Some 2 years later when all the periodontal and conservative treatment had been completed and seen to be satisfactory the temporary bridge was removed and an overall impression taken for the construction of the permanent prosthesis. No further tooth preparation proved to be necessary and thus the dies from the original model, provided they were undamaged, could have been used, and transferred to the new impression prior to casting. However in practice it is probably safer and easier to make an entirely new model on which to construct the permanent prosthesis.

Bibliography

Impression Techniques

Bell J. W., Davies E. H. and von Fraunhofer J. A. (1975) The dimensional changes of elastomeric impression material under various degrees of humidity. *J. Dent.* **4**, 73.

Bell J. W. and von Fraunhofer J. A. (1975) The handling of elastomeric impression materials. A review. *J. Dent.* **3**, 229.

Ellam A. H. and Smith D. C. (1966) The relative effectiveness of adhesives for polysulphide impression materials. *Br. Dent. J.* **120**, 135.

Ferguson N. C. and Strode J. (1970) Accurate thiokol impressions for crown and bridge prosthodontics. *J. Can. Dent. Assoc.* **36**, 336.

Joseph E. K. (1965) Gingival retraction in conservative dentistry. *Dent. Practnr Dent. Rec.* **15**, 359.

Scrivner E. I. (1971) Gingival tissue management during fixed prosthodontic procedures. *Dent. Clin. North Am.* **15**, 587.

Wilson C. A. and Tay W. M. (1977) Alum solution as an adjunct to gingival retraction. *Br. Dent. J.* **142**, 155.

(*See also* references in Chapter 4, under Impression Materials)

Shade Taking and Temporary Bridges

Armstrong S. R. (1971) Dentist-laboratory communications. *Dent. Clin. North Am.* **15**, 577.

Braden M. and Causton B. E. (1970) Epimine temporary denture material. *J. Dent. Res.* **50**, 690.

Dahl B. L., Tronstad L. and Spangberg L. (1974) Biological tests of a temporary crown and bridge material. *J. Oral. Rehabit.* **I**, 299.

17

OCCLUSAL RECORDS

Simple Bridges . Extensive Bridge Prostheses . Bite Transfers
Combined Reconstruction of Opposing Quadrants
Wax Additive Techniques
Fully Adjustable Articulator

BRIAN J. PARKINS

Having obtained an accurate impression of the prepared bridge abutments, the pontic area, the occluding surfaces of all the teeth in both arches and the whole of the crowns of the teeth which may be required to assess the correct morphology of the pontic, it is then necessary to record the occlusion. Not only is it desirable to do this with the mandible in centric relation but also in other pertinent maxillo-mandibular positions.

The presence of any interferences or prematurities in the finished bridge would greatly jeopardize the life of the restoration by increasing its liability to cementation failure and by producing a breakdown of the supporting tissues of the abutment teeth.

The interferences in lateral excursions result in a most damaging stimulus to the periodontium. Lateral forces applied to the teeth will eventually bring about both qualitative and quantitative changes in the supporting tissues which will manifest themselves clinically as increasing mobility.

The degree of accuracy required of the occlusal recordings varies with the complexity of the case. Thus with a relatively simple three-unit bridge with standing teeth both in front and behind, a fairly straightforward procedure may be adopted. However, with a complex bridge involving, say, 7–8 teeth and particularly when the entire occlusal anatomy will be lost and have to be rebuilt on one side, a far more elaborate technique has to be employed in order to reproduce the various relationships of the occlusal surfaces in the laboratory.

SIMPLE BRIDGES

It can be said, with little definite evidence but a great deal of experience, that most single-unit, three-unit, and to a lesser extent even larger restorations, have in the past been made successfully without using any form of articulator.

The probable explanation is the care which has been taken to ensure that there were no 'high spots' in the intercuspal position, and no interferences on either the working or non-working sides of the arch in both right and left lateral excursions.

It would therefore appear that this technique should be considered adequate for simple bridges and quite rightly so in view of the success of the restorations made in this way. However, it must be pointed out that although they conform to the physiological adaptation of the patient, and are therefore within 'normal' limits, they almost certainly do not provide the 'ideal' restoration of the occlusal anatomy necessary for maximum functional efficiency.

Bearing these points in mind in the construction of a three-unit posterior bridge, it is doubtful if much improvement can be made in their construction if the following approach is used as a guideline:

1. Preparation of the Whole Occlusion

A mouth which requires a bridge will almost certainly have a deranged occlusion because of the loss of continuity of one of the arches. This will mainly be due to the teeth adjacent to the space tilting and producing interferences (*see Fig.* 2.2, p. 8).

Thus prior to any preparation of the abutment teeth, the entire occlusion should be examined and if necessary corrected. The reader is referred to more extensive works for a detailed description of these techniques, as only a brief outline can really be given in a book of this nature.

Basically the aims of all equilibration techniques are to produce:

a. Maximum contact of the teeth when the mandible is in the most retruded position. Often the intercuspal position is about 1 mm anterior to the most retruded position, and is considered acceptable provided this shift is no greater than about 1·5 mm and in a straight line in an antero-posterior direction.

In such cases there must be good support for the mandible in the most retruded position, though of course this will not now be intercuspation, to permit other oral physiological functions such as deglutition.

b. There must be no interferences to mandibular movement in any direction, either lateral, protrusive, and, in the cases described in (*a*), 'retrusive', so that the patient can pass from one position to another at will.

c. The contact area on the cusps should be as small as can be attained and as near as possible towards the tip of the cusp.

d. There should be no cross-arch contact. In left lateral excursions of the mandible there should be no contact on the right side of the arch, and similarly there should be no contact on the left side of the arch in right lateral excursions.

If the foregoing procedures are followed correctly the mouth will then present a favourable 'occlusal environment' for any restoration. The intercuspal position will coincide with the most retruded position of the mandible (centric relation) and there will be no interferences in lateral excursions.

2. Preparation of the Abutment Teeth and Retainers

The abutment teeth are next prepared in the usual way, ensuring that sufficient occlusal reduction is carried out to allow for the correct thickness of material to cover and protect the teeth both in centric and lateral excursions of the mandible.

Impressions are taken of both arches, and mounted in the intercuspal position, which should coincide with centric relation if the equilibration has been properly executed.

A plane line articulator can be used for this procedure and the cuspal inclinations required estimated from those present on the existing natural teeth. Occasionally difficulty may be experienced in accurately locating the two models. In these cases use may be made of bite transfers which are mentioned later in this chapter.

The bridge is now constructed, care being taken to attain the correct cusp/fossa/ridge relationship of the restorations with regard to the opposing teeth.

3. Cementation of the Bridge

When the completed restoration is offered to the mouth, it is better to leave the gold occlusal surfaces unpolished (sandblasted) and the porcelain occlusal surfaces unglazed. This makes the marking of the occlusal anatomy with articulating papers or crayon far easier.

It should be realized that the final bridge will only be an approximation of the true occlusal anatomy and cuspal inclines, no matter how much care has been taken up to this stage. With the best will in the world nothing more can be hoped for when using the plane line articulator.

A final readjustment of the occlusion is now carried out using the same 'laws' of equilibration as when preparing the whole of the mouth. After this the bridge is polished or glazed and finally cemented, when the occlusion is checked once again.

EXTENSIVE BRIDGE PROSTHESES

If the restoration or restorations are going to re-establish an entire quadrant or the anterior portion of either arch, a semi-adjustable articulator should be used. Examples of these include the Dentatus (*Fig*. 17.1*a*), Hanau Model H, and the Whip-Mix.

They are termed 'semi-adjustable' because they cannot reproduce the exact movements executed by the mandible. The technique of obtaining records (to be described later) includes only the registration of the centric position, the protrusive position, and both lateral excursions. Although these will be correct for the commencement and completion of each excursion, it assumes that the paths between the recordings are straight lines. We are now able to show by using a pantograph that this is not true. The excursions, excepting perhaps the protrusive one, consist of curved paths.

This is why these instruments must be regarded as only semi-adjustable, although to be fair their design was originally intended for use in the construction of complete denture prostheses.

Dentatus Articulator

The use of the Dentatus instrument (*Fig*. 17.1*a*) will be described here to illustrate the principles involved in the use of a semi-adjustable articulator.

The treatment of a case needing a

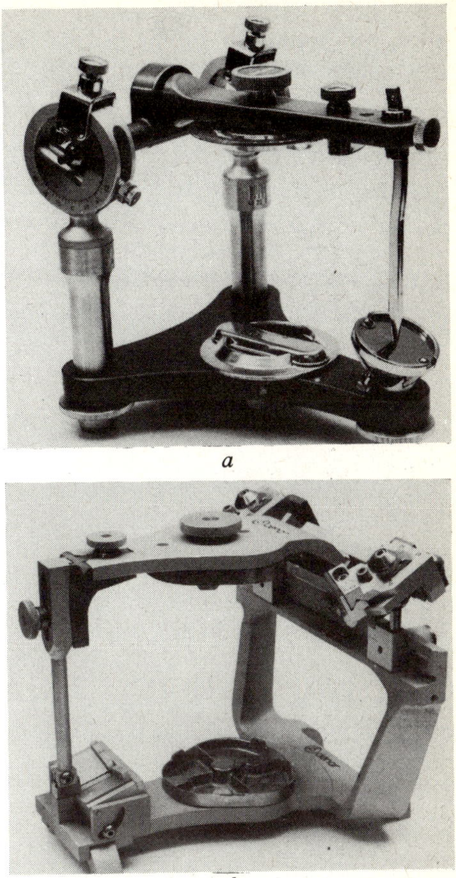

a

b

Fig. 17.1. *a, The Dentatus ARL model. An example of a semi-adjustable articulator. b, The Denar Instrument, which is a fully adjustable articulator.*

quadrant reconstruction requires an initial approach similar to that described earlier for three-unit restorations.

Face Bow Recordings

Face bow recordings are taken only for orientation of the maxillary cast on the instrument. This is achieved by using a point 13 mm anterior to the tragus of the ear on a line joining this with the outer canthus of the eye. This should be marked on the skin and then the earpiece of the face bow centred over it (*Fig*. 17.2*a*).

This is easier said than done because the adjustment of this type of face bow is difficult. It is necessary to locate the earpieces in a position where they exactly centre over the marks on the skin (*Fig.* 17.2*b*).

At the same time even pressure must be exerted on these sites and identical numerical readings obtained on the adjustments on both sides. Everything has then got to be maintained in its correct relationship whilst the locking nuts are tightened, which is no easy task and makes it difficult to obtain accurate recordings.

The procedure has now been made simpler and more convenient by the introduction of a face bow which utilizes the external auditory meatus as the location point. The Whip-Mix articulator is designed to be used with such a face bow.

Either wax or impression compound may be used on the bite fork, although it is best to keep the amount employed to a minimum and the indentations of the teeth as shallow as is compatible with retaining the upper model in a stable position when it is being mounted.

The infra-orbital pointer is used to form a third point of reference on the Frankfurt plane, before the face bow is removed from the patient. It is centred on the infra-orbital notch.

Face Bow Transfer

The face bow is now transferred to the articulator (*Fig*. 17.2*c*) and the maxillary cast mounted on this. The lower model is then located using a suitable material (*see later*) to record centric relation, with no tooth contact but minimal opening of the vertical relationship. This is the most important transfer record and, if the initial equilibration has been correctly followed, should coincide with the intercuspal position. If this is not so, and one is sure of the equilibration procedure, an error has occurred in the face bow transfer. However, an error in the recording of centric relation is far more serious than a mistake in transferring the face bow.

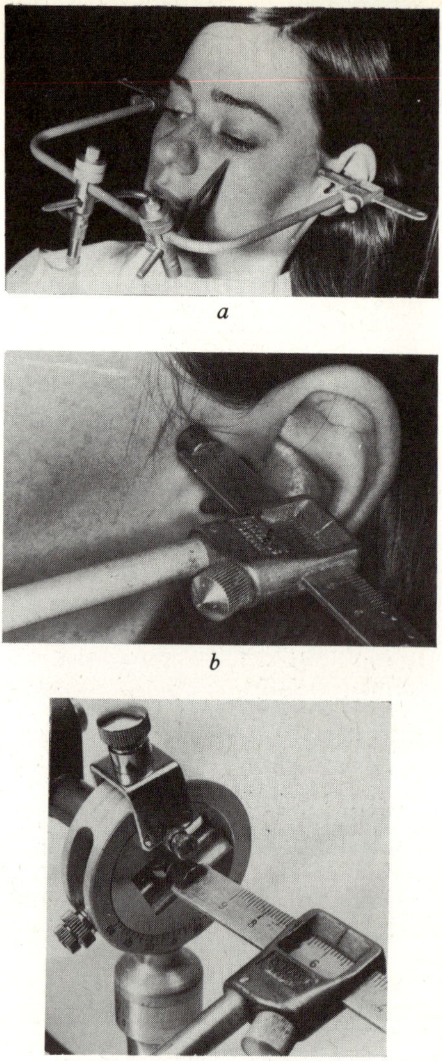

a

b

c

Fig. 17.2. *a, The Dentatus face bow. b, The location point is 13 mm anterior to the tragus along the line joining the tragus to the outer canthus of the eye. c, The face bow location on the articulator.*

A more accurate method of transferring the face bow recording than the foregoing is to locate, mark and transfer the retruded hinge axis of the patient.

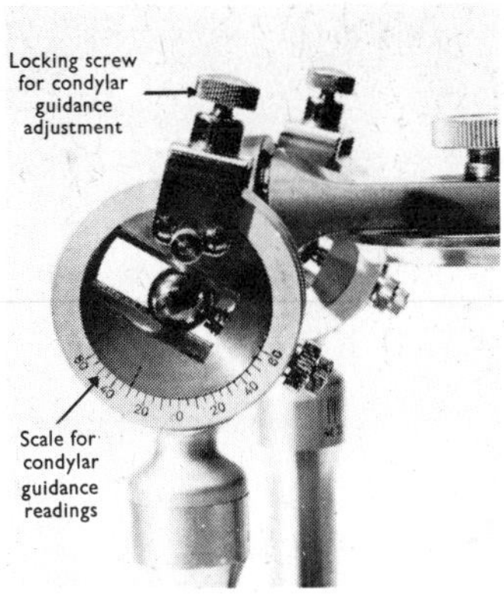

a

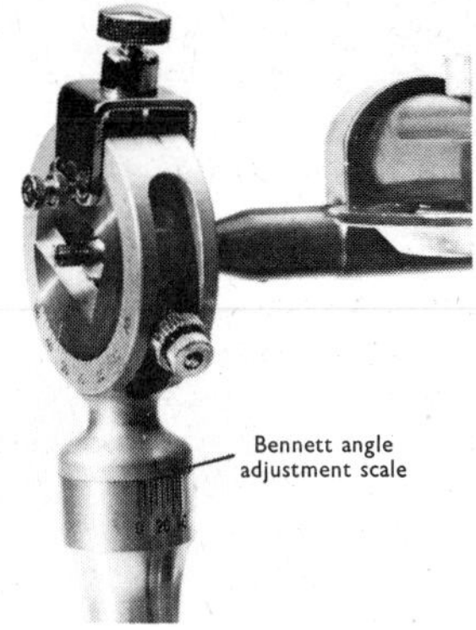

b

Fig. 17.3. *a, The condylar guidance adjustment mechanism on the Dentatus articulator. The figures on the scale are only arbitrary numbers which can be noted and reproduced at a later stage in the treatment. b, The Bennett angle reading is taken from the scale.*

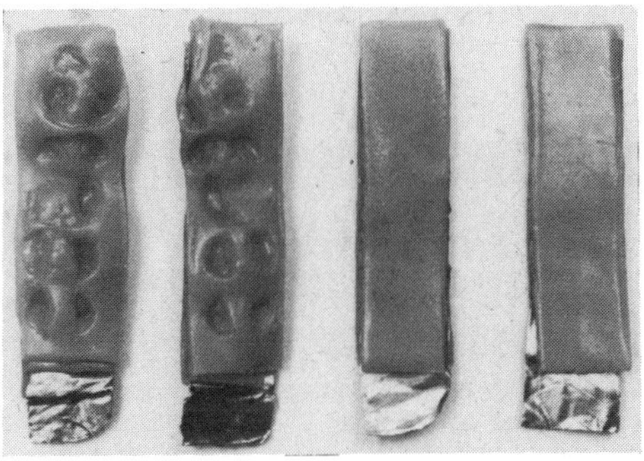

a

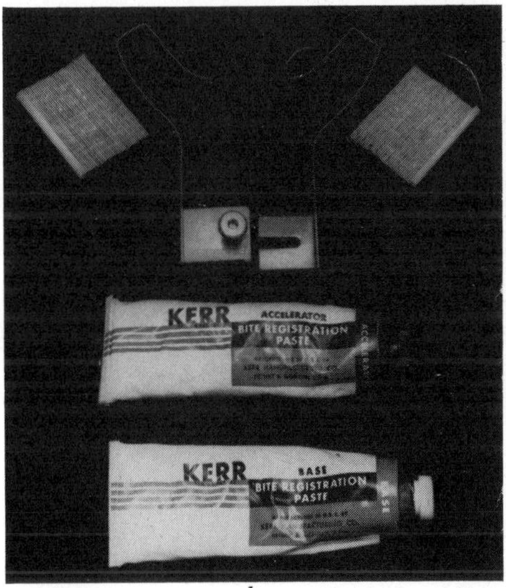

b

Fig. 17.4. *a, Wax wafers made by placing a sheet of hard wax (Moyco) on each side of a piece of 0·003 in foil or X-ray film lead sheet. b, The Kerr Bite Registration paste and frame.*

Once the lower cast has been mounted, other recordings are taken from which the articulator is set. The patient is requested to protrude to bring the anterior teeth edge to edge. The position is recorded and transferred to the articulator. With all adjustments loosened, the models are then inserted into the protrusive record and the condylar guidance adjusted (*Fig*. 17.3*a*) so that the casts seat well into the bite transfer. The condylar guidance is then locked.

A left lateral record is taken in a similar way, and the models are inserted into it on the articulator. The contralateral Bennett angle adjustment is set (*Fig*. 17.3*b*), during which care must be taken to see that the casts seat well into the record. A similar set of readings are taken on the right side and the process repeated. The articulator is now ready for use.

It should be pointed out that sometimes the lateral records cannot be accommodated by the articulator without disturbing the condylar guidance which has already been set. A compensating adjustment to the condylar guidance may then be made, but the techniques involved in these refinements are beyond the scope of this text.

BITE TRANSFERS

Many materials can be used for recording the transfers, that most commonly employed being wax. A specially hard type (such as Moyco Beauty wax) is ideal for this purpose. It is very easily handled if a single piece is placed on either side of a sheet of 0·003 in (0·08 mm) tin-foil, thus producing a sandwich. This can be cut into strips and heated in a water bath at 53°C (120°F) before use and afterwards cooled in iced water (*Fig.* 17.4*a*).

An alternative to wax is to use a zinc oxide based impression paste on a frame covered with gauze. Kerr's Bite Registration Paste is an example of this (*Fig.* 17.4*b*).

Other materials such as self-curing resin may also be employed, although this has the disadvantage that it takes a relatively long time to set and is very exothermic. Impression plaster used with a slurry (water from the model trimmer) can also be of value because it gives an almost constant setting time.

■ Anterior Bite Stop

A small anterior bite stop made of acrylic or composition can be of assistance in maintaining the mandible in centric relation to the maxilla after the occlusal surfaces of the posterior teeth have been prepared, thus preventing overclosure (*Fig.* 17.5*a*).

The bite stop is made on the lower incisor teeth and provides a permanent record of centric relation and, in the case of overclosure, the new occlusal vertical dimension, which can be referred to at any time during the reconstruction.

It is fixed to the lower incisors and plaster may then be injected into the space between the upper and lower posterior teeth and allowed to set with the arches held in a rigid relationship.

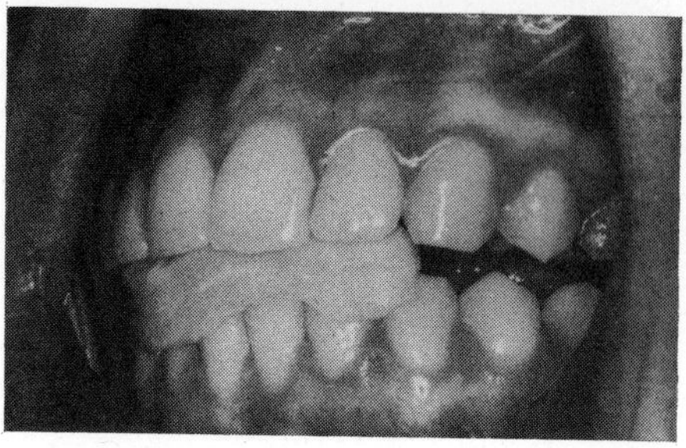

a

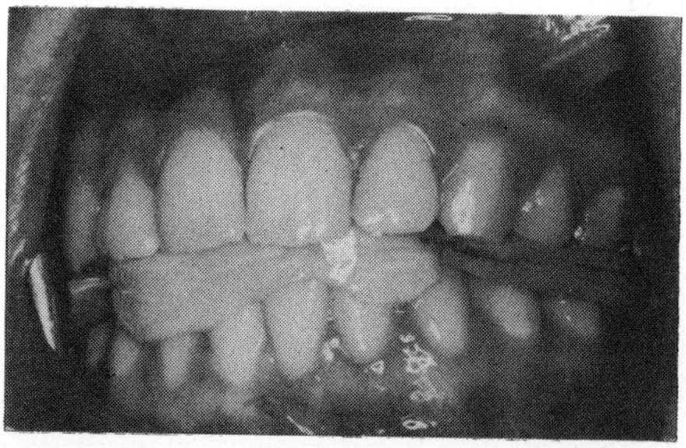

b

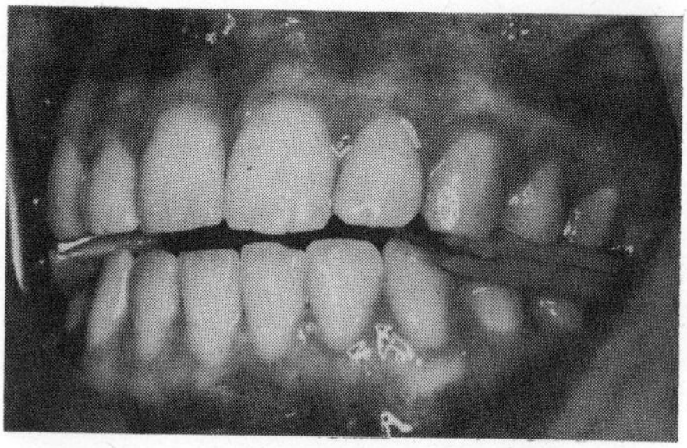

c

Fig. 17.5. *a, A small acrylic bite stop in position. This maintains the vertical dimension and centric relation. b, Wax wafers in position to record the vertical dimension in the posterior region. c, The recorded position with the bite stop removed.*

Alternatively, wax wafers can be employed (*Fig.* 17.5*b*, *c*).

Many other materials besides those already mentioned have been tried for bite transfers, rejected, and retried again. probably the age-old adage that any material will work provided it is properly handled is applicable in this case. The hard wax is possibly the easiest and most reliable, although plaster and the zinc oxide pastes will serve the purpose well.

There is one set of circumstances which deserves a mention in this context: a case which presents with a complete upper dentition and requiring a bridge from, say, the lower first and second premolars to the lower third molar, with the remainder of this arch intact.

One often notices that although much attention is paid to the occlusal reduction of the last standing molar in the bridge preparation, when the patient is requested to close, the space between the preparation and the upper teeth is much less than would be expected, and sometimes the opposing tooth and the preparation are even in contact. This is due to either a slight displacement of the joint or to a frank bending of the mandible across the midline.

In such cases the recording material should only be placed over the preparation. The patient is then instructed to 'close' so that the teeth on the opposite side of the arch just touch, without any degree of clenching at all.

Obviously the recording material must be extremely soft to permit this to occur. Zinc oxide impression paste on a bite frame is probably the best in such circumstances although a wash to Aluminax (Aluwax, USA) on a hard wax template can also be used satisfactorily.

Once the models have been set on the articulator the bridge is made and offered to the mouth. It must be stated yet again that the use of these types of articulator does necessitate a reappraisal of the occlusion at this stage.

Their limitations will almost certainly lead to the building of interferences in lateral excursions in the bridge, which must be corrected by equilibration techniques.

COMBINED RECONSTRUCTION OF OPPOSING QUADRANTS

It is possible to construct opposing quadrants on the same articulator at the same time.

Preoperative procedures are carried out as explained earlier and the quadrants prepared. When constructing such large restorations it is best to locate the terminal hinge axis and use these recordings for the mounting of all casts on the articulator (*Fig*. 17.6).

The upper teeth are prepared, a full arch impression taken, and the model transferred to the articulator.

The lower teeth are then prepared and an impression taken of these. A model is made from this which is now located to the upper teeth on the articulator using hard (Moyco) wax for the bite transfer as explained previously. A bite stop may be of value in this procedure.

WAX ADDITIVE TECHNIQUES

It is recommended that the more sophisticated wax additive techniques are used when the pattterns for the bridges are prepared so as to ensure a good functional and anatomical relationship between the two arches.

These were first employed by Everett Payne and have more recently been modified by Peter K. Thomas. The technique is to gradually build up the wax patterns by adding small increments rather than starting with a large amount and cutting this back. The cusps are placed first, then the functional fossa, triangular ridges and marginal ridges. In this way each increment can be shaped to function in all excursions with the opposing arch until the full anatomy of the tooth is completed.

It must be stressed that a final intraoral equilibration will still be necessary, although with experience the amount of chairside time required is greatly reduced.

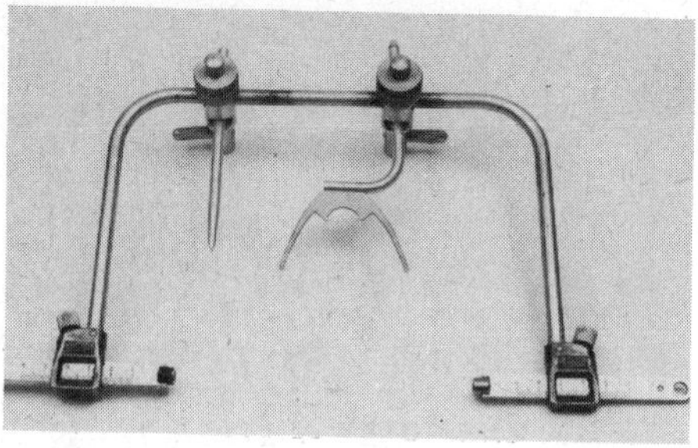

a

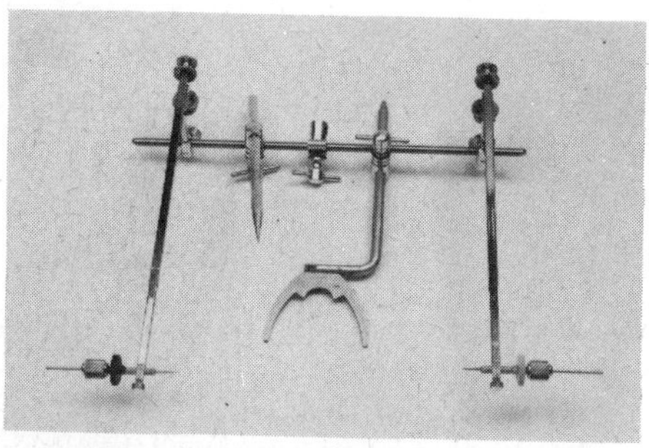

b

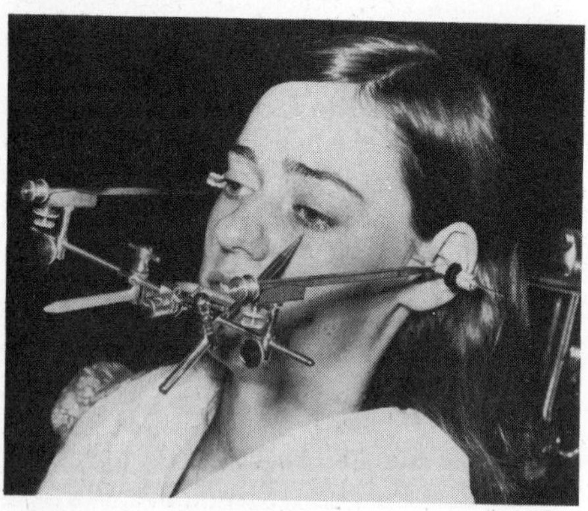

c

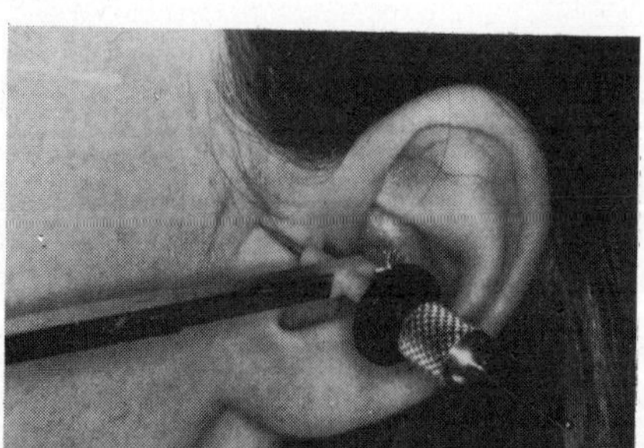

d

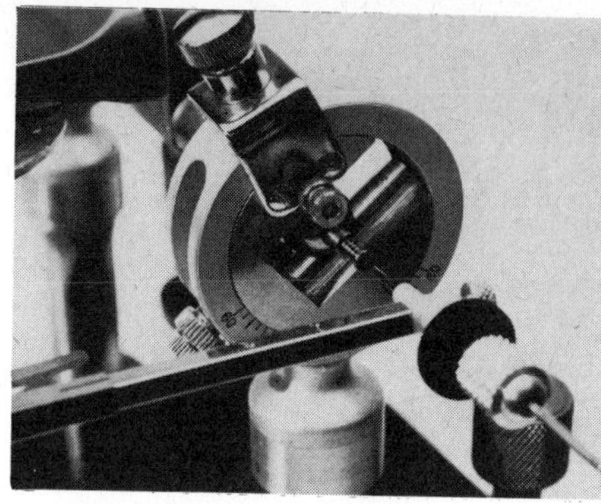

e

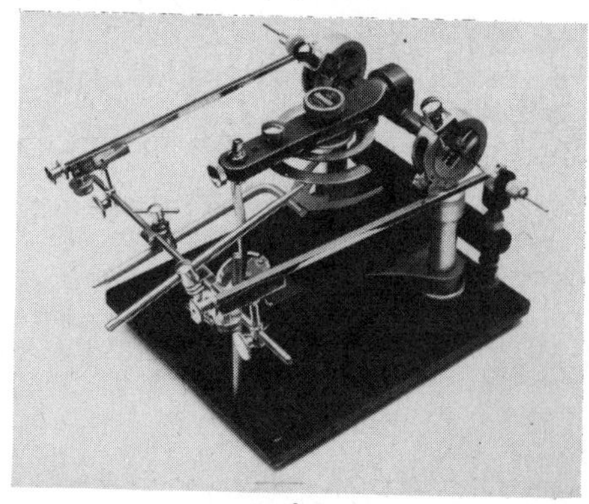

f

Fig. 17.6. *a, The Dentatus face bow. b, The Almore hinge axis transfer bow. c, The Almore transfer bow on a patient. d, The hinge axis location point. e, The location point on the ARL model Dentatus articulator. f, The Almore face bow on the mounting frame on the Dentatus articulator.*

FULLY ADJUSTABLE ARTICULATOR

The fully adjustable instrument, that is, one which can be made to follow all paths of every excursion of the mandible, is of great value when restoring a large number of units. Its correct use, together with the employment of the wax additive techniques, can enable the operator to construct all four quadrants at one and the same time.

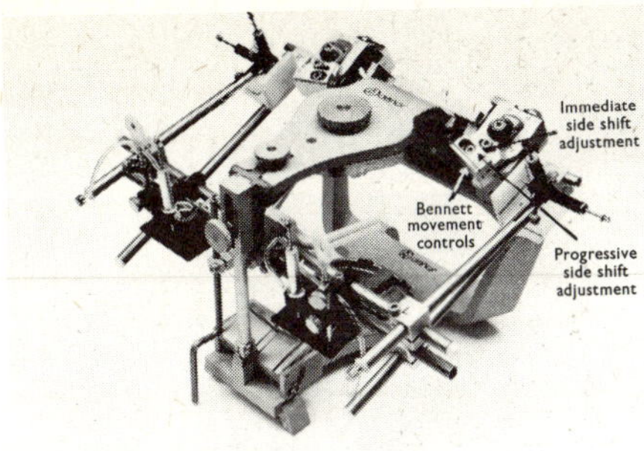

a

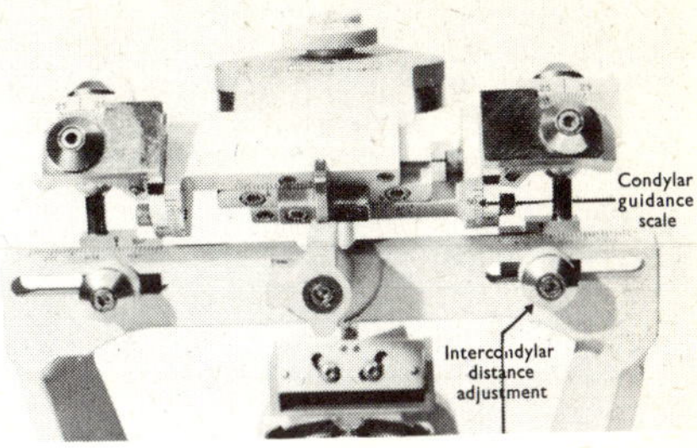

b

Such instruments include the Gnathascope, the De Pietro (Ney), the Stuart, and the Denar (*Fig.* 17.7). Recordings are carried out using a pantograph which registers all jaw movements and scribes them on pressure-sensitive paper.

It is essential that the operator fully understands the workings of both pantograph and articulator before attempting a clinical case. The instrument is often blamed for errors when in fact the operator has been at fault.

In such articulators jaw movements can be followed very closely, and the equilibration necessary on completion is minimal. This is because the immediate side shift—a functional jaw movement at the commencement of the Bennett shift—can be reproduced on the articulator.

Once set by the operator, the technician has the closest record of mandibular movements yet attained by any design of instrument.

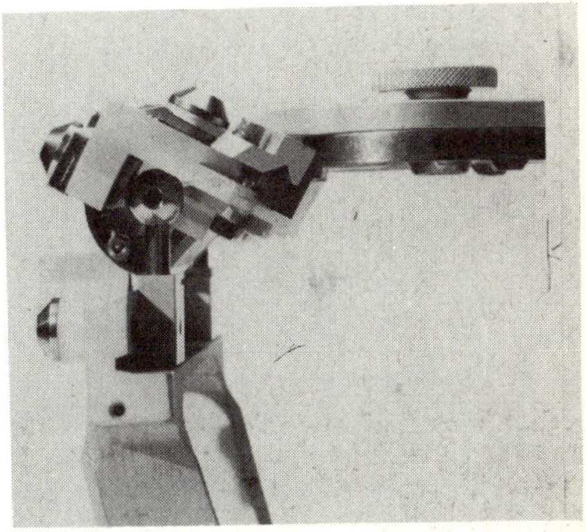

c

Fig. 17.7. *a, The Denar Pantograph mounted on the Denar instrument. Note the adjustment for Bennett movement. Compare with the semi-adjustable instrument in Fig. 17.3b, c. The adjustment for the condylar guidance on the Denar fully adjustable articulator. Compare with the semi-adjustable instrument in Fig. 17.3 a.*

Bibliography

Occlusal Records

Getz E. H. (1971) Functional 'Checkbite-impressions' for fixed prosthodontics. *J. Prosthet. Dent.* **26,** 146.

Guichet N. F. (1969) *Procedures of Occlusal Treatment; a Teaching Atlas.* Anaheim, California, Denar Corporation.

Lauritzen A. G. (1951) Function: prime object of restorative dentistry; a definite procedure for obtaining it. *J. Am. Dent.* **42,** 523.

Le Pera F. (1964) Determination of the 'hinge axis'. *J. Prosthet. Dent.* **14,** 651.

Mann A. W. and Pankey L. D. (1963) Concepts of occlusion. The P.M. philosophy of occlusal rehabilitation. *Dent. Clin. North Am.* November, p. 621.

Posselt V. (1957) Terminal hinge movement of the mandible. *J. Prosthet. Dent.* **7,** 787.

Thomas P. K. (1967) *Syllabus on Full Mouth Waxing Technique for Rehabilitation Tooth-to-tooth Cusp-fossa Concept of Organic Occlusion.* San Francisco, University of California.

18

BRIDGE PLACEMENT AND CARE

Try-in of Goldwork
Tissue Contact . Occlusion
Morphology and Shade
Trial Cementation . Permanent Cementation
The Patient's Care of a Bridge
Review of Case
Routine Bridge Check

Ideally, a bridge should always be checked in the laboratory by the operator before the patient's appointment to make certain that he is satisfied with the overall design, occlusion, fit on the model, aesthetics and strength of the prosthesis. In this way any alteration may then be carried out before the patient arrives, thus preventing wasting their time and possibly avoiding some loss of confidence in the operator.

If this is not practical, then at least it should be checked carefully in the dental surgery before trying it in the mouth. Often considerable chairside time can be saved by carrying out minor adjustments before the patient attends.

Particular factors which are sometimes easier for the operator to adjust than the technician, because of his more intimate knowledge of the patient, are the aesthetics and the occlusion. A further factor to be borne in mind is the strength of the prosthesis and its ability to stand up to the stresses of the occlusion for a long period of time. It is most distressing to have an otherwise satisfactory bridge fail after 2–3 years because, for instance, a solder joint fails. When in doubt, it is far better to get a bridge modified or remade rather than take a chance and fit it.

With bonded bridges it is often difficult to assess the thickness and strength of the underlying gold. This may be checked quite easily by taking X-rays of the bridge in two different planes, using an intra-oral film and a standard exposure (*see Fig.* 7.4, p. 132). Very little time is involved and a potential failure may well be avoided. Should the bridge be weakened by adjustments to the occlusion after trying it in, then a further X-ray may prove necessary.

When a patient attends to have a bridge cemented, before commencing any clinical procedures it is best to take a brief history to make certain that the abutment teeth have settled down completely after their preparation. If there is any indication that a pulpitis has occurred in one of the teeth this should be investigated further. It may prove advisable to delay placing the bridge for a week or two until the tooth is completely sign and symptom free. To cause further irritation to an already inflamed pulp by removing the temporary bridge, drying the teeth, and then cementing the prosthesis may well make all the difference as to whether or not the tooth remains vital. Should there be any doubt regarding the vitality of one of the abutment teeth this should be checked.

The use of local analgesia is nearly always indicated when placing a bridge on vital abutment teeth. Considerable pain will otherwise be caused when the dentine is exposed on removal of the temporary bridge and further pain will result when the teeth are dried and when actually cementing the prosthesis. Even the checking and adjustment of the margins of the retainers will cause appreciable discomfort. All the foregoing is likely to be carried out less efficiently if the operator is aware that he is hurting the patient.

Having removed the temporary bridge, which may possibly be best achieved with a crown remover (*see Fig.* 19.14, p. 256), the teeth should then be isolated and checked very carefully to see that none of the temporary cement remains.

Similarly, the pontic area and gingival margins will require examination to see that they are not inflamed and thus possibly of a different shape or contour to that present when the impression was taken.

TRY-IN OF GOLDWORK

Having cleaned the teeth the gold work may be tried in without, when practical, any relevant facings. If it is of the fixed-movable type or possibly if it incorporates precision retainers, the castings may be assessed as separate units. However, if it is of the fixed-fixed variety then this is not possible. Should the casting not seat fully then:

a. Check the Contacts

This may sometimes be done visually but is generally best carried out by feeling how readily a piece of dental floss passes through the mesial and distal contact points. Occasionally a patient will be able to tell you, particularly if local analgesia is not used, that the bridge is pressing too hard on one or both of the adjoining teeth. Where necessary the contacts should be eased after having carefully assessed where the exact point of initial contact is. This may be done either by direct vision, scratching the gold to note the spot, or by painting the contact area of the neighbouring tooth with graphite, which will then leave a mark on the gold of the retainer where it first touches it when inserted.

b. Examine Model

Careful examination of the model and, where necessary, comparing this with the original impression may indicate that it has been damaged during the laboratory procedures. If there are signs of model damage then providing it does not affect the marginal fit of the retainer, the gold may be eased where the model is defective, but in all other instances the only course available is a remake of at least the retainer involved and possibly of the entire bridge.

c. Examine Fit Surface of Castings and the Teeth

By careful examination of the fit surface of the castings it may be possible to see the spot which is binding; alternatively a mark may be seen on the prepared surface of the tooth. Graphiting of the fit surface of the casting or the use of lipstick may occasionally make this easier to observe.

d. Check Alignment of Retainers

In the case of a fixed-movable bridge the castings may be tried-in individually, and thus it will be known if each retainer fits correctly. If they do so but the bridge will not seat fully, their relationship with each other must be incorrect. This may be either because of a poor impression, because one of the abutment teeth has moved, or because the various parts of the bridge have been incorrectly related in the laboratory. In any case the simplest procedure, unless the misalignment is slight, is to unsolder the various components of the bridge, take a plaster or rubber base localizing impression, which need only involve the occlusal surfaces, and then resolder them. Alternatively, the various parts of the bridge may be separated and then refixed together in the mouth with a plastic such as Duralay and the whole removed in one piece, invested, and soldered. However, it must be remembered that the occlusion may also be deranged because of the incorrect alignment.

In the case of the fixed-fixed bridge it is more difficult to assess why a bridge is not seating, as it is by no means easy to differentiate between the bridge which will not go right home, because of a faulty fit, from the one in which the alignment of the retainers relative to each other is incorrect. The only difference which may sometimes be apparent is that in the case of misalignment the bridge will have some 'spring' in it and tends to seat further on pressure due to the abutment teeth moving slightly, whereas in the case of a defective fit the resistance felt will be solid.

Where it is felt that the problem is one of misalignment and the bridge seats almost fully with pressure, then by merely leaving it in place for ½–1 hour and getting the patient to exert gentle, continuous pressure on it, it will often seat completely. If it has not done so within 1 hour but shows signs that it may do so over a longer period it is best to cement the bridge temporarily to whichever abutment it will seat on to fully, and then send the patient away for a day or two. It is unwise to do this without fixing the bridge to one of the retainers. In many instances what appears to have been a very tight fitting bridge becomes a very loose one after the teeth have moved back to their correct positions. The author has knowledge of at least two instances when patients have swallowed bridges which were placed uncemented. One of these consisted of five units and posed no mean problem to the alimentary tract, taking a full ten days to complete its journey.

If the bridge still does not fit after having been left in the mouth for a day or two, or if it seems unlikely that it will do so in the first instance, then the bridge should be unsoldered and the separate components tried in. If these then seat correctly it is only a matter of taking a locating impression and resoldering them, but should one of the castings still fail to fit it may be examined to see if there is any obvious reason for this. However, in the majority of cases a fresh impression and a new retainer will be required. The impression should be taken with the satisfactory part of the bridge in situ. This will usually be removed with the impression and the dies can then be seated in the castings before pouring the model.

Electropolishing and Electrostripping

Some authorities recommend the use of a stripping device when a casting fails to fit. This consists of an electrochemical bath which may be used either for polishing or reducing a gold casting.

Electropolishing is a non-abrasive process whereby the surface of a metallic specimen is made smooth and brought up to a specular finish. The specimen is the anode of an electrochemical cell and in most dental electropolishing units the metal container for the electrolyte is used as the cathode.

The process is considerably influenced by temperature; below 60°C little happens whereas above 80°C severe etching occurs. If it is desired to reduce the fit surface of a casting the margins must first be protected with varnish. Wax is contraindicated as it will not withstand the temperatures involved. After this the restoration is placed in the bath at a constant temperature. The gold will then be removed from the fit surface at an even and predetermined speed, the amount actually taken away being gradually increased until the casting seats completely.

The disadvantages of this method are:

a. That it is often a defect at the margin of the retainer, which cannot be altered, which is preventing the casting from seating.

b. That the overall fit of the retainer will be spoilt and thus retention will be bound to suffer.

When the bridge is fully seated the following should be checked:

a. The Contacts

If they are too tight they may be eased. When they are too light they may be added to at the chairside providing they are of gold by using solder of the appropriate melting range. This may be limited to the contact area by painting the surrounding gold with graphite.

b. The Margins

With the latest impression materials and casting techniques the fit of the retainers should be excellent and require little attention. However, where the margins are accessible they may be finished up with sandpaper disks and stones, using the finest grades last. Following this, rubber wheels or cups and finally rouge may be employed.

If the margin is a feather or chamfer this can often be burnished with a suitable instrument. In these cases one is probably bending rather than burnishing the gold. Where necessary the margin of the gold may be thinned down to simplify this procedure.

TISSUE CONTACT

The pontic should exert only light pressure on the tissues; if it presses sufficiently hard to cause blanching it must be eased, otherwise undue gingival proliferation will take place around the pontic (*Fig*. 18.1 and *Fig*. 5.10, p. 72). If it fails to touch the mucosa, then provided this gap is minimal, i.e. not more than 0·1 mm, the tissues will proliferate to establish a good contact. However, if the gap is more than this they may not do so, particularly if the patient's oral hygiene is excellent. An addition will thus be required. This is relatively simple to carry out with the bonded porcelains and facings such as the long-pin pontic, but with a gold to tissue contact either a new pontic will be necessary or an addition will have to be made with solder.

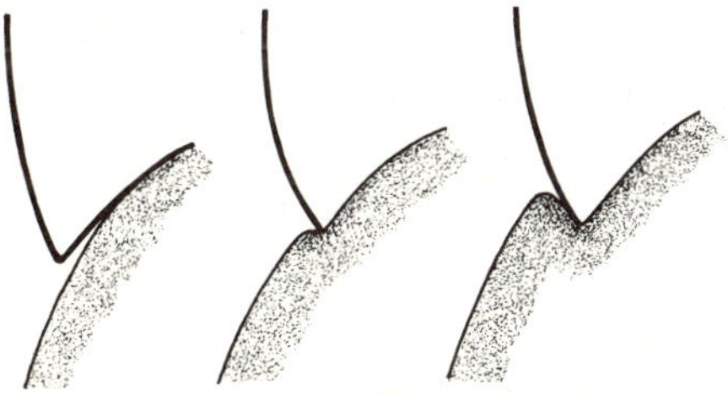

Fig. 18.1. *Pontic-tissue contact. If this is too light a permanent space will remain between the tissues and the pontic. If too heavy, gingival proliferation will occur, preventing the use of dental floss and making the undersurface difficult to clean.*

The surface contact area covered by the pontic should be checked and, if this is too much, reduced. This has already been discussed in pontic design.

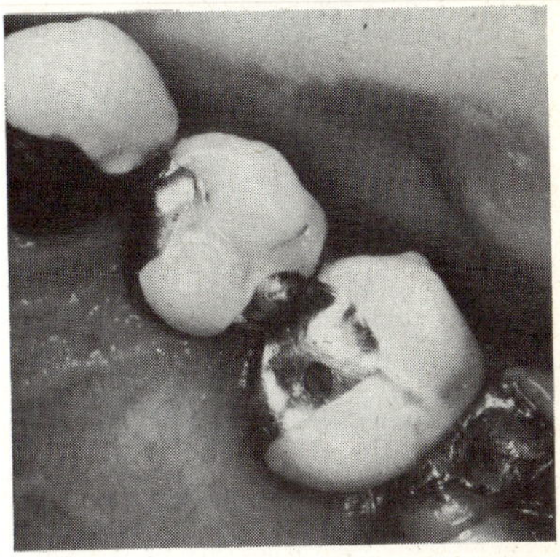

Fig. 18.2. *A localized 'high spot' marked on a tooth by using thin red articulating paper.*

OCCLUSION

The occlusion should now be checked. This has already been discussed in the section on occlusal records in Chapter 17. The principal methods used are:

1. *Touch*. By placing a finger on the buccal or labial aspect of the tooth and feeling if the occlusion is too heavy on any particular tooth during closing and the various excursions of the mandible.
2. By the use of thin articulating paper which will leave a mark on the 'high spots' (*Fig*. 18.2). This will work satisfactorily on tooth tissue and also sandblasted gold, but will not mark highly polished surfaces very well.

A range of plastic articulating strips, available in three different colours and only 20 µm thick, has recently been marketed by Hanel-Medizinal.* It is stronger, thinner and cleaner to use than the articulating papers.

* Hanel-Medizinal D7440, Würtingen, Germany.

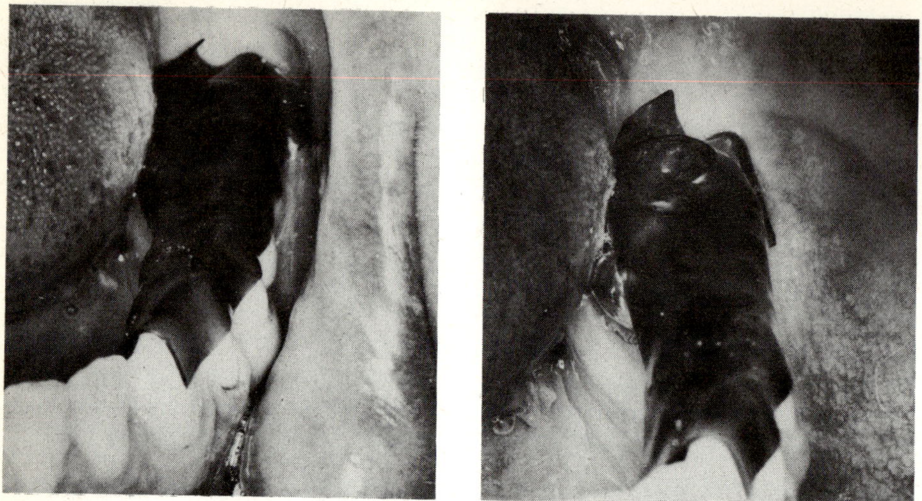

a *b*

Fig. 18.3. *The use of occlusal indicator wax to disclose 'high-spots' on a bridge. a, Before and b, after occluding.*

3. By using occlusal indicator wax (*Fig.* 18.3). With this technique a thin sheet of wax is moulded over the teeth or bridge one requires to check. The patient is then asked to bite into this. Where the restoration shows through the wax is the point which needs easing. If required this can be marked with a crayon or, alternatively, red articulating paper may be laid over the wax and the patient asked to occlude again. It will only produce a mark where no wax covers the occlusal surface.

4. Where gold occlusal surfaces are employed, these are best sandblasted first so that high spots may be detected with the minimum of difficulty with or without articulating paper. However, whereas gold may be sandblasted and even if left in this condition will do little harm, a rough porcelain occlusing surface should never be left unglazed as it is highly abrasive and will wear the opposing teeth.

5. The placing on of an extremely thin (12 μm), but strong strip of plastic shimstock (Huffman et al., 1969)* between the teeth on either side of the bridge when they are firmly occluded and then trying to pull it out will indicate whether or not the bridge is preventing the patient from closing completely.

It is important to adjust the occlusion not only in centric but also the lateral and protrusive excursions, otherwise either the pontic (*Fig.* 18.4) or the retainers may fail or periodontal problems may ensue.

MORPHOLOGY AND SHADE

In the case of a bonded bridge or one employing pontics such as porcelain jackets the overall form is first adjusted where necessary, as with a porcelain jacket crown. After this the characterization is obtained. Finally the shade can be checked and any surface stains added. The fit surface of the pontic should now be polished or glazed as required.

If gold is visible it is advisable to try the bridge in with the patient sitting upright. The position of the light should be varied to see which aspects of the gold reflect the light and the angulation of these should be gradually adjusted until

* The Artus Corporation, Englewood, New Jersey 076321, USA.

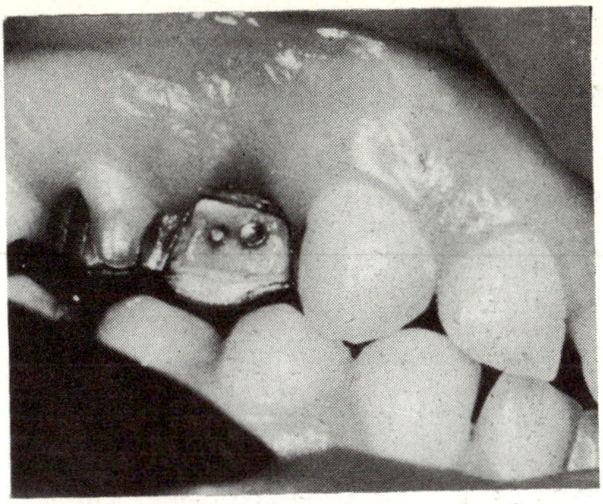

Fig. 18.4. *Facing failure due to inadequate clearance of the occlusion in right lateral excursions.*

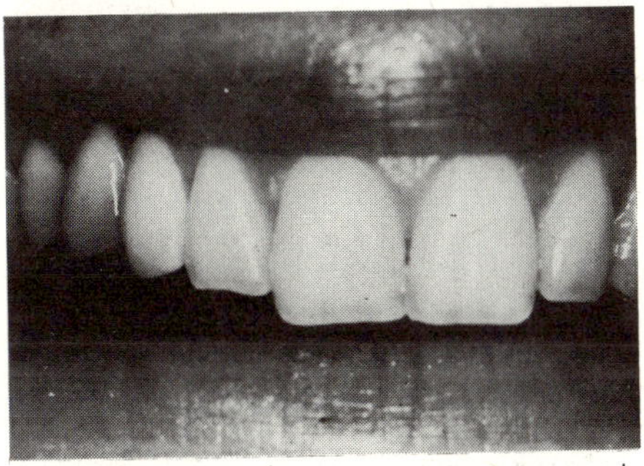

Fig. 18.5. *A cantilever bridge replacing* 3| *by a bonded pontic, with three-quarter crowns on* 54|. *Note minimal 'awareness' of the gold incisal edges on these teeth.*

they are no longer noticeable. In this way any display of gold may be reduced to a minimum (*Fig.* 18.5). The gold is then finally polished and if necessary the porcelain reglazed. At this stage the patient should be shown the bridge, preferably with them out of the chair and in front of a full-length mirror. It can then be ascertained that they are satisfied with its appearance prior to cementing it.

TRIAL CEMENTATION

Should there be even the slightest doubt that the patient is happy with the bridge or the operator has any reservations, then it is best to put the bridge in place with a 'trial' cement made of silicone paste, such as that marketed by Opotow * (Griffith and Cannon, 1974). This permits both the patient and, sometimes more important, their relatives and friends to see it and to make certain that they are happy with it before it is permanently cemented in place.

The use of trial cement is also of value if one or more teeth have moved slightly and time is required for them to realign prior to permanent cementation of the prosthesis.

A specially formulated material is to be preferred to most temporary cements as it simplifies removal of the prosthesis and is also relatively easy to remove from the teeth and the fit surface of the retainers. To cement temporarily an extensive prosthesis in place with quick-setting zinc oxide and eugenol is fraught with danger, particularly if long and retentive full crowns are employed, as it may well be impossible to remove it at a later date. If this material is used only the margin and a little of the fit surface should ever be coated with it.

PERMANENT CEMENTATION

■ Factors Determining which Cement to Use

The properties of the various media which may be employed for cementing a bridge have already been considered in Chapter 4. However, there are four main considerations when deciding which should be used in any given case:

1. The degree of retention required.
2. The materials to be joined.
3. The depth of the preparations.
4. The number of retainers involved.

Thus where retention is of paramount importance zinc phosphate is probably the material of choice. It is also generally best where high load factors are concerned (e.g. with post crowns) as its crush

* Dental Mfg Corp., Brooklyn, New York, NY 11208, USA.

strength is higher than polycarboxylate. However, it is undoubtedly more irritant having a pH of around 3·5 on cementation, and thus where the preparations are deep and good retention is available, the polycarboxylates are to be preferred. Although their pH of 4·8 at cementation is fairly low, it appears to result in relatively little pulpal irritation, possibly because the large molecules of polyacrylic acid are unable to penetrate the dentinal tubules (Going and Mitchem, 1975).

Theoretically, when the preparations are very deep, the bridge should be cemented with a substance that is virtually non-irritant, such as the EBA Cements which are accelerated zinc oxide and eugenol materials, with part of the eugenol being replaced by ethyl benzoic acid. Unfortunately, however, their high solubility usually contraindicates their use for this purpose.

For the cementing of facings zinc phosphate is still the most suitable material. Polycarboxylates should not be used for this purpose.

■ Cementation of Bridge

The facings where applicable, should always be cemented to the bridge before it is finally placed, so that their margins may be checked and finished outside the mouth. The abutment teeth should now be isolated and carefully dried. However, this should not be carried to excess as dehydration may make the tooth more susceptible to any irritation from the cementing media.

At this stage, cavity varnish should be applied to try and prevent the cement causing pulpal irritation via the dentinal tubules (Swartz et al., 1966).

It is essential that the correct proportioning and mixing of the cement is always carried out if the minimal film thickness and maximum working time, which are essential for extensive prostheses, is to be achieved (Eames et al., 1977). The liquid is thus best dispensed from a graduated syringe and the powder measured by using one of the dipsticks or scoops available from the manufacturers. On checking, it has been found that the weight of powder dispensed by this means is remarkably constant. With phosphate cement 0·5 ml of liquid will normally be used in conjunction with 1·00 g of powder. The optimum mixing time, which should always be measured, is 90 sec.

The cement should be mixed over as large an area of the slab as possible to assist heat dissipation and thus make certain that the optimum working time is achieved. For the same reason, the powder should be added to the liquid in increments spread over the whole mixing period. Although the slab should be cool, it should not be too cold, otherwise condensation may occur on it and adversely affect the mix.

When maximum working time is required, a *little* powder may be added to the liquid before the main mix is commenced. This will slow the reaction time by buffering the acid, but it will not permit any more powder to be incorporated in the mix. The bridge is placed using continuous pressure which is exerted for at least one minute to allow the excess cement to flow out and the castings to go fully home. When almost fully seated an automatic mallet

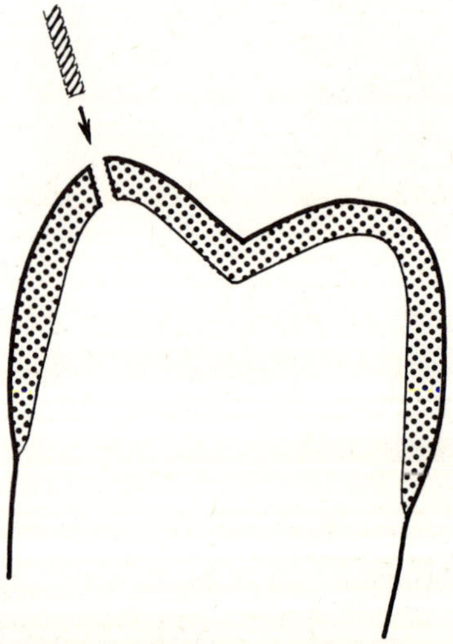

Fig. 18.6. *The use of a threaded screw to provide a vent-hole for the cement when placing a full crown.*

may be used to complete the positioning of the bridge. A suitable biting pad may then be placed in the mouth and left there until the cement is set.

There should be a considerable excess of cement which will be left around the margins of the teeth until it is fully set. This will prevent any moisture reaching the cement at the edge of the retainers.

It is particularly important to have a very slow setting mix of cement when placing full crowns as they may prove difficult to seat. One way of overcoming this is to provide a vent hole (*Fig*. 18.6) which may subsequently be sealed with cohesive gold, a threaded pin, or amalgam.

Considerable research has been carried out on venting and it has been shown that it enables full seating to be achieved on average in 15 sec, whereas with unvented crowns it takes one minute (Dimashkieh and Davies, 1974). Interestingly, whereas with crowns with a 2–5° taper, venting was essential if a minimal cement film thickness was to be achieved, when the tapers were 10° or more full seating of the crown was obtained, even without venting. Jørgensen (1960) noted a reduction in cement thickness to only a little more than half when venting was carried out.

After the cement has fully set all the excess must be removed, taking particular care that none remains subgingivally. Dental floss may be used interstitially and a probe should be passed around all the margins.

The edges of the retainers are then checked and refinished again as necessary. Usually only fine sandpaper discs are required. Finally the occlusion is rechecked and then the patient instructed in the routine care of the bridge.

THE PATIENT'S CARE OF A BRIDGE

Patients should already be aware of the ways of caring for their teeth in general, including the correct method of tooth brushing, the use of interdental stimulators, floss, and disclosing solutions. Of these latter the fluorescent varieties used by the operator in conjunction with a plaque light have the advantage that they do not stain soft tissues.

However, more specific methods are required for the care of a bridge. Thus if there is a relatively large amount of soft-tissue coverage an oral irrigator which will pulsate water beneath the prosthesis and keep the fit surface fairly clean may be indicated. However this will not remove plaque and it must be remembered that if used at too high a pressure it may damage the periodontal tissues, particularly if they are weak.

The use of dental floss or tapes beneath the pontics and, in the case of the spring bridge, the bar, is of use in keeping the fit surfaces clean and free from plaque (*see Fig*. 5.6, p. 71). These may be difficult to pass interdentally and in these cases they can sometimes be passed through with an Interdens, a ZON* plastic needle (*Fig*. 18.7) a plastic loop, such as the Ezz-Thru †(*Fig*. 18.8), fuse wire twisted around the end of the dental floss, or even a blunt darning needle. Once passed interstitially the floss or tape is held tight and passed over the fit surfaces several times.

In the case of the spring bridge the dental floss is passed through one of the contacts adjoining the pontic and then the buccal or labial end is passed below it and through the second contact. The floss can then be moved distally beneath the bar as far back as the retainer. This régime should be carried out daily.

Other methods of removing plaque from the mesial and distal surfaces of the teeth involve the use of a small interdental or 'proxy' brush and wood sticks. The undersurface of sanitary pontics and the distal aspects of the last molars may be cleaned by using a strip of gauze.

If any pontics are liable to fracture, for instance the all-porcelain occlusal and porcelain jacket types, the patient should

* Johnson & Johnson Co., East Windsor, New Jersey, USA.
† John D. Butler Co., Chicago, Illinois, USA.

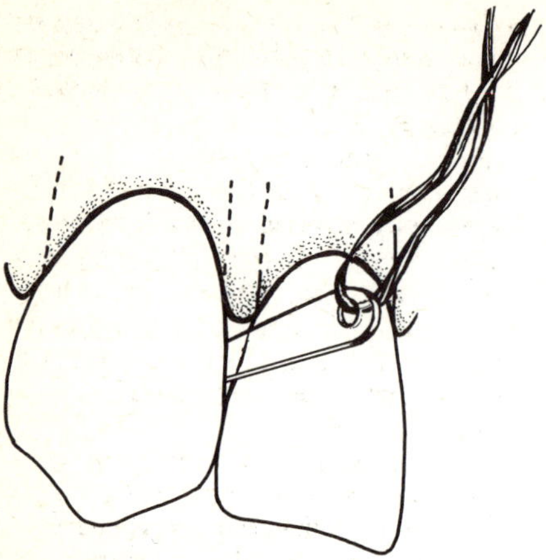

Fig. 18.7. *ZON plastic needles threading floss silk interdentally so that the undersurface of the pontic may be cleaned.*

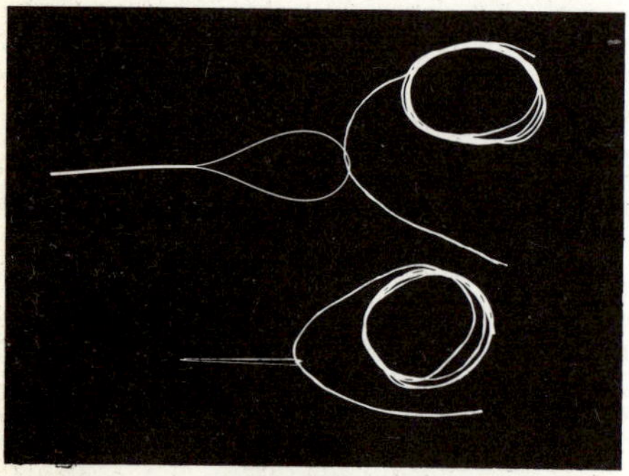

Fig. 18.8. *Top, The Ezz-Thru plastic loop for threading dental floss interproximally. Bottom, The ZON plastic needle.*

be advised of this and told to avoid any sudden impact on these such as that caused by biting a nut or a metal object. Similarly the bar of a spring bridge may fracture if excess leverage is put on it, as for instance when biting a piece off a hard apple.

There is always the risk of bridges being damaged, usually by the anaesthetist, during an operation and the patient should be advised to tell him beforehand if he has a fixed prosthesis or indeed even a crown.

The patient may now be dismissed and an appointment made for 3–4 weeks time. If there is likely to be any cervical sensitivity he should be advised to use a desensitizing toothpaste, such as Sensodyne or Emoform. The patient should always be told that bridges take a considerable time to settle in and that complete comfort will not be achieved for some while.

REVIEW OF CASE

When the patient returns he should be asked if he has experienced any discomfort. He may, for instance, have noticed that the occlusion is incorrect. Any defect of which the patient has become aware should be dealt with first and then the bridge checked in detail.

The bridge should be examined to see how well the patient is carrying out his oral hygiene routine. He should be told of any areas where plaque is being retained, preferably, where practical, by having it demonstrated to him and advised on how best these areas may be kept clean. The articulation can then be checked and in particular any gold occlusal surfaces should be examined for wear facets which may indicate the need for an adjustment.

The margins of the preparations should again be viewed and an examination made to ensure that there is no cement remaining sub-gingivally. An indication of this may often by gained by a localized area of gingival inflammation.

Finally, fullest details of the bridge should be recorded for comparative purposes in future years. This should include the condition of the crowns and apices of the abutment teeth and their pocket depth and mobility; the adequacy of retention; colour match and tissue contact of the pontic, and such other factors as may be considered of value. Unless, for instance, mobility is recorded at the outset, it is extremely difficult to tell in future years, if it is noticed that a tooth is mobile, whether this has always been the case or whether it is due to periodontal breakdown, possibly because of overloading. Photographic records may well prove an asset in the years to come.

After all the foregoing checks have been carried out the patient may be dismissed, but only after emphasizing to him how important it is that the prosthesis be checked every six months and that he should contact you immediately if he is in any way concerned about it. If he does not do so, for instance in the case of partial cementation failure, the results may well be disastrous.

ROUTINE BRIDGE CHECK

Every bridge should be examined at maximum intervals of six months. At this stage the following should be checked for:

a. Caries. Bite-wing X-rays are always indicated.

b. Cementation failure. It is extremely important to make certain that all the retainers are firmly fixed to the abutment teeth. This is particularly true with fixed-fixed designs. The following methods may be employed to detect cementation failure:

1. Pull down firmly on each of the retainers, when one of them may be seen to move. There is no risk of uncementing a retainer by this method. Tests have shown that the average posterior three-quarter crown, for instance, needs a force of approximately 29·5 kg (65 lb) before it is displaced.
2. Press up on each retainer in turn, when a bubble may appear at the margin, indicating cementation failure.
3. In the case of post crowns and box-type preparations it may sometimes be possible to pass a probe under the margin of the restoration. This may either be because the fit is defective or the casting uncemented. However, these may be differentiated between by exerting firm pressure on the retainer when the probe is under the margin. If it is felt that the probe is held in place by the pressure and freed as soon as it is released, the casting is uncemented.

Partial cementation failure of a retainer such as an MOD may sometimes be detected by placing a metal instrument on its occlusal surface and getting the patient to bite hard on it. It may then be seen that the casting is flexing, or it may be possible to pass a probe under a margin which has been opened up (*see Fig.* 6.9, p. 88).

c. Mobility, pocketing and bleeding index of abutment teeth. Check and record the foregoing to make certain that there is no sign of overloading of the abutment teeth, or localized gingival irritation. If there is any doubt reference may be made to the original bridge records and also to the corresponding teeth on the other side. The latter will indicate whether any periodontal deterioration is localized to the bridge or if it involves the whole mouth. In particular it is important to check that the patient's oral hygiene is good.

d. Occlusion. A patient's articulation is by no means constant for life and a bridge which may be correct when fitted may come into traumatic occlusion a few years later. If it is the first check after a bridge has been placed then wear facets on the gold may indicate any adjustment needed.

e. Wear. Examine the gold to see that there is no sign of flexion, tearing or undue wear. In particular the solder joints should be examined to see that there is no bending taking place at this point.

The occlusal surfaces need to be checked to see that they are not perforated. Similarly the bar of a spring bridge must be examined carefully to see that there is no sign of cracking or fatigue.

f. Vitality. If there is any doubt regarding the vitality of the abutment teeth or if they have been previously root-filled, X-rays will be required to make certain that the apical condition is satisfactory. Electric pulp tests may sometimes be indicated, although they will prove difficult when full coverage is used.

If all the foregoing are satisfactory the patient may be dismissed, but the importance of attending quickly should any disaster befall the bridge should again be stressed.

Bibliography

Balshi T. J. (1977) Maintenance procedures for patients after complete fixed prosthodontics. *J. Prosthet. Dent.* **37**, 420.

Dahl B. L. (1974) Some biological considerations in crown and bridge prosthetics. *J. Oral Rehabil.* **1**, 245.

Dimashkieh M. R., Davies E. H. and von Fraunhofer J. A. (1974) Measurement of cement film thickness beneath full crown restorations. *Br. Dent. J.* **137**, 281.

Eames W. B. et al. (1977) Proportioning and mixing of cements: A comparison of working times. *Op. Dent.* **2**, 97.

Going R. E. and Mitchem J. C. (1975) Cement for permanent luting: a summarizing review. *J. Am. Dent. Assoc.* **91**, 107.

Griffith J. R. and Cannon R. W. S. (1974) Cementation—materials and techniques. *Aust. Dent. J.* April, 93.

Huffman R. W., Regenos J. W. and Taylor R. R. (1969) *Principles of Occlusion, a Laboratory and Teaching Manual.* Columbus, Ohio, H & R Press.

Jones M. D., Dykema R. W. and Klein A. I. (1971) Television micromeasurement of vented and non-vented cast crown marginal adaptation. *Dent. Clin. North. Am.* **15**, 663.

Jørgensen K. D. (1960) Factors affecting the film thickness of zinc phosphate cements. *Acta Odontol. Scand.* **18**, 479.

McLean J. W. and von Fraunhofer J. A. (1971) The estimation of cement film thickness by an in vivo technique. *Br. Dent. J.* **131**, 107.

Paffenbarger G. C. (1972) Dental cements, direct filling resins, composite and adhesive restorative materials: A résumé. *J. Biomed. Mater. Res.* Symposium No. 2 (Part 2), 363.

Swartz et al. (1966) Role of cavity varnishes and bases in the penetration of cement constituents through tooth structure. *J. Prosthet. Dent.* **16**, 963.

19

CAUSES AND TREATMENT OF BRIDGE FAILURES

Causes of Bridge Failure
Treatment of Bridge Failures

CAUSES OF BRIDGE FAILURE

After discussing bridge maintenance and care it is as well to consider the various causes of bridge failure and how some of these may be avoided.

Faults which may occur are:

1. Cementation failure.
2. Mechanical breakdown.
3. Gingival irritation or recession.
4. Periodontal breakdown.
5. Caries.
6. Necrosis of the pulp.

These may be due to faulty bridge design or execution either in the laboratory or at the chairside, poor maintenance by the patient or even the operator, or to fair wear and tear.

1. Cementation Failure

Cementation failure may be either partial (*Fig*. 19.2; *see also Fig*. 6.9, p. 88) or complete, and is normally the result of retainers which are inadequate for the bridge in question. This has already been discussed in some detail in Chapter 6; suffice it to say here that too much rather than too little retention should always be provided. With fixed-fixed designs if there is any doubt regarding the adequacy of retention and particularly if the clinical crowns are short, full crowns should be employed. It is worth remembering that the sides of the preparation should be as near parallel to each other as possible, the ideal being a convergence angle of 5–6°.

Another important factor is the rigidity of the casting. Even slight flexion will cause cementation failure and this can only be prevented by using a hard gold and making certain that it has been correctly heat-treated and is of sufficient

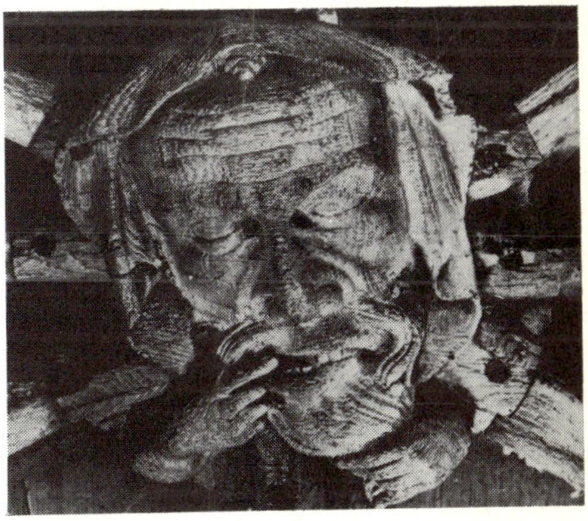

Fig. 19.1. *Toothache depicted on the carved wooden roof of Lincoln Cathedral. Motto: A bridge should never be embarked on unless you are reasonably sure of the prognosis. The results of failure are nearly always disastrous.*
(By courtesy of the Wellcome Trustees.)

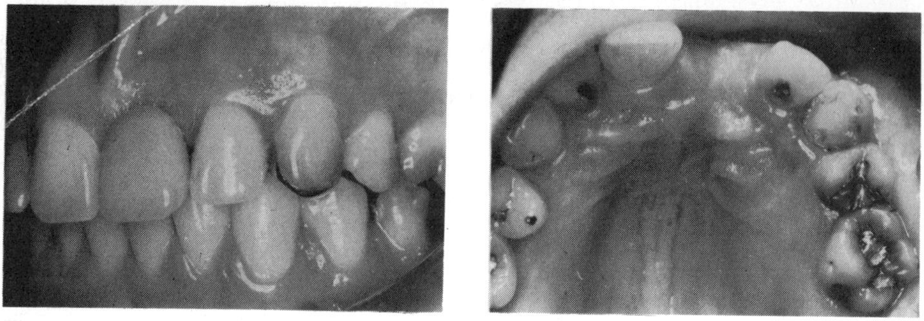

Fig. 19.2. *The three-quarter pinlay on* $\lfloor 3$ *was held in situ by only one of its pins. Caries around the uncemented pins necessitated devitalization.*

thickness. The detection of cementation failure has already been discussed on p. 247.

Besides an inadequate retainer, failure can also occur because of a poor cementation technique. This may be due to the wrong choice of material, failure to observe the manufacturer's mixing instructions, the use of old or contaminated stock, an inadequate powder/liquid ratio, or the insertion of the prothesis when the cement has started to set. This latter may result in a weak cement and a casting which is incompletely seated. Likewise if the teeth are not dried off carefully before cementation the bond will be weakened. Where full crowns are being employed, venting is usually indicated.

■ 2. Mechanical Breakdown

Mechanical failures which may beset a bridge are:

a. Flexion, Tearing or Fracture of the Gold

These may of themselves result in failure of the bridge. They may also result in cementation failure of the retainers or the loss of a facing.

Most of these disasters may be avoided by providing gold of adequate thickness, using a careful casting technique to ensure freedom from porosity (*Fig.* 19.3), carrying out the heat treatment advised

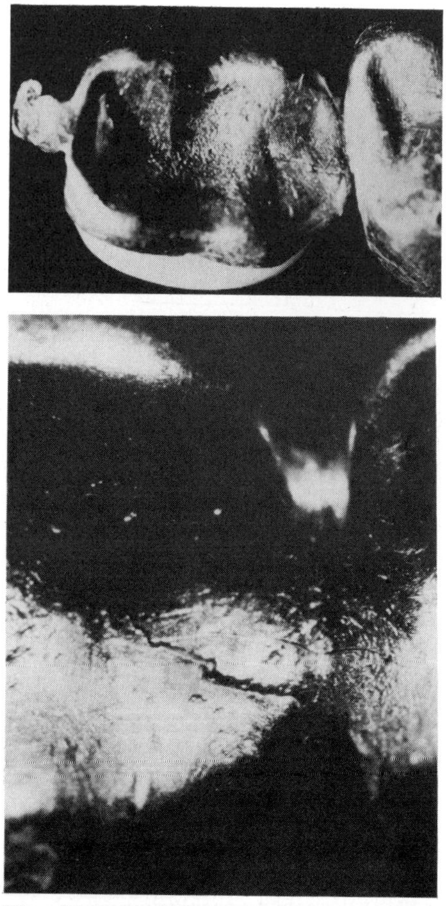

Fig. 19.3. *A thick but porous gold casting resulting in tearing of the occlusal gold and failure of the facing.*

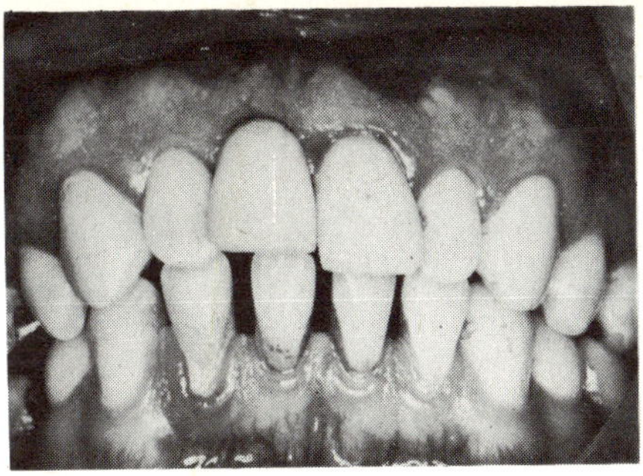

Fig. 19.4. *Bending of the gold bar of a spring bridge resulting in upwards and outwards displacement of the pontic.*

by the manufacturers, and making certain that the occlusion is correct. It is also necessary to remember that the longer the span the stronger and thus the thicker the gold will have to be.

In the case of spring bridges, if gold is used for the bar and particularly if there is porosity then permanent bending may occur, resulting in the pontic moving labially and upwards,. when the only remedy is a remake (*Fig.* 19.4).

b. Solder Joint Failure

There are several points to watch if a breakdown of the solder joint is to be avoided:

i. It is important that it has not only adequate width, but also depth, as it is the latter which provides the resistance to occlusal stresses. The contour should be roughly as shown in *Fig.* 19.5 with the lower surface well clear of the gingivae so as to allow an adequate interdental space.

ii. A sufficient bulk of gold must be provided in the region of the solder joint. If this is not done then although the joint itself may not fail the metal adjoining it will tear. For this reason it is necessary to carry out a box-type preparation in the region where the joint will be so as to reinforce the gold (*see Fig.* 6.46, p. 106).

iii. Different soldering techniques are required when joining different alloys and materials, and the correct soldering flux must always be used. This is particularly important when joining the nickel-chrome alloys to gold.

c. Pontic Fracture

Mechanical failure of the pontic may occur because of inadequate strength. Thus an all-porcelain occlusal pontic should never be used unless the occlusion is favourable. Similarly the gold framework must always be of adequate rigidity. Even slight flexion will cause cementation failure or fracture of the porcelain facing.

Probably one of the commonest causes of pontic failure is a faulty occlusion, particularly in lateral excursions, which was not corrected when the bridge was placed (*Fig.* 19.6).

An acrylic facing will wear and discolour quite rapidly. This will usually necessitate a remake of the bridge in 5–7 years if it is in the anterior region, or possibly 7–10 years for a posterior bridge.

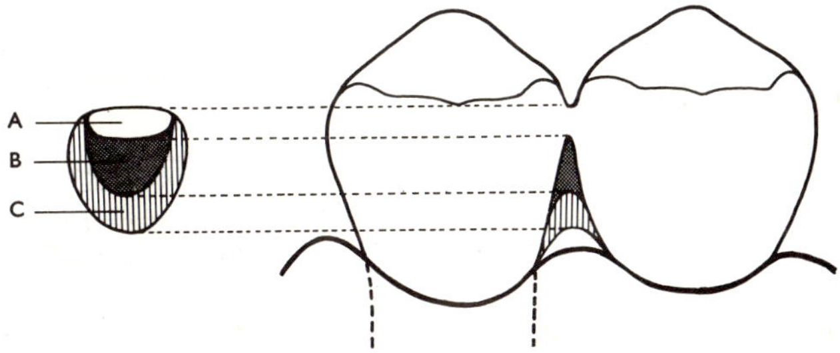

Fig. 19.5. *The solder joint.* A *Inadequate depth to resist occlusal stress.* B *Correct size and shape for both adequate strength and good oral hygiene.* C *Too deep a solder joint which will result in poor interproximal embrasures.*

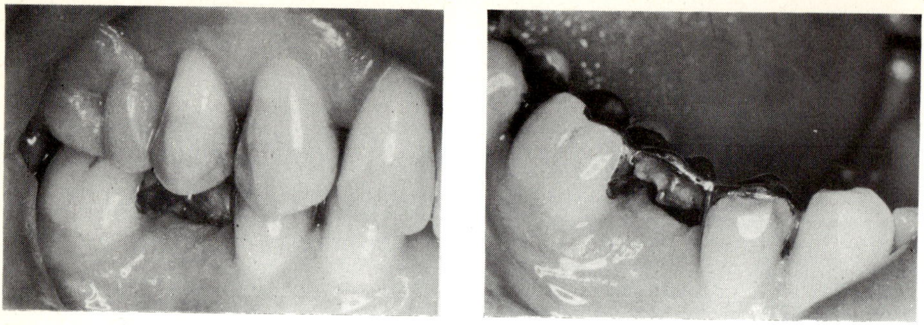

Fig. 19.6. *Pontic failure due to a heavy occlusion. Note wear facet on* 4⌉ *which is causing a breakdown of the enamel at the margin of the retainer.* (*See also* Fig. 6.62, p. 116)

d. Bonded Porcelain Failure

The failure of porcelain bonded to gold is usually due to faulty design. Thus, incorrect preparation of the occlusal surfaces of posterior teeth may well result in uneven, and in places, excessive thicknesses of porcelain (*see Fig.* 5.19, p. 77) which will be liable to fracture, particularly in the case of molar cusps. Should this occur, the replacement of the missing porcelain will prove difficult. The only technique with which some measure of success may be achieved is to remove all the porcelain overlying the gold in the region of the fracture; thread pins into the metal and, if this is thin, extend them into the dentine and then use these to retain a composite restoration.

Where the problem can be foreseen, it is sometimes practical to make the pontic section or even possibly the whole bridge, removable, usually by means of screws which are fixed in place by the operator. In this way the damaged section may be removed, returned to the laboratory and repaired and then refitted with the minimum of inconvenience to both operator and patient. Where porcelain is becoming detached because of flexion of the metal, then the only recourse is a remake.

The various other causes of bonded porcelain failure, such as inadequate strength of the interproximal metal (*see Fig.* 6.8, p. 88), have already been dealt with in Chapter 6.

■ 3. Gingival Irritation

Probably the commonest cause of gingival irritation around a bridge is plaque retention because of the patient's poor oral hygiene, possibly because they have never been instructed in its special care or because the design of the bridge makes this difficult. Other factors may be faulty margins of the retainers (*Fig.* 19.7), incorrect occlusal anatomy, over contouring of the buccal or lingual aspects, or inadequate interproximal embrasures.

Irritation of the mucosa by the pontic may also be due to the wrong choice of material for its fit surface. Acrylic is a particularly bad offender in this respect

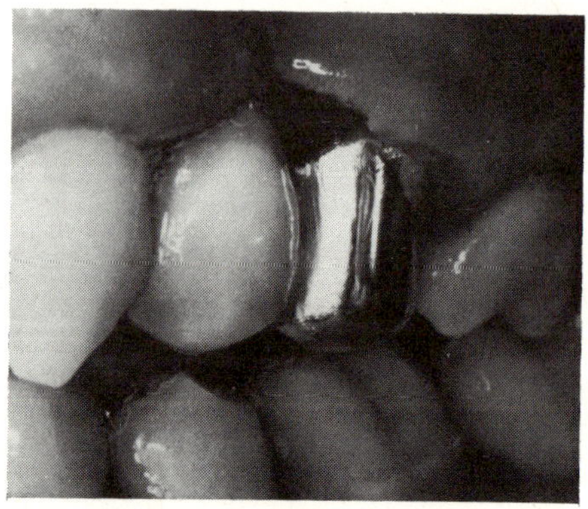

Fig. 19.7. *A poorly fitting full crown abutment and lack of a satisfactory interproximal embrasure, causing acute ulcerative gingivitis.*

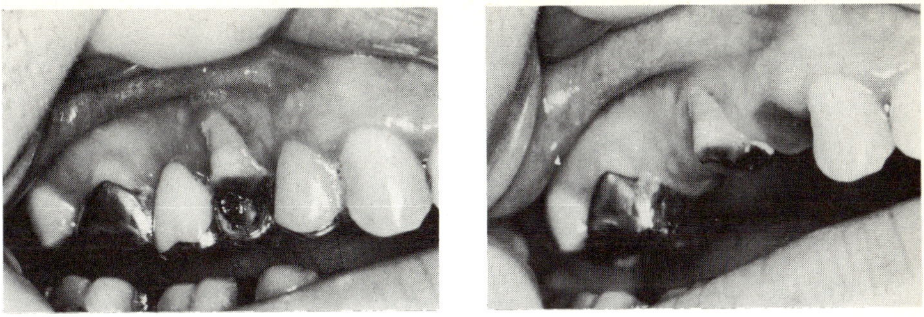

Fig. 19.8. *Periodontal breakdown of 5| and finally cementation failure of the retainer due to periodontal overloading. 64| are pontics.*

and the gingival irritation it causes may be further aggravated by the deposition of calculus on it (*see Fig.* 5.8, p. 71).

Gingival Recession

This may be local or general. If the former, the reason should be assessed and if possible eliminated. If the latter and there are no aesthetic considerations, such as the exposed, discoloured root of a non-vital tooth, the situation may be acceptable as it stands. However, generalized periodontal therapy may be indicated.

■ 4. Periodontal Breakdown

This can be either a general periodontal breakdown of the whole mouth, which may be associated with drifting of teeth, or it may be localized to the bridge abutments. The latter will usually be due to poor bridge design or execution, such as the incorrect assessment of abutment strength (*Fig.* 19.8) and possibly the number of teeth to be incorporated in a bridge.

Traumatic occlusion may be related to periodontal breakdown and should be eliminated as soon as it is evident. A bridge must always be reassessed and probably remade at the first sign of periodontal overloading of the abutment teeth.

It is important to realize that a patient's occlusion may change, sometimes very slowly as the result of wear and sometimes rapidly after a tooth is lost. It is thus essential to constantly review the occlusion of a bridge. Because it is correct when the prosthesis is fitted it does not mean to say that it will be satisfactory five to ten years later.

■ 5. Caries

Caries may affect a bridge in several ways, either directly at the margins of the retainer, indirectly by starting elsewhere on the tooth and spreading to the fit surface of the castings, or it may follow cementation failure (*Fig.* 19.9). The latter is by far the most rapid and will often result in pulpal exposure within 3–4 months.

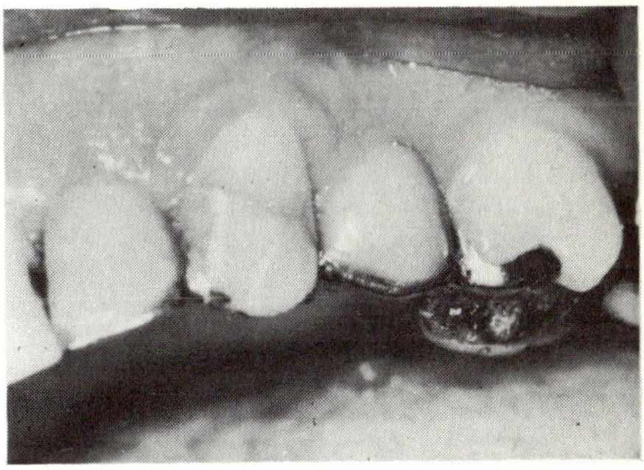

Fig. 19.9. *Caries at the margin of an uncemented retainer repeatedly treated by placing silicate fillings with the resultant loss of most of the tooth tissue.*

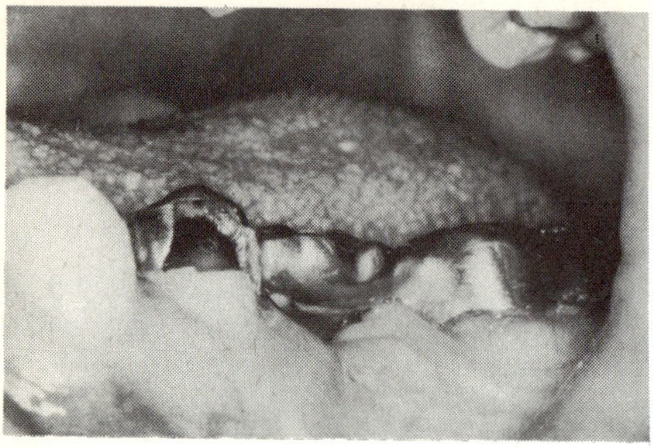

Fig. 19.10. *A fixed-fixed bridge with cementation failure of the three-quarter crown on* ⌈5 *and rampant caries. Note also the gingival proliferation below the sanitary pontic due to failure to provide adequate clearance.*

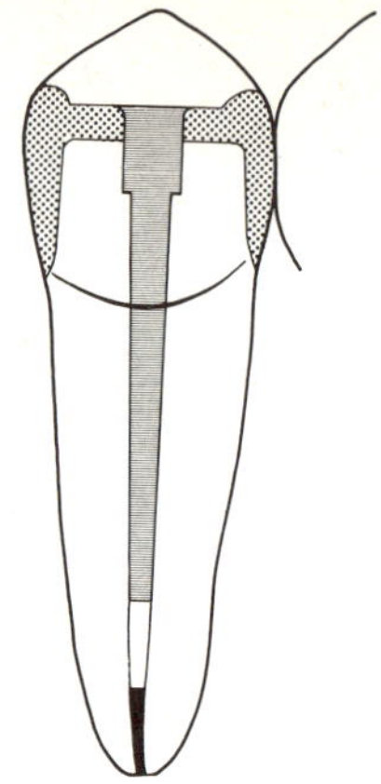

Fig. 19.11. *A cast post used to reinforce a bridge abutment following root-canal therapy. The bridge is not disturbed.*

Caries at the margins of the retainer may usually be dealt with by the use of conventional filling materials. Cohesive gold may be indicated on the occlusal surfaces; elsewhere amalgam is satisfactory or, if aesthetics demand it, composite or a similar material may be used.

Because of the rapid caries which occurs beneath a loose casting this must be removed as quickly as possible (*Fig.* 19.10). A remake is nearly always required.

■ 6. Pulpal Necrosis

If a bridge abutment dies and the tooth involved is an anterior one the case may be treated by apicectomy and the placing of a retrograde amalgam, thus avoiding disturbing the bridge at this stage. However, reinforcement of the tooth with a post will nearly always be indicated to prevent a fracture.

Should a posterior tooth be involved it will usually be necessary to gain access to the pulp chamber through the retainer to carry out the root-canal therapy. Rarely, if ever, is there any point in removing the bridge at this stage. It will serve no useful purpose and merely complicate the root treatment. After this has been carried out the tooth will require reinforcing either by a cast post (*Fig.* 19.11) or by other means, if its subsequent fracture is to be avoided (*Fig.* 19.12). Should this occur a remake is inevitable and caries in the root canal will often necessitate extraction of the abutment involved.

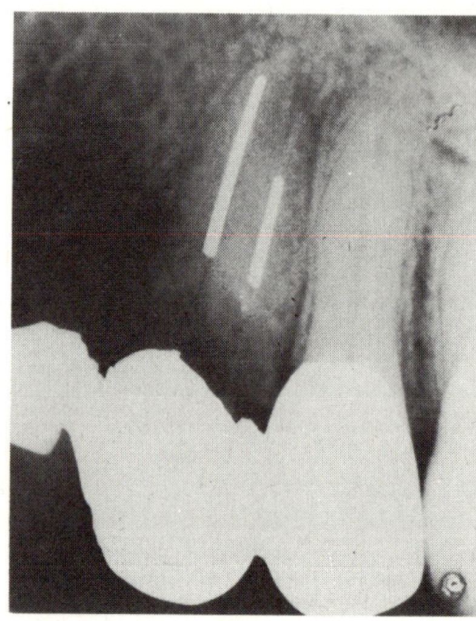

Fig. 19.12. *Non-vital bridge abutment at* ⌊4 *has fractured at the cervical margin. This has resulted in gross caries and necessitated extraction of the tooth.*

TREATMENT OF BRIDGE FAILURES

By examining and checking a bridge regularly it is frequently possible to pick up minor faults such as a premature contact or caries commencing at the margin of a retainer before they have caused any serious trouble. Their treatment is often simple and may prolong the life of the bridge by many years. Even if the fault is discovered at a later stage prompt treatment may make the difference between being able to make another bridge using the same abutment teeth and having to extract one or more teeth and fitting a partial denture. A typical example of this is cementation failure.

■ Cementation Failure

If a bridge becomes partially uncemented it is extremely important that it be removed as soon as possible, otherwise rapid caries will ensue beneath the loose casting (*Fig*. 19.13).

Before deciding on the method of removing a bridge, it is best to consider whether or not the abutment teeth may be damaged in the process. If there are any doubts on this score, it is far better to destroy the bridge during its removal than risk adversely affecting the abutment teeth and possibly rendering the construction of a further bridge impossible. An example of this is the removal of an MOD inlay, particularly in a premolar. Any attempt to remove it intact is almost bound to result in fracture of either the lingual or buccal cusp, unless the preparation is of minimal depth. The same remarks apply in varying degree to all other intracoronal retainers and even to extracoronal restorations where a deep box has been incorporated in the preparation. Thus it is always best to refer to the old X-rays and working models before proceeding, so as to get some idea of the strength of the underlying abutment tooth and of the type of preparation that was carried out.

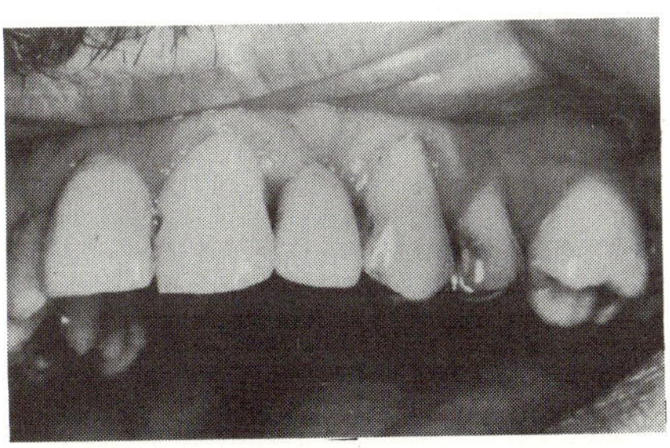

a

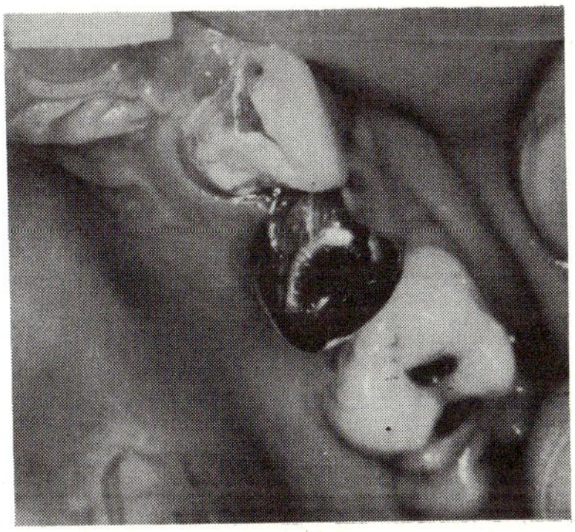

b

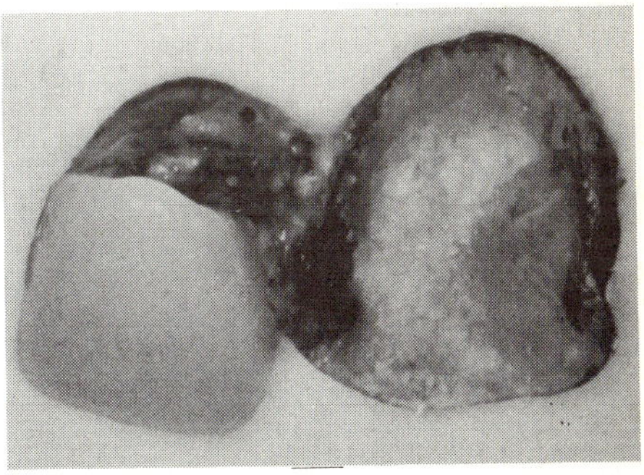

c

Fig. 19.13. *a, b, A cantilever bridge replacing ⌊2, supported by three-quarter crowns on ⌊34. The anterior retainer, being the weaker of the two, has become uncemented and rapid caries has ensued. However, by prompt treatment devitalization was avoided. The mesial shadow on ⌊4 is due to an underlying amalgam. The silicate in ⌊3 is unconnected with the retainer. c, The uncemented casting. Note the plaque on its fit surface.*

Where the tooth has appreciable mobility, the periodontal membrane may be unable to withstand the force required to dislodge the retainer intact, and thus in these instances also it is better to sacrifice the bridge.

Having decided that it is desirable to remove the prothesis intact and that this can be safely carried out, four different methods may be employed, three of which involve the application of a sudden blow in the line of withdrawal of the retainer. It is absolutely essential that the force be applied in the correct direction if fracture of the abutment teeth is to be avoided.

1. Crown Remover

When this instrument can be applied it is probably the best method of removing a fixed prosthesis. It has the advantage that it is relatively easy to see that force is being exerted in the correct direction.

There are several types of crown remover (*Fig*. 19.14). One consists of a hooked bar to which is attached a sliding weight. The hook is applied to the cervical margin of the retainer (*Fig*. 19.15) and the weight is then thrown down against a knob on the end of the handle, thus applying a sudden blow to the retainer. With some types it may also be used below the pontic.

Initially, after placement of the hook at the cervical margin, a few light blows are given to flatten the edge of the gold and provide a surface onto which the hook can engage. Before trying to remove the bridge, the second retainer should be held firmly in place by an assistant, particularly if it is uncemented. If this is not done, then when the bridge is finally dislodged a rotating force will be applied to the other retainer and thus to its abutment tooth, which may well fracture (*Fig*. 19.16). A sudden fairly hard blow is normally required to dislodge a bridge retainer. Repeated applications of a lesser force will never succeed and be far more likely to create a periodontitis. If the prosthesis is not loosened fairly readily, it is pointless to continue with the crown remover; alternative methods should be employed.

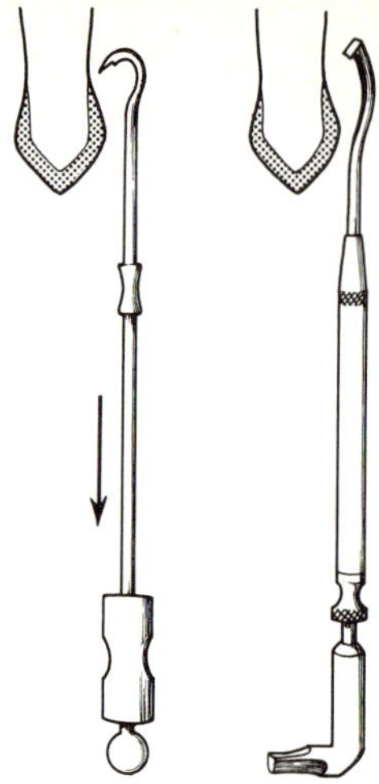

Fig. 19.14. *Two different types of crown remover. Both have a hook to engage the margin of the retainer. The left one has a sliding weight, which when thrown against the end of the handle results in a sudden blow being applied to the retainer. The right instrument is operated by jerking the handle, which passes through the body of the instrument, up and down.*

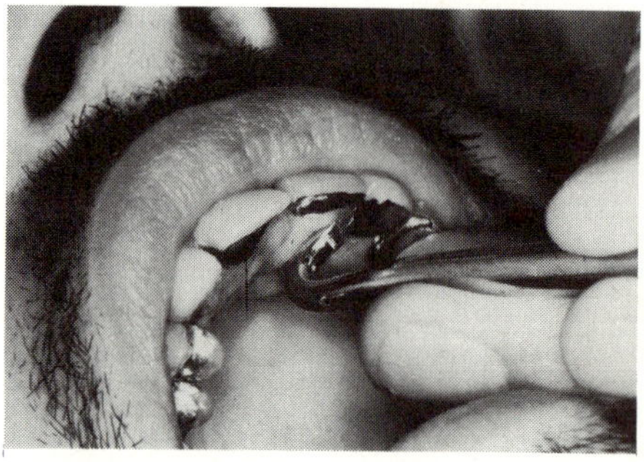

Fig. 19.15. *A crown remover being applied to the cervical margin of a retainer. The sliding weight is thrown down to remove the retainer.*

2. Use of a Straight Chisel

This is generally used as a means of applying force to a retainer on which one cannot use a crown remover. Initially the chisel is placed, either mesially or

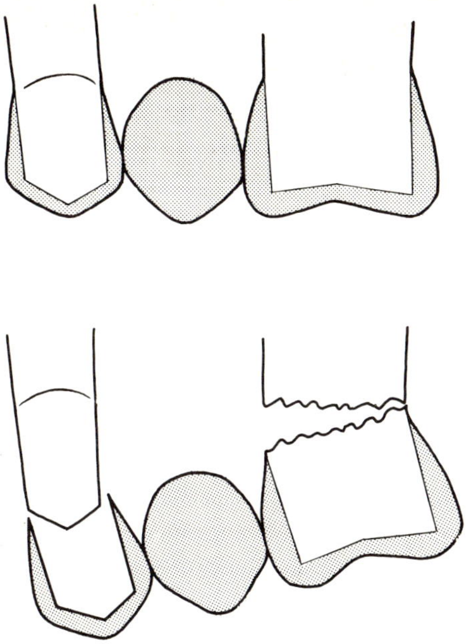

Fig. 19.16. *It is very important that the other end of a fixed-fixed bridge is held firmly in place when the second casting is being removed. Otherwise, if this suddenly becomes displaced, the resultant rotating force may cause fracture of the other abutment.*

distally, at an angle of 45° to the surface of the gold and tapped sufficiently to create a facet (*Fig.* 19.17). The point of the chisel is applied to this and the instrument positioned parallel to the line of withdrawal of the retainer. A sudden fairly hard blow, of which the patient should have warning, is then applied. Generally, it will only be necessary to apply force on one aspect of the retainer, but occasionally a blow will be required both mesially and distally.

3. Use of Brass Ligature Wire

This method may be of use where it is impossible to apply the crown remover or a chisel. A 4 ft length of wire is threaded between the pontic and the retainer which needs to be dislodged and then tied so that a loop is created (*Fig.* 19.18). A metal bar is put through this loop, one end of it held firmly, and a sudden blow applied to the other end. Great care must be taken when using this method to make certain that the wire does not cut the patient's lip. The nurse should always be instructed to guard against this occurrence.

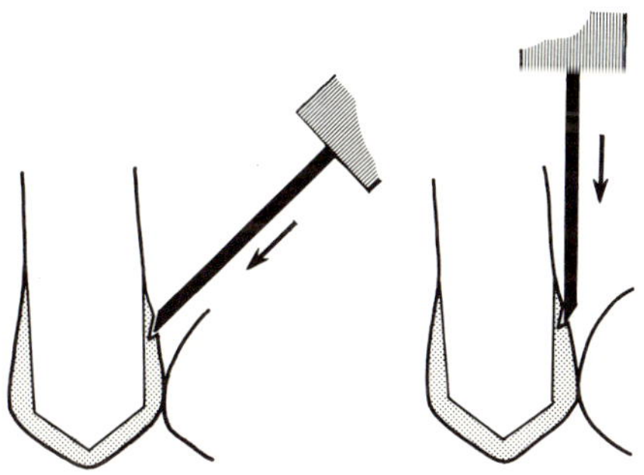

Fig. 19.17. *To remove the retainer, a straight chisel is first tapped at 45° to the surface of the casting to create a facet. It is then moved to align it with the line of withdrawal of the retainer, and hit firmly.*

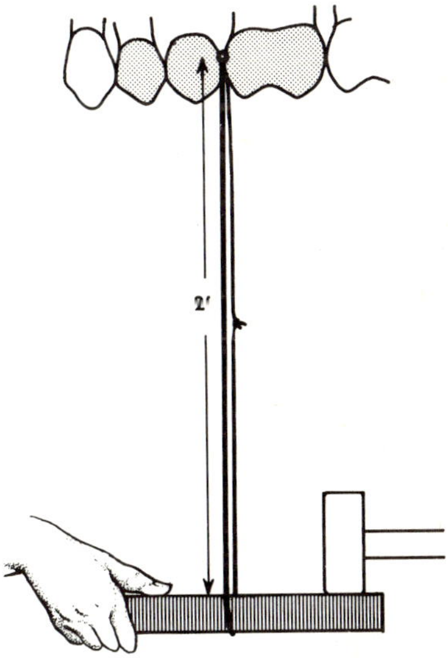

Fig. 19.18. *A wire is threaded between the pontic and the retainer and a 4 ft loop formed. A metal bar is passed through this, which is then tapped to dislodge the bridge.*

4. Use of Screw Thread
Where the retainer has a gold occlusal surface, a small hole may be drilled in this and then tapped. A threaded bolt is now inserted into the hole until it reaches the bottom. If the bolt continues to be turned, its base will then press on the tooth tissue and, with a little good fortune, will elevate the casting from the tooth. Obviously, the bolt will only be able to exert sufficient force if the casting is reasonable thick, otherwise the thread in the gold will merely strip with the pressure.

Should all the above methods fail, the retainer must be weakened, in the case of a full crown by cutting up its side (*Fig.* 19.19) and in the case of a three-quarter crown by cutting across the occlusal surface. It will then be possible to apply an instrument which will spread the crown slightly and break the cement seal. Occasionally a point of application will have to be created with a small round bur.

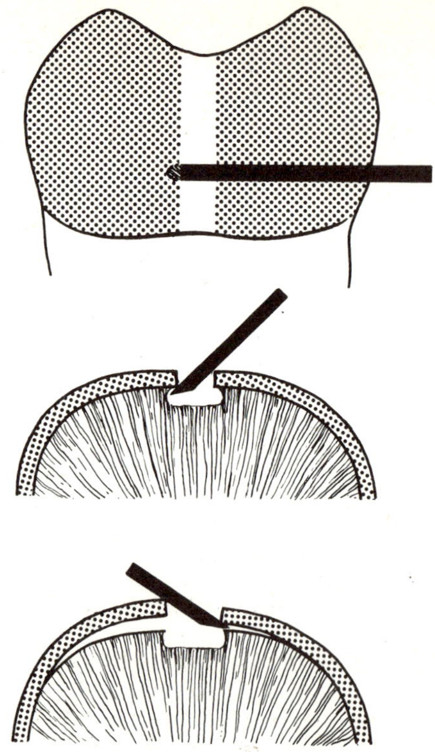

Fig. 19.19. *A full crown weakened by cutting a slot in its buccal surface. Points of application are created with a small bur and then an instrument is used to lever-up the gold and break the cement seal.*

Great care must always be taken when cutting gold with tungsten carbide burs as the head is liable to fly off and can impact in the throat or be inhaled if rubber dam is not being used. Either tungsten burs such as the 'Beaver' marketed by Jet* which are specially designed for cutting gold should be employed or diamond stones, preferably with a coarse grit.

When the operator needs to replace the bridge, the damaged crown can often be made good with a little gold and solder. In these cases it is best to wax up the defect and to check the fit in the mouth prior to investing and rebuilding it. Alternatively, an overall impression may be taken with the casting in situ.

Removal of Post Crown Retainers
If it is necessary to remove a post-retained restoration complete with post intact, the only method is the use of brass ligature wire. However, this should not normally be necessary. Where a post crown is used as a retainer, then it should always be made with a post/core unit (*see Figs*. 6.64, 6.65, p. 117) so that, if required, the separate overlying crown and thus the bridge can be removed without disturbing the post. Whenever a post is removed from a root canal, the tooth is liable to be damaged to some degree and the root can easily be split. Thus rather than trying to remove a one-piece post crown it is often best to treat it as tooth tissue and reduce it sufficiently for a full crown to be placed over it.

Where it is essential that a post is removed from a root canal then this may sometimes be achieved, provided some of the post protrudes from the root face, by

* Beaver Dental Products Ltd, P.O. Box 900. Morrisburg, Ontario, Canada KOC1X6

using a post puller such as the Eggler* which acts rather like some corkscrews. It has one pair of jaws to clamp onto the post and a second pair which press onto the root face. Thus when the screw is turned the post is elevated away from the root.

Where a post is sheered within the root canal its removal is always a slow process. Either instruments have to be gradually worked down around the post, making certain that only a minimal amount of tooth tissue is lost, until it can be removed, or it has to be drilled out.

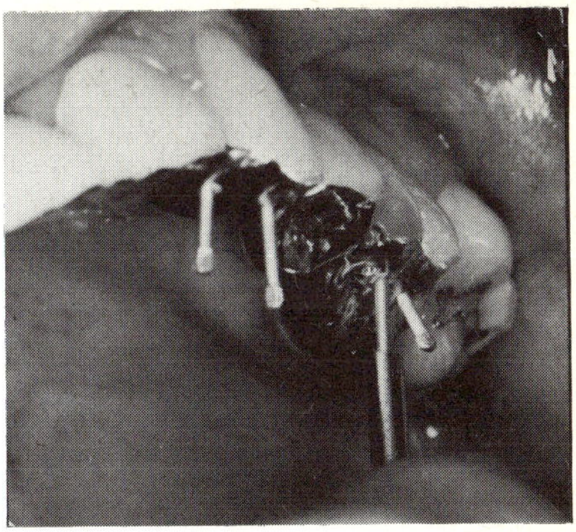

Fig. 19.20. *The bridge shown in Fig. 19.15 is being replaced and additional support obtained by using non-parallel pin fixation.*

■ Replacement of Bridge

If the bridge has been removed intact and no caries is present beneath it then it may be recemented, but before doing so the reason for the failure should be assessed. If it was due to a faulty cementing technique then it can be replaced immediately. However, the articulation should be checked to see whether or not a premature contact, for instance, has been a contributory factor. Should the failure have been due to an inadequate retainer a remake is usually indicated, but occasionally, if the casting is sufficiently rigid, it may be recemented and additional support obtained by using a method of non-parallel pin fixation, such as the threaded steel pins (*Fig.* 19.20). However, it must be remembered that this is by no means the ideal way of incorporating pins in a casting (*see* pp. 93–96).

If caries has occurred beneath the casting, this should be removed and the bridge replaced as a temporary measure with a quick setting zinc oxide and eugenol cement. If a large amount of tooth tissue has been lost it may be necessary to refit the bridge first with a self-curing acrylic prior to replacing it.

Should the pulp be exposed this will have to be removed and root-canal therapy carried out before remaking the bridge. The failed bridge will require refitting with acrylic and a post will have to be incorporated. This temporary bridge should be fabricated as carefully as possible as it will be required not only until the root-canal treatment is carried out but preferably until it can be seen that this has been successful.

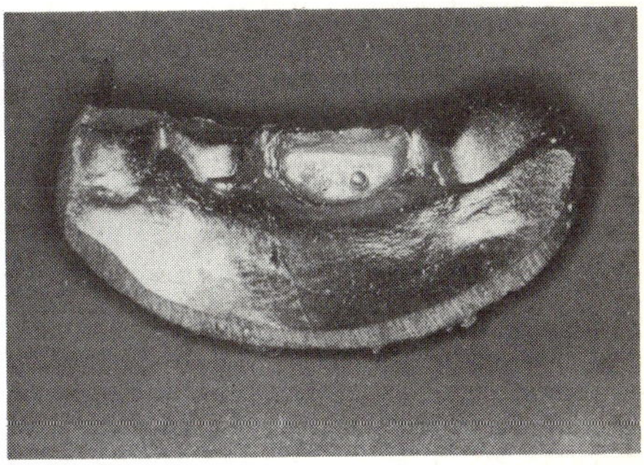

Fig. 19.21. *A rubber base impression material used on a wooden spatula has been employed to make this localized model for the construction of a new bridge pontic.*

■ Pontic Failure

Discoloration

The treatment of pontic failure depends on the cause. Thus if an acrylic facing becomes discoloured it may be possible to remove it and take an impression of

* Percy J. Clark & Co. Ltd, 1–6 Speedy Place, 118 Cromer St. London, WC1H 8BX.

the gold work still in situ, using an impression technique with a buccal or labial line of withdrawal, such as Impregum on a wooden spatula. A model is then made (*Fig*. 19.21) on which new facings may be constructed, preferably by grinding manufactured teeth to fit. These can then be cemented in place with a self-curing acrylic.

Repeated Loss of a Facing

If a porcelain facing such as the long-pin pontic repeatedly fails this is nearly always due to flexion of the gold framework breaking down the cement seal. Where the gold work seems reasonably satisfactory and flexion is minimal the porcelain facing may sometimes be replaced with an acrylic one, which is relatively flexible and not so prone to cementation failure. It may then be fixed in place with a quick-curing material, after having roughened the gold and if possible created undercuts. If retention is likely to be lacking, additional support for the facing can be gained with self-tapping screws such as the TMS.

When the gold of the pontics is thin or appreciably worn a new bridge may be necessary. However, on occasions the existing retainers can be removed, cleaned, replaced, and then an impression taken for a new pontic which can be constructed and soldered to the existing retainers.

Irritation of the Mucosa or Gingivae

If the pontic is causing gingival irritation the reason for this must be ascertained. Quite often this is due to poor oral hygiene which can be remedied by suitable instruction. However, on occasions the stage may be reached where a local gingivectomy has to be carried out before satisfactory maintenance of the gingivae in the region of the bridge can take place. This is particularly true in the case of the sanitary pontic where gingival proliferation is likely to occur beneath it. But on these occasions, unless there is a good clearance between the pontic and soft tissues, it will probably recur. Other causes of gingival irritation are defects in the design of the pontics or retainers. Faults in design include lack of adequate interproximal embrasures, excess ridge coverage, and a faulty occlusal contour, all of which can only be cured by a remake.

Calculus is liable to form on the fit surface of acrylic and, to a lesser extent, of gold. This should always be removed regularly. In many cases a remake will be indicated, with a different type of pontic, preferably with porcelain to tissue contact.

Solder Joint Failure

If a solder joint fails, the bridge should, if possible, be removed without damaging it. Should it have any separate porcelain facings these must then be detached from it by boiling in acid. The components of the bridge are then cleaned and relocated in the mouth before they are resoldered. The occlusion should be carefully checked to see that it has not been a contributory factor in the failure. Similarly the gold in the region of the solder joint should be assessed to see that it is sufficiently thick.

Periodontal Overloading

If mobility of one of the abutment teeth is noticed it is important to check the original records and X-rays to see whether or not this was present when the bridge was first fitted. If it was not, the whole mouth should be examined and in particular the corresponding teeth on the other side to try to assess if the periodontal breakdown is confined to the bridge abutments or whether it affects the whole mouth.

If it is found that it is confined to the bridge abutments this will often be due to overloading. This may be the result of faulty design, for instance incorporating too few abutment teeth in the prosthesis, or it may be due to an incorrect occlusion. Should the former be the case a remake will always be necessary, but if the latter, occlusal equilibration may provide the answer.

If the bridge has to be remade the effective root surface area and bony support of all the relevant abutments must be assessed before proceeding. In the majority of cases a fixed-fixed bridge will be indicated.

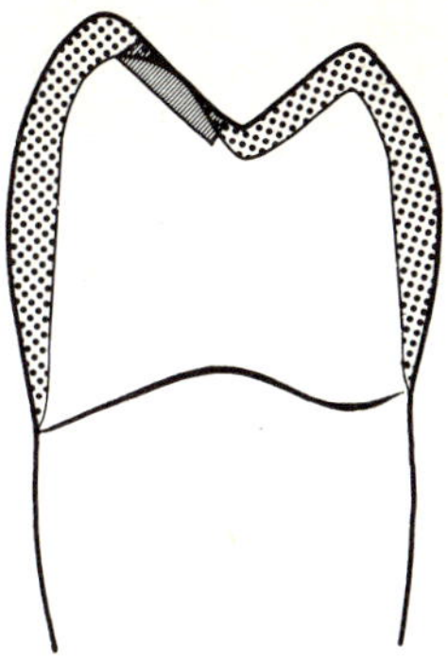

Fig. 19.22. *Perforation of the occlusal surface treated by cutting back the gold until a reasonable thickness is obtained and then plugging the cavity with amalgam or cohesive gold.*

Occlusal Adjustments

The articulation of the bridge should be checked regularly and any premature contacts, interferences, etc., eliminated. If they are allowed to persist for too long periodontal breakdown may result.

It is important that not only the bridge but also the opposing teeth be maintained in their correct articulation. Thus any restorations placed in the other arch should always be accurately contoured, any denture regularly relined, and worn teeth replaced so as to maintain the articulation in its correct relationship. If this is not done over-eruption of the bridge abutments may take place which will result in a loss of bony support and occlusal disharmony.

Caries

If caries occurs at the margin of one of the retainers then, provided it is reasonably accessible, it may be removed and a conventional restoration, usually amalgam, placed. However, if the removal of the caries has appreciably reduced the retention of the casting a remake is usually indicated. Likewise if it is impossible to be certain that all the caries has been eliminated it is better to remove the bridge and probably remake it rather than risk the loss of an abutment tooth.

Where the caries commences elsewhere on the tooth than at the margin of the retainer it can be dealt with as a conventional filling. However, the most permanent restoration possible should always be placed, otherwise the bridge will be 'at risk'. Thus a gold restoration is often to be preferred to amalgam or silicate.

If caries is secondary to cementation failure then the bridge must always be removed and the sooner the better, before it is treated. Shown in *Fig.* 19.9 (p. 253) is a bridge in which three successive silicates have been placed at the margin of an uncemented retainer to try to control the caries. The result has been the progressive loss of the majority of the tooth tissue of the canine.

Perforation of Occlusal Gold

If the occlusal gold becomes perforated it should be cut back until a reasonable thickness of metal is reached and then plugged with either cohesive gold or amalgam (*Fig.* 19.22). If, however, when the gold is taken back in the region of the perforation it proves that a large part of the occlusal coverage is very thin, a remake is indicated.

Bibliography

Harty F. J., Parkins B. J. and Wengraf A. M. (1970) The success rate of apicectomy. *Br. Dent. J.* **129**, 407.
Kantorowicz G. F. (1971) The repair and removal of bridges. *Dent. Practnr Dent. Rec.* **21**, 341.
Rajczak E. J. (1971) Trouble shooting with pins. *Dent. Clin. North. Am.* **15**, 711.

20

SPECIFIC REPLACEMENTS

Single-unit Replacements
Multiple-unit Replacements
The Treatment of a Patient

In this chapter the various ways of replacing the individual teeth will be discussed and a few multiple replacements described to illustrate some of the basic principles involved.

With the designs suggested it is assumed that all the indications for a fixed bridge prothesis are present and furthermore that there are no specific contraindications to the types described. However, the replacements suggested can never be any more than an indication of what is likely to prove most successful in any one case. No specific design for any particular missing tooth can always be applicable. It is only by considering all the factors involved in every instance that the correct type of replacement can be decided on.

To try and illustrate the way in which a case may be managed, Mr Parkins describes, at the end of this chapter, the treatment of a lady who was experiencing pain due to a faulty occlusion and who required fixed prostheses in the lower arch.

SINGLE-UNIT REPLACEMENTS

■ Upper Central Incisor

1. Spring Bridge

If the teeth adjoining the space are sound and aesthetically pleasing it is often desirable to avoid having to use them as bridge abutments. This may be achieved by replacing the central with a spring bridge (*see Fig*. 10.1, p. 152).

The abutment tooth of choice is usually the first premolar, but if this is contraindicated for any reason the second premolar may be used instead. Should the effective root surface area of these teeth be low both premolars may have to be employed, in which case the bar will be taken off the more posterior one.

A three-quarter crown is usually the most suitable retainer, but if the clinical crown is short and lacking retention a full crown may be advisable.

The pontic of choice is nearly always the porcelain jacket crown, but where the bite is very close a metal-ceramic one may be indicated. In cases where there has been appreciable soft-tissue loss a removable pontic with labial gumwork may be desirable. This can be held in place by a precision retainer, for example a Hüser.

The bar is best made of a nickel-chrome alloy, but a hard gold may also be used if laboratory facilities for producing high-temperature castings are not available.

The only real contraindications to a spring bridge are a steeply vaulted palate, which would give inadequate tissue support for the bar, and unsuitable abutment teeth.

2. Fixed-fixed Bridge

a. If there are indications for placing full crowns on the teeth on either side of the central, an all metal-ceramic bridge is the restoration of choice (*see Fig*. 7.2, p. 130). In the most favourable of cases where minimal demands will be made on the strength of the bridge aluminous porcelain may be contemplated, reinforced with discs or rods of pure alumina. However, the relatively small saving in cost is seldom justified in view of the relatively high failure rate of this type of bridge. Alternatively, a bridge comprising a gold subframe and porcelain jacket type pontics may be used (*see Fig*. 5.15, p. 75). This latter is capable of producing an excellent aesthetic result and is of particular use in the young patient. Unfortunately, it is difficult to cleanse (*see Fig*. 5.17, p. 76) and the pontics are relatively fragile. For all these reasons it is seldom employed nowadays.

b. Where it is desirable to avoid full crowns and a spring is contraindicated, a fixed-fixed bridge may be placed which is retained by pinledge preparations on 1⌋⌊2. However, great care must be taken to obtain adequate retention, particularly where the crowns of the teeth are at all short.

Summary

1. Spring Bridge

⌊1 Porcelain jacket pontic
Nickel-chrome bar
⌊4 Three-quarter gold crown

2a. Fixed-fixed Bridge

1⌋ FC
⌊1 Pontic
⌊2 FC
} All bonded porcelain

2b. Fixed-fixed Bridge

1⌋ Three-quarter pinledge
⌊1 Bonded, or possibly a long-pin pontic
⌊2 Three-quarter pinledge

■ Upper Lateral Incisor

The upper lateral is one of the commonest teeth to be lost and also, fortunately, one of the easiest to replace by means of a bridge. This is because one has an excellent abutment tooth in the form of the canine next to it.

1. Cantilever Bridge

a. Where aesthetics is of prime importance and the occlusion is favourable the best design is an all-porcelain cantilever bridge with a full crown preparation on the canine (*see Fig*. 9.1, p. 147). This has little more chance of fracture than a simple porcelain jacket crown. However, where the occlusion is heavier, bonded porcelain should be used (*see Fig*. 9.2, p. 148).

b. If the aesthetic demands of the patient are less critical, a three-quarter crown may be used on the canine and a bonded or possibly a long-pin pontic employed to replace the lateral. Less tooth tissue loss and gingival irritation will be caused by this design than by the previous one.

2. Spring Bridge

Where a simple cantilever bridge is contraindicated a spring bridge may be used, the retainer being a three-quarter crown on either the first or second premolars. The latter is preferable if its root surface area is adequate, as a more favourable line will be achieved for the bar.

3. Fixed-fixed Bridge

If both the central and canine require full crowns a three-unit metal-ceramic bridge would normally be employed.

4. Fixed-movable Bridge

Should one of the retainers be weak—e.g. a post crown may lack retention because there has been extensive caries in the root canal prior to its construction—then a fixed-movable design will be indicated using the post crown as the minor retainer. The stress-breaking effect of the dovetail and slot will appreciably reduce the likelihood of cementation failure.

Summary

1a. Cantilever Bridge

⌊2 pontic
⌊3 FC
} All porcelain or bonded porcelain

1b. Cantilever Bridge
⌊2 Long-pin or bonded pontic
⌊3 Three-quarter crown
2. Spring Bridge
⌊2 Porcelain jacket pontic
Nickel-chrome bar
⌊5 Three-quarter gold crown
3. Fixed-fixed bridge
⌊1 FC
⌊2 Pontic
⌊3 FC
} All bonded porcelain

■ Upper Canine

The loss of an upper canine is far more serious than the loss of a lateral. The occlusion is heavy in this region and the tooth mesial to it is a poor abutment because of its relatively small clinical crown and low root surface area. To gain adequate support it is necessary to extend the design distally to involve both premolars or mesially to involve not only the lateral, but also the central.

1. Cantilever Bridge
The design of choice for the replacement of the canine, providing the abutment teeth are suitable, is the use of three-quarter crowns on both premolars and a bonded pontic soldered to these (*see Fig.* 9.3, p. 149). If it is particularly important to avoid any display of gold or the clinical crowns are short, then bonded full crowns may be employed on the premolars and a three-unit metal-ceramic bridge placed.

2. Fixed-fixed Bridge
When the lateral requires crowning and particularly if this form of treatment is indicated on the central as well, a four-unit bonded bridge may be placed using full crowns on the central, lateral, and first premolar. If the occlusion is favourable then it may only be necessary to use the lateral mesially.

3. Spring Bridge
If the premolars are weak and unsuitable as abutments a spring bridge, using the first molar as a retainer, may be employed, providing that the shape of the palate is acceptable. However, the replacement of the canine by a spring bridge is not nearly so satisfactory as the use of this design for the central.

Summary
1. Cantilever Bridge
⌊3 Bonded pontic
⌊4 Three-quarter or FC
⌊5 Three-quarter or FC
2. Fixed-fixed Bridge
⌊1 FC
⌊2 FC
⌊3 Pontic
⌊4 FC
} All bonded porcelain
3. Spring Bridge
⌊3 Porcelain jacket pontic
Nickel-chrome bar
⌊6 Three-quarter gold crown

■ Upper First Premolar

This tooth probably requires replacement more often than any other and because of its proximity to the anterior region good aesthetics is usually required.

1. Fixed-movable Bridge
This replacement of the first premolar has the merit of being simple, reliable, and aesthetically pleasing.

a. A Selberg modified three-quarter crown, which will not involve any display of gold, or occasionally a conventional three-quarter crown is employed in the canine and a slot cut in the distal aspect of this to house the dovetail attached to the pontic. A three-quarter crown is generally used on the second premolar. However, if a bonded full crown is indicated this may be provided and the pontic made of the same material.

b. If the canine requires restoring with a full crown the design is usually reversed, a bonded full crown being employed on this tooth. The pontic is made of a similar material and the three-quarter crown in the second premolar becomes the minor retainer, a box being incorporated in the mesial aspect of the preparation to accommodate the slot.

2. Cantilever Bridge
In rare instances where the canine is unsuitable as an abutment, a cantilever bridge using both the second premolar and first molar may be indicated.

3. Fixed-fixed Bridge
Should bonded full crowns be necessary to restore the canine and second premolar then a fixed-fixed bridge may be placed.

Summary

1a. Fixed-movable Bridge

|3 Selberg modified three-quarter crown with distal slot
|4 Bonded pontic
|5 Three-quarter crown

1b. Fixed-movable Bridge

|3 FC } Both bonded
|4 Pontic } porcelain
|5 Three-quarter crown with mesial slot

2. Cantilever Bridge

|4 Bonded or possibly long-pin pontic
|5 Three-quarter crown
|6 Three-quarter crown

3. Fixed-fixed bridge

|3 FC } All
|4 Pontic } bonded
|5 FC } porcelain

■ Upper Second Premolar

Fixed-movable Bridge
The replacement of the upper second premolar is relatively straightforward, a fixed-movable design being the method of choice in the majority of cases. The tooth used as the major abutment is the first molar. This is well able to withstand the additional load placed on it and provides excellent retention. A three-quarter crown is usually employed as the retainer. However, if the molar requires restoration with a full crown this will usually be of the metal-ceramic type and the pontic will then be of a similar material.

The minor retainer is usually a three-quarter crown in the first premolar with a distal slot. However, if the caries rate is low and the mesial contact of the tooth is sound a modified distal-occlusal inlay may be employed. Alternatively, an MOD may be indicated in cases where this restoration is necessary to restore the tooth. Both these have the advantage that they avoid any display of gold incisally. However, no Class II inlay is as reliable as a three-quarter crown.

Summary

1a. Fixed-movable Bridge

|4 Three-quarter crown with distal slot
|5 Bonded or long-pin pontic
|6 Three-quarter crown

1b. Fixed-movable Bridge

|4 DO or MOD gold inlay with distal slot
|5 Pontic } Both bonded
|6 FC } porcelain

■ Upper First Molar*

The replacements indicated for this tooth are similar to those used for the second premolar, a fixed-movable design being employed with three-quarter crowns on the teeth on either side. An intracoronal inlay is rarely indicated as the minor retainer as aesthetics is of less importance in this region.

If the periodontal condition is doubtful it may prove necessary to use both premolars mesially or employ a fixed-fixed design.

A bonded pontic is generally employed, but occasionally where there has been extensive soft-tissue loss a sanitary design may be of value.

Should the prognosis of the second molar be doubtful and the third molar missing, it may be desirable to use full crowns on both premolars mesially and incorporate a precision retainer such as the rigid Crismani in the distal aspect of the second premolar. Should the second molar be lost at a later stage then it and the pontic can be removed without

* Second molar has similar design

disturbing the other retainers. A free-end saddle supported by a movable Crismani fitted into the matrix of the original rigid Crismani can then be placed.

Summary
Fixed-movable Bridge
⌊5 Three-quarter crown with distal slot
⌊6 Metal-ceramic pontic
⌊7 Three-quarter crown

■ Lower Central Incisor

This is a difficult tooth to replace by any form of prothesis, fixed or removable. The small size of the lower anterior teeth makes their preparation and also the housing of any dovetail very difficult and generally precludes the use of precision retainers. An alternative to conventional bridge work is the use of horizontal pin fixation.

1. Fixed-fixed Bridge

a. The best method of replacing the lower central is usually by means of a three-unit bonded bridge with full crowns on the neighbouring teeth. However, the aesthetic results achieved are often poor as it is impossible to reduce the tooth tissue sufficiently to provide an adequate thickness of porcelain over the gold (*see Fig.* 6.48, p. 108).

b. An alternative to the bonded bridge is the use of three-quarter pinlays on the abutments. However, these preparations are by no means easy to carry out on lower incisors; a lot of gold will often be displayed, particularly if the teeth are fan shaped, and the retention obtained is likely to be inadequate.

2. Cantilever Bridge

An alternative to the fixed-fixed bridge is a simple cantilever design extending from the lateral. Whether or not this will be satisfactory depends on the root surface area of the abutment tooth and the occlusion. However, if both these are acceptable a very satisfactory bridge can result. In its favour is the fact that the lateral is normally a larger tooth than the central with a bigger root surface area. A metal-ceramic bridge is usually indicated. Alternatively, if the crown is reasonably large and aesthetics is not critical, a three-quarter crown may be used as the retainer.

3. Horizontal Pin Fixation

This has already been described in detail in Chapter 6. Providing their periodontal condition is good the use of just the neighbouring teeth as abutments is satisfactory. A bonded or long-pin pontic is generally employed.

Summary
1a. Fixed-fixed Bridge
1⌉ FC
⌈1 Pontic
⌈2 FC
} All bonded porcelain
1b. Fixed-fixed Bridge
1⌉ Three-quarter pinlay
⌈1 Long-pin pontic
⌈2 Three-quarter pinlay
2a. Cantilever Bridge
⌈1 Bonded or long-pin pontic
⌈2 Three-quarter crown
2b. Cantilever Bridge
⌈1 Pontic
⌈2 FC
} All bonded porcelain
3. Horizontal Pin Fixation
1⌉ Horizontal pin
⌈1 Bonded or long-pin pontic
⌈2 Horizontal pin

■ Lower Lateral Incisor

1. Cantilever Bridge

a. The lower lateral is a far easier tooth to replace than the central, a simple cantilever bridge from the canine being all that is required in the majority of cases. A bonded full crown may be used on the canine and the pontic constructed from a similar material. The all-porcelain cantilever bridge which is so successful in the upper arch is not satisfactory here because it is too prone to fracture.

b. Where aesthetics is of less importance a three-quarter crown may be used on the canine with a long-pin pontic for the lateral.

2. Fixed-fixed Bridge
If the bite is very heavy then a three-unit all metal-ceramic bridge may be indicated.

3. Horizontal Pin Fixation
A similar design may be used to that described for replacing the central.

Summary
1a. Cantilever Bridge

⌈2 Pontic	All bonded
⌈3 FC	porcelain

1b. Cantilever Bridge
⌈2 Bonded or long-pin pontic
⌈3 Three-quarter crown
2. Fixed-fixed Bridge

⌈1 FC	All
⌈2 Pontic	bonded
⌈3 FC	porcelain

3. Horizontal Pin Fixation
⌈1 Horizontal pin
⌈2 Bonded or long-pin pontic
⌈3 Horizontal pin

■ Lower Canine

1. Cantilever Bridge
The replacement of this tooth is similar to the upper canine, the most usual method being a cantilever bridge from both lower premolars. However, the shape and size of the lower premolars, particularly the first, is not so favourable, sufficient retention being far more difficult to achieve. Thus, whereas a three-quarter crown is usually adequate on the upper first bicuspid, a full crown is often needed on the corresponding lower tooth. The most suitable pontic because of the heavy occlusion in this region is a metal-ceramic one.

2. Fixed-fixed Bridge
Where a cantilever bridge is contra-indicated a fixed-fixed design may be used, with full crowns on the lateral and first premolar, the bridge being constructed of porcelain bonded to gold.

Summary
1a. Cantilever Bridge
⌈3 Bonded or long-pin pontic
⌈4 Three-quarter crown
⌈5 Three-quarter crown
1b. Cantilever Bridge

⌈3 Pontic	All
⌈4 FC	bonded
⌈5 FC	porcelain

2. Fixed-fixed Bridge

⌈2 FC	All
⌈3 Pontic	bonded
⌈4 FC	porcelain

■ Lower First Premolar

1. Fixed-movable Bridge
a. If the angulation of the teeth is favourable the lower first premolar may be replaced by a fixed-movable design using a three-quarter crown on the second premolar as the major retainer. In the canine a Selberg modified three-quarter crown is usually satisfactory. However, the canine is frequently inclined lingually and, because of this, it is impossible to prepare an adequate box in its distal aspect at the correct angulation to house the dovetail, which must have the same line of withdrawal as the major retainer. This may sometimes be overcome by using a three-quarter crown on the canine.
b. Occasionally it may be necessary to go to a full crown on the canine, but in these instances the design may be reversed, using a bonded full crown on the canine as the major retainer and constructing the pontic of a similar material. The dovetail attached to this will rest in a three-quarter crown in the second premolar.

2. Cantilever Bridge
Where incorporation of the canine in the bridge is contraindicated, usually because of its unfavourable angulation, a cantilever design may be employed using three-quarter or full crowns on both the

second premolar and first molar. The pontic of choice would be either one made of bonded porcelain or possibly a long-pin facing. It is desirable to keep the occlusal surface to a minimum to avoid any overloading of the second premolar.

Summary

1a. Fixed-movable Bridge

⌈3 Selberg modified three-quarter crown. (Occasionally three-quarter crown is indicated)
⌈4 Bonded or long-pin pontic
⌈5 Three-quarter crown

1b. Fixed-movable Bridge

⌈3 Full crown } Bonded
⌈4 Pontic } porcelain

⌈5 Three-quarter crown with mesial slot

2. Cantilever Bridge

⌈4 Bonded pontic
⌈5 Three-quarter or full crown
⌈6 Three-quarter or full crown

■ Lower Second Premolar

Fixed-movable Bridge

A fixed-movable design is generally indicated for this replacement.

The major retainer would be a three-quarter crown on the first molar with a similar restoration in the first premolar as the minor retainer with a slot in its distal aspect to house the dovetail. Alternatively, a distal occlusal inlay with a mesial countersink in the lock may be satisfactory if the caries rate is low, and will be better aesthetically. A bonded or long-pin pontic is usually employed. On occasions a sanitary pontic may be used if it is aesthetically acceptable, but it must be possible to design it so that there is plenty of space between it and the soft tissues so that it can be easily cleaned.

Summary

Fixed-movable Bridge

⌈4 Three-quarter crown (or DO or MOD gold inlay with distal slot)
⌈5 Bonded or possibly sanitary pontic
⌈6 Three-quarter crown

■ Lower First Molar*

1. Fixed-movable Bridge

Here again a fixed-movable design is indicated, with three-quarter crowns on the second molar and second premolar as the major and minor retainers respectively. Occasionally the second molar may be badly tilted and inadequately erupted, particularly at its distal aspect. In these instances a full crown may be required to make certain of sufficient retention.

If there is plenty of vertical clearance a sanitary pontic is preferable, but if the space is at all limited then a bonded pontic will be best.

2. Fixed-fixed Bridge

With nearly all the posterior single-unit replacements a fixed-fixed all metal-ceramic bridge may be employed and this will avoid any display of gold. However, it must be borne in mind that a far more drastic reduction of tooth tissue will be necessary. The occlusal reduction required, for instance, will be approximately 2 mm and this will appreciably reduce the retention available.

Summary

1. Fixed-movable Bridge

⌈5 Three-quarter crown with distal slot
⌈6 Sanitary or bonded pontic
⌈7 Three-quarter or sometimes FC

2. Fixed-fixed Bridge

⌈5 Full crown } All
⌈6 Pontic } bonded
⌈7 Full crown } porcelain

MULTIPLE-UNIT REPLACEMENTS

Some of the bridge replacements suitable for multiple tooth loss will now be described. It is impossible to enumerate all the combinations and permutations of missing teeth here. Similarly, the designs

* Second molar has similar design.

may well vary more with each individual case than those of the single-unit replacements. However, some idea should be obtained of the possibilities involved. Where practical it is nearly always desirable to break down a large bridge, for instance one involving the whole upper arch, into several smaller units. Reliability is improved thereby and if a failure should result then it will probably only affect one part of the total restoration, thus saving both time and expense in its repair.

■ Upper Central and Lateral Incisors

Fixed-fixed Bridge

Here a four-unit all-bonded bridge is usually indicated, with full crowns on the other central and the canine. If the clinical crowns are fairly long, three-quarter pinlays may prove satisfactory, but should be used with care.

■ Replacement of Upper Lateral and Canine

1. Fixed-fixed Bridge

This is a difficult replacement because of the weight of the occlusion on the canine. Usually both centrals and both premolars will have to be involved and in the majority of cases full crowns will be indicated on these teeth to make certain of adequate retention.

2. Compound Bridge

An alternative is the use of two separate bridges, a cantilever bridge from the premolars to replace the canine and a spring bridge from the first molar carrying the lateral.

■ Upper First and Second Premolars

1. Fixed-movable Bridge

Here a fixed-movable bridge is usually indicated. The major retainer would be a three-quarter crown on the first molar and the minor retainer a three-quarter crown or possibly a full crown on the canine.

2. Fixed-semimovable Bridge

Instead of the conventional dovetail and slot connecting the two parts of the bridge a covered dovetail may sometimes be preferable to limit vertical movement, particularly if the bridge is opposed by a denture.

■ Both Upper Premolars and the First Molar

1. Fixed-fixed Bridge

Because of the length of the span a fixed-fixed design is usually desirable in this instance. A full crown will be required on the canine and a strong three-quarter or full crown on the second molar. If there is any doubt regarding the ability of the second molar to carry the load the third molar, where present, may also be involved in the design.

Should there be difficulty in aligning the preparations on the abutment teeth a rigid retainer (attachment) such as the Bayeler may be incorporated in the design.

2. Fixed-semimovable Bridge

If it is desirable to avoid a full crown on the canine a three-quarter crown may sometimes be employed, but in these instances a covered dovetail should be used at the distal aspect of the canine to allow of limited vertical movement so as to provide some stress breaking, thus reducing the chance of cementation failure.

■ Upper Second Premolar and First Molar

The design indicated here may be:

Fixed-semimovable Bridge

This will have a strong three-quarter crown on the first premolar, a covered dovetail in its distal aspect, and a good three-quarter or full crown on the second molar. Alternatively, a fixed-fixed design may be used with a full crown on the premolar and a very strong three-quarter or a full crown on the second molar.

In a large number of cases the first premolar will not be strong enough to carry the load mesially, particularly if there has been no forward drift of the second molar. In these instances both the canine and premolar should be used with full crowns on these teeth and a fixed-fixed design employed.

■ Both Upper Centrals

1. Spring Bridges

If all the other anterior teeth are sound and aesthetically pleasing two individual spring bridges may be the best replacement if there is no specific contra-indication to this type of prothesis (*see Fig.* 10.10, p. 156). However, they should always be kept entirely separate and adequate clearance must be provided between the two bars.

2. Fixed-fixed Bridge

Alternatively a fixed-fixed design may be employed. However, the laterals are not usually able to carry the additional load on their own and thus the canines have to be incorporated in the design also. The bridge will usually be constructed with full crowns on the abutment teeth and the whole made in a bonded porcelain.

If three-quarter pinlays are used the crowns should be of a reasonable length and great care taken to make certain that retention is adequate.

■ All the Upper Incisors

1. Fixed-fixed Bridge

In the majority of cases the canines are strong enough to support a bridge replacing the four incisors. The commonest restoration would be an all-bonded bridge with full crowns on the canines.

Where there is any doubt regarding the ability of the canines to carry the load either one or two premolars on either side of the arch should also be involved in the design.

2. Compound Bridge

An alternative is to use three-quarter crowns on both premolars on either side, soldered together. Slots will be provided in the mesial aspect of the first bicuspids into which dovetails will sit which are fixed to the full crowns on the canines. In this way additional support is gained for the canines and any mesial displacing force will be resisted, without fixing the three-quarter crowns to the canines and thus risking cementation failure.

■ Both Lower Centrals or the Central and Lateral Incisors

1. Fixed-fixed Bridge

The best replacement in these instances is usually a four-unit bonded bridge with full crowns on the teeth on either side as retainers. However, because of the lack of space for the porcelain and metal the aesthetic result will usually be inferior to that achieved in the upper arch. It is extremely difficult in the average case to obtain sufficient retention from conventional pinlays. It is only when the crowns of the abutments are larger and longer than average that these prove feasible.

2. Horizontal Pin Fixation

The only other alternative is horizontal pin fixation, again using one tooth on either side as abutments, unless the periodontal condition of these teeth is in doubt, or where there is an unfavourable arch form, when additional abutments will have to be employed.

■ All the Lower Incisors

1. Fixed-fixed Bridge

A fixed-fixed bridge is indicated here, using bonded full crowns on both canines. These teeth are generally able to carry the load without any additional support, although occasionally the design may have to be extended to involve the premolars.

2. Precision-retained Prothesis

Should there be extensive soft-tissue loss

a removable prosthesis will have to be provided. This may be achieved by using a conventional denture, or, in suitable cases, either precision retainers in the canines or a milled bar fixed between them (*see Fig.* 12.7, p. 170).

■ Both Lower Premolars

Fixed-movable Bridge

The design of choice here is usually a fixed-movable one, the major retainer being a three-quarter crown on the first molar and the minor one a three-quarter crown on the canine with a slot in its distal aspect to incorporate the dovetail. Sometimes, because of the unfavourable angulation of the canine, a full crown will be required. If this preparation on the canine will align with that on the molar without sacrificing retention on either tooth, consideration may be given to a fixed-fixed bridge. However, it is important to be certain that there will be sufficient retention from the three-quarter crown on the molar and if there is any doubt a full crown should be used.

■ Lower Second Premolar and First Molar

Fixed-fixed or Fixed-movable Bridge

Here the choice is fairly evenly balanced between a fixed-fixed and fixed-movable design and it is local factors such as the angulation of the teeth and their periodontal condition that will determine which is the more desirable.

A strong three-quarter or full crown is used distally; mesially it will often be best to incorporate both the canine and premolar in the design to provide adequate support. If the design is fixed-fixed a full crown will be required on the premolar, but if it is fixed-movable a three-quarter crown may prove adequate as the minor retainer if it is used on its own. However, when the canine and first premolar are splinted together it will often be necessary to use full crowns on both teeth to ensure adequate retention. If there is any doubt regarding the prognosis of the molar, continuity of treatment may be provided for by using two full crowns as retainers mesially and placing a rigid Crismani in their distal aspect, which could later be replaced by a movable Crismani should the molar be lost and a free-end saddle be required.

■ Both Lower Premolars and the First Molar

Fixed-fixed Bridge

A fixed-fixed design is indicated here, providing the operator is certain that the abutment teeth are capable of withstanding the very considerable strain imposed by a span of this length. Full crowns should be used as retainers on the canine and second molar and it may even be desirable to involve the third molar, if present. The whole of the bridge, except possibly the full crown on the second molar, is best constructed of bonded porcelain.

If there is extensive soft-tissue loss a sectional or conventional chrome-cobalt denture will usually be the best form of replacement.

■ Lower Second Premolar and First and Second Molars

Fixed-fixed Bridge

Because of the length of the span, bridgework will often be contraindicated and a sectional denture will be the best replacement, particularly if the teeth are badly tilted. However, if the abutment teeth are strong, and particularly if there has been some mesial drift of the third molar, a fixed-fixed bridge should be placed with full crowns on the canine and first premolar mesially and the third molar distally.

With this replacement and also occasionally with the ones described previously for the lower posterior region, unfavourable angulation may make the provision of a conventional fixed-fixed bridge impossible. In these instances a precision retainer may solve the problem as it will permit different lines of insertion for the retainers whilst still keeping the advantages of a fixed-fixed bridge. A Beyeler is suitable for this purpose.

However, it must be remembered that a deep box will have to be cut in the distal aspect of the relevant tooth to house it, and this may not always be possible.

If there is any doubt regarding the prognosis of the third molar the placing of a rigid Crismani in the distal aspect of the premolar may be indicated. If at some future date the third molar is lost the male component of the Crismani can be changed from a rigid to a movable type and then incorporated in a free-end saddle prothesis. The retainers in the canine and first premolar will not have to be disturbed as the male components of the rigid and movable Crismani are interchangeable.

In conclusion it must be emphasized that no one bridge design will always be the correct one, particularly for multiple unit replacements. However, it must always be right to break down extensive bridgework into several small units, thus simplifying and improving the preparation of the abutment teeth. Furthermore, should any one component fail only a relatively small part of the whole bridge will be affected.

Continuity of treatment should always be carefully considered at the design stage and the prognosis of each of the abutments evaluated. Thus if a tooth is lost a few years after the bridge is placed this should already have been allowed for and will be treatable with the minimum of disturbance of the existing restorations and inconvenience to the patient.

THE TREATMENT OF A PATIENT

BRIAN J. PARKINS

The treatment of one particular case will be described to illustrate how some of the basic principles of bridgework and, indeed, restorative dentistry in general may be applied.

It is important that with all restorative dentistry the approach must always be flexible and take into account the individual requirements of the patient. It is also necessary to understand that a treatment plan is pieced together over several consultations spanning a period of time which is sufficient to permit all investigative tests to be applied and assessed (and, if necessary, reassessed) in the areas where the prognosis is not as obvious as one may wish.

A good premise is the maximum conservation of tooth tissue compatible with the long-term prognosis of any restorations which may be cemented. For example, when one is assured of a satisfactory prognosis, three-quarter crowns should be used in preference to full crowns because less tooth tissue is destroyed during preparation and because a large part of the margin is supragingival—a great advantage in itself—a better finish can be obtained. Obviously, if it is felt that a three-quarter crown may not provide sufficient retention, then it must never be used. Likewise, it is desirable, where practical, to have margins which are just subgingival in areas where the aesthetic considerations are critical, as with the labial surface of upper anterior teeth.

When carrying out occlusal equilibration, although in many ways it may prove simpler to crown all or a large number of teeth, thereby enabling the control of the reconstruction of the occlusal surfaces, it is often far better to make adjustments to the natural teeth. It is wise, when a patient is symptom-free but exhibits a less than textbook occlusion, to leave well alone. It must be remembered that in the vast majority of cases the natural dentition is, in the unrestored state, infinitely better than one where the operator has imposed his own parameters as to the necessities of an ideal occlusion.

■ Case History

The patient who presented for treatment was a very pleasant, sensible lady aged 37 years. She was a dental receptionist and had been referred by the principal of the practice in which she was employed, because of difficulties in movements of the lower jaw and associated problems, in particular with the muscles of mastication.

History of the Present Condition

The patient said that she always had a 'strange bite'. Orthodontic therapy had never been suggested although the upper second premolars had been extracted 'in an attempt to clear up sinus problems'.

During the last five years, the patient had developed a click in the left temporomandibular joint and was able to 'dislocate' the condyle on yawning first thing in the morning. Sometimes the pain radiated to the area over the insertion of the temporalis muscle, and sometimes presented as toothache on the upper left side, however, there was still an awareness of maxillary sinusitis which it was thought could present as toothache.

Previous Medical History

Nothing relevant.

Discussion So Far

There are various important implications which can be of great assistance in forming a provisional diagnosis.

First, the patient was sensible. It is not at all uncommon that patients suffering from muscle dysfunction syndrome are emotionally disturbed and insecure, thus making the interpretation of their description of the symptoms difficult.

Second, the occupation of the patient is such that motivation of the practice of preventive measures and procedures, and the understanding of the nature of the treatment, were facilitated.

Third, from the history there could be a strong indication that even at this stage the presence of attrition required examination of the muscles of mastication as well as the teeth and supporting tissues.

■ On Examination

The patient was able to open to about two fingers height in the incisor region. This was in a straight line until the final phase when there was a deviation to the left.

Palpation of the muscles revealed tenderness in the region of the insertion of the left temporalis and left lateral pterygoid muscles. The gingival contour was very good and the oral hygiene was of above average standard but could be improved, especially on the lingual aspect of the lower incisors. There was an adequate band of attached gingivae around the teeth requiring restorations and over the edentulous areas where pontics would be placed. There was, however, a high attachment of the frenum in the lower left premolar region which could give trouble by retracting the attached margin, should hygiene control fall below par.

Teeth Standing

8765 321	123 5678
87 54321	12345 8

Radiographic examination showed that the supporting tissues were healthy and favourable root anatomy was present in all posterior teeth, especially the molars. The amalgam restorations in the upper teeth had good marginal integrity and the contours interproximally were favourable to gingival health. The contour of the occlusal aspects were, however, a little flat (*Figs*. 20.1, 20.2). There was no apparent necessity for endodontic therapy.

The restorations in the anterior teeth, although a little discoloured, were satisfactory in terms of marginal integrity and contour. Gingival health was above average and there was no region where introduction of a pocket depth probe led to subsequent bleeding or where the sulcus depth was more than 3 mm.

Occlusion

The skeletal base was Class 1. The patient had complained of severe limitation of movement which had been treated by her general practitioner who prescribed the use of a bite guard. Following regression of the symptoms, the retruded contact was seen to be only

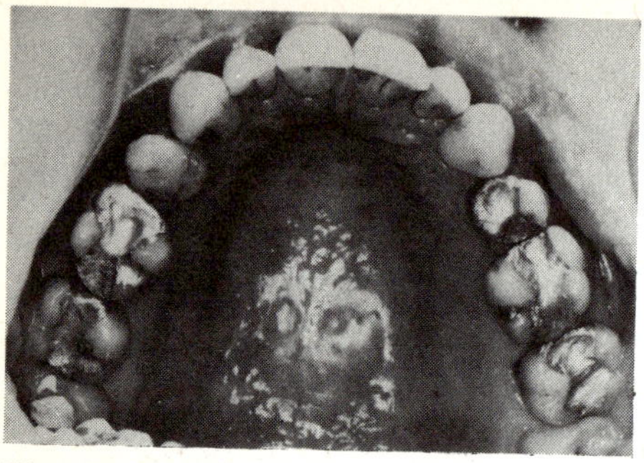

Fig. 20.1. *Upper arch. Note relatively flat occlusal surface of the amalgams and the extensive and inadequate composite restoration in 4⌋ which had been placed in an effort to maintain good aesthetics.*

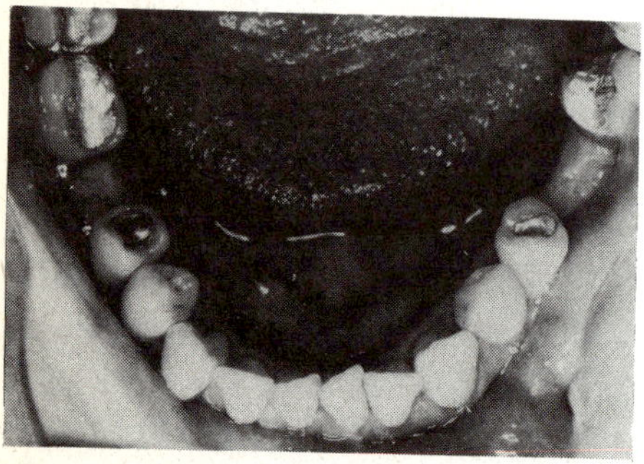

Fig. 20.2. *Lower arch. Note absence of 6|67 and rotation of ⌈5 which complicated the preparation of this tooth.*

on posterior teeth, there being an anterior open bite.

In protrusion there was no anterior contact, all potential incisal guidance being eliminated by the contact of interferences on the posterior teeth.

In left lateral excursion the patient exhibited a good cuspid rise, there being no posterior contact. On executing the right lateral excursion there was a slight cuspid contact at the commencement of the movement, but free progressive lateral movement was hindered by interfering contacts in the right molar region. It is possible, though not admitted by the patient, that she went into extreme right lateral excursion to achieve contact on these molar teeth.

On close questioning the patient was aware that most masticatory activity took place on the left side of the mouth.

Discussion So far

The palpatation of the muscles revealing tenderness strongly confirms that there was a muscle dysfunction present in this case which had to be dealt with before the teeth were even considered. It would seem that the problem would then be to restore the occlusion in the most conservative method incorporating an incisal guidance and stabilizing the posterior occlusion against further deterioration. This could be accomplished by the restoration of the occlusion of the teeth in both upper and lower arches using a pantographic recording device and a fully adjustable articulator. However, in view of the satisfactory condition of the amalgams in the upper teeth and the degree of destruction which the extensive crowning would produce, it was decided to restore only the lower arch and modify the upper amalgams. The 8⌋ required an occlusal amalgam restoration and a provisional restoration was placed at the time of examination. The 4⌋ had been restored with a composite material and it was decided that later this tooth should be restored, probably by means of a full crown.

■ Summary of Treatment Procedure

1. Medical and dental histories. Full mouth radiographic survey using periapical and bite wing films. Alginate impressions for two sets of study casts.

Oral examination included muscle palpation, observation of abnormalities of opening the mouth, examination for caries, lost restorations, missing teeth together with altered relationships following the loss of these teeth, gingival bleeding, open contacts, tooth mobility and pocketing. Vitality tests were carried out where any doubt existed.

Finally a face-bow recording and a retruded jaw registration was required.

2. One set of casts was marked and examined for degree and direction of shift (if present) from retruded contact to the intercuspal position. On the second set of casts a diagnostic preparation was carried out of the stone teeth and a diagnostic wax-up completed. Meanwhile the patient underwent some hygiene instruction and curettage.

3. The proposed treatment plan was explained to the patient as far as had been decided.

4. The contour of the occlusal surfaces of the amalgam restorations in the upper teeth was modified to create the cusps and fossae relationship in alignment with the modified mounted study casts.

5. To overcome alignment problems and reduce the retention required, particularly on the premolars, fixed-movable bridges were decided on. Bonded full crowns were employed on the premolars as the patient had requested porcelain occlusal surfaces for these teeth. However, as only a small part of the buccal surfaces were visible during conversation, the buccal margins of these preparations were kept supragingival (*Fig.* 20.3*b*, *c*). Usually, the molars would have been used as the major retainers, however, in this instance the designs were reversed with dovetails in the mesial aspects of $\overline{7|7}$. This avoided any over preparation of $\overline{5|5}$ when cutting the boxes to house the dovetails, which would have been aggravated by the mesial angulation of the molars and thus the line of withdrawal of the full crowns on these teeth which would have had to be copied by the dovetails. A further consideration was the rotation of $\overline{|5}$ (*Fig.* 20.3*a*).

Although bonded full crowns were employed on $\overline{5|45}$ gold crowns were used on $\overline{7|7}$, because aesthetic considerations were of no importance here. This reduced the amount of tooth tissue which had to be removed and simplified the production of a crown of satisfactory contour. There is always a temptation with bonded full crowns to overbuild and over contour them to provide an adequate thickness of porcelain for aesthetic reasons. This will inevitably have an

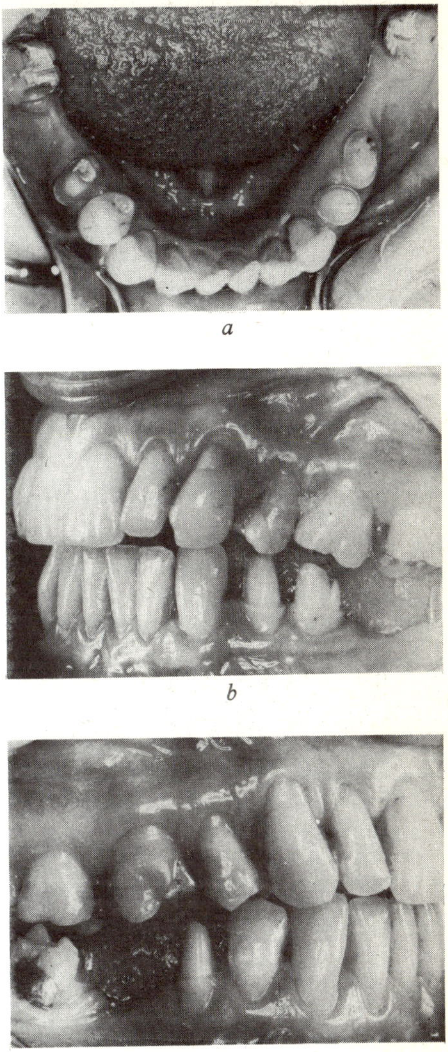

Fig. 20.3. *a, Preparation of abutment teeth for fixed movable bridges. To avoid having to cut boxes to house the dovetails in the distal aspects of* $\overline{5|5}$, *which might have resulted in pulpal involvement because of the unfavourable morphology and position of these teeth, the designs were reversed, dovetails being cut in the mesial aspects of* $\overline{7|8}$ *instead. b, c, The buccal margins of* $\overline{5|45}$ *were made supragingival to avoid overpreparation of these teeth and minimize gingival irritation. For aesthetic reasons porcelain finishing margins were employed.*

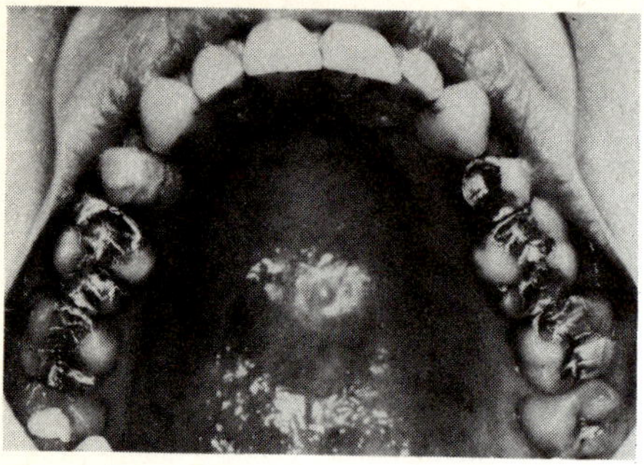

Fig. 20.4. *The occlusal contour of the existing amalgam restorations was altered to provide better marginal ridge contour and improved occlusal relationships.* 4| *has been restored with a bonded full crown. It was appreciated that at a later stage the teeth which were heavily filled could require further treatment because of the extent to which some of the cusps may have been undermined. Should this situation occur it would be a relatively simple matter to restore the individual units as the dentition has already been stabilized.*

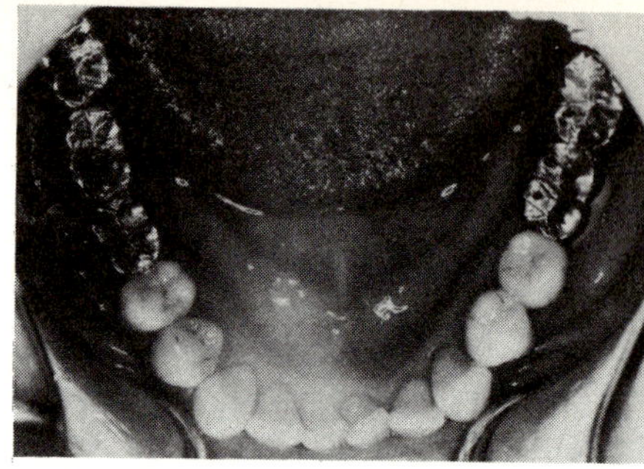

Fig. 20.5. *Occlusal view of finished fixed-movable bridges. Note how patient is now, following oral hygiene instruction, maintaining the lingual aspects of the lower incisors correctly.*

adverse effect on the periodontium. The alternative, which is equally undesirable, is over reduction of tooth tissue.

6. Once completed, an alginate impression of the modified upper arch was made and the cast transferred to the articulator.

7. The teeth were prepared as indicated and quadrant impressions as well as full arch impressions were made. The transfer of the full lower arch was facilitated by the use of five registrations and a split cast. The occlusal vertical relation at this stage could be established by the contact of the incisor teeth and therefore a split cast could be employed using an arbitrary face bow without recourse to a kinetic face bow.

Examination at this stage revealed that on closure without the presence of provisional restorations, the incisal and canine relationships in protrusive and lateral excursions now showed sufficient incisal and cuspid guidance.

8. Restorations were fabricated and provisionally cemented using Temp-Bond.* Minor occlusal corrections were made at this stage.

9. Two weeks later the restorations were permanently cemented.

10. Minor retainers in this case were finished supragingivally with a porcelain finish line to maintain the aesthetics (*Figs.* 20.3*b*, *c* and 6.55, p. 113).

11. The 8| was restored with an occlusal amalgam and 4| with a bonded crown (*Figs.* 20.4, 20.5).

12. Final occlusal correction was carried out and the patient went to the hygienist for evaluation and remotivation of plaque control.

13. The patient was initially put on a 4-monthly recall, this period being lengthened when full support from the patient was attained.

After one year the patient reported that all discomfort associated with limitation of movement had abated and she could eat food of all consistencies without any discomfort or tiredness. The hygienist had not found any area related to the restorations where their contour had led to plaque accumulation. The patient is now on a regular 6-monthly recall.

*Kerr Mfg 6, Romulus, Michigan 48174 U.S.A.

Appendix

METRIC AND ENGLISH EQUIVALENTS

1. Length

SI	English	English	SI.
1 μ (micron)	0·000039 in	$\frac{1}{64}$ in	0·397 mm
1 mm	0·039 in	$\frac{1}{32}$ in	0·794 mm
2 mm	0·079 in	$\frac{1}{16}$ in	1·588 mm
3 mm	0·118 in	$\frac{1}{8}$ in	3·175 mm
4 mm	0·157 in	$\frac{1}{4}$ in	6·350 mm
5 mm	0·200 in	$\frac{1}{3}$ in	8·700 mm
6 mm	0·236 in	$\frac{1}{2}$ in	12·700 mm
7 mm	0·276 in	1 in	25·400 mm
8 mm	0·315 in	2 in	50·800 mm
9 mm	0·354 in	3 in	76·200 mm
1 cm	0·394 in	4 in	101·600 mm

2. Weight

SI	English	English	SI
1 mg	0·000035 oz	1 oz	28·350 g
1 g	0·035 oz	2 oz	56·700 g
2 g	0·071 oz	3 oz	85·049 g
3 g	0·106 oz	4 oz	113·340 g
4 g	0·141 oz	5 oz	141·748 g
5 g	0·176 oz	6 oz	170·100 g
6 g	0·212 oz	7 oz	198·447 g
7 g	0·247 oz	8 oz	226·796 g
8 g	0·282 oz	9 oz	255·146 g
9 g	0·317 oz	10 oz	283·495 g
1 kg	2·205 lb	1 lb	0·454 kg

3. Volume

Note: Except in measurements of high precision, when the cubic centimetre is the preferred unit, 1 cc is equal to 1 ml.

SI	English	English	SI
1 cc	0·061 c in	0·25 c in	4·097 cc
2 cc	0·122 c in	0·50 c in	8·149 cc
3 cc	0·183 c in	0·75 c in	12·290 cc
4 cc	0·244 c in	1·00 c in	16·387 cc
5 cc	0·305 c in	2·00 c in	32·770 cc
6 cc	0·366 c in	3·00 c in	49·160 cc
7 cc	0·427 c in	4·00 c in	65·548 cc
8 cc	0·488 c in	5·00 c in	91·936 cc
9 cc	0·549 c in	6·00 c in	98·323 cc
10 cc	0·610 c in	7·00 c in	114·710 cc

English	SI
1 fl oz	30 ml
2 fl oz	60 ml
4 fl oz	115 ml
5 fl oz	140 ml
6 fl oz	170 ml
8 fl oz	230 ml
10 fl oz	280 ml
20 fl oz (1 pint)	568 ml
1 gallon	4·546 litres

INDEX

Abrasive discs, 180
Abutments, 238
in acid-etch technique, 174
alignment of, precision retainers in, (*Fig.* 12.3) 168
anterior region, 130, 137
arch curvature and, (*Fig.* 6.5) 85
bridge type factor, 81, 137, 147, 164
caries in, 82, (*Fig.* 6.6) 85, 140–1, (*Fig.* 19.12) 254, 261
changing morphology of, 34
compound bridge, 162
contraindications, (*Figs.* 3.7–3.9) 39–42
fixed-fixed bridge, 81, (*Fig.* 6.4*a*) 84, (*Figs.* 6.12–6.13) 90, 130, 200
fixed-movable bridge, 81, (*Fig.* 6.4*b*) 84, 86, (*Fig.* 6.13) 90, (*Fig.* 20.3*a*) 275
fractured, (*Fig.* 19.12) 254
long-span bridge, 81, 39–41, 140
multiple, 163
multirooted, 186–7, 196
overloading, 69, 85, 260
periodontal condition, 37, 82, 86–7, 161, 186
premolar, 153, 265, 267–8, 270–1
preparation of, 202, (*Figs.* 15.21–15.35) 203–9, 230
reinforcement of, (*Fig.* 19.11) 254
restoration, 34, 82, 105, (*Figs.* 15.11–15.15) 196–8
root condition of, 39, 83, (*Fig.* 6.3) 84
root surface area, 81–2
rotated and tilted teeth, 41, 84–5, 136, (*Fig.* 15.18) 200
routine check, 247
selection of, 195
spring bridge, 81, 90, 151, 153, 161
strain on, 86
reducing, by precision retainers, 170, (*Fig.* 12.9) 171
for temporary bridge, 222, 223
treatment of, 195, (*Figs.* 15.11–15.17) 196–9
unopposed, 152
See also Crown as abutment
Accelerators, 63
Acid, leachable free, in phosphate cement, 64
Acid-etch technique, 32, 173–4, (*Fig.* 13.9) 178
Acrylic
bite stop, (*Fig.* 17.5*a*) 234
bridge, 222–3, 251
cold-curing, 72, 222
copings, 53–4
in crown removal, 54
denture, tissue-borne, festooned, (*Fig.* 2.19) 18–20
facing, 68–9, 220, 251, 259
fit surface, 260
gold and, 49–50, 68, 107, 132, 227
jacket, 87
pontic, 77–9, 170, (*Figs.* 13.3–13.4) 175–6, 252–3
prostheses, (*Fig.* 2.19) 18–20, 32, 43, (*Figs.* 4.1–4.5) 44–5
quick-curing, 223, 225
resin
auto-polymerizing, 226
bonded, 173, 180
impression, 52–3
self-curing, 126, 174, 222–3, 234, 259
variable appearance of, 219, 251
Acrylic-headed screws, (*Fig.* 6.27) 97, 100
Adhesive bridges, 173–4, (*Figs.* 13.1–13.15) 175–9, 180
Adrenaline, 211
Aesthetics, 12, 68–70, 77, (*Fig.* 15.3) 192, 263, 266
anterior bridge, 129, (*Figs.* 7.2–7.3) 130–1, 133
cantilever bridge, (*Fig.* 9.1) 147, 263
gold, (*Figs.* 6.41–6.42) 102–3, (*Fig.* 15.27) 204
of retainer, 102, (*Figs.* 6.41–6.42) 103, (*Fig.* 6.48) 105, 111, 115
spring bridge, 151, (*Fig.* 10.1) 152
Age of patient
bridge failure rate and, (*Fig.* 3.4) 35–6, 38
caries rate and, 37
Airotor, 202, 204
Alginates, 57, 276
Alignment
abutments, (*Fig.* 12.3) 168
multiple pinlays, 120, (*Figs.* 6.69–6.76) 121–6
multiple pins, 123, (*Figs.* 6.71–6.72) 124
problems, 239–40, 275
All-acrylic pontic, 78

All-gold pontic, sanitary, (*Figs*. 5.20–5.21) 78–9
All-porcelain bridges, 46, 133, (*Figs*. 7.5–7.7) 134–5, (*Fig*. 9.1) 147–9, 263, 266
  pontics, (*Fig*. 5.14) 74–5, 78, 251
Allergy
  to local analgesia, 38
  to polyether rubber, 61
  zinc chloride, 211
Alloys, 47–8
  alternative to Type III gold, 48
  base metal, 48, 51
    and porcelain, (*Fig*. 4.9) 50–1, 77
  chromium, 50
  gold, 46, 48, 107, (*Fig*. 4.8) 49–51, 109
  semi-precious, 176
Almore face and transfer bows, (*Figs*. 17.6*b*, *c*, *f*) 236
Alumina reinforcement, (*Fig*. 4.6) 46, (*Figs*. 7.5–7.7) 134–5
Aluminax, 235
Aluminium trichloride, 2, 11
Aluminous porcelain, 46, 133, 135, 263
Anaesthesia, 246
  contraindications to, 35
Analgesia, 5, 238
  contraindications, 38
Ancient dental appliances, (*Figs*. 1.1–1.10) 1–6
Ankylosis, 178
Anterior bridge, 129–45
  aesthetics, 129, (*Figs*. 7.2–7.3) 130–1, 133
  all-porcelain, 46
  cantilever, rotation of, 146
  fixed-fixed, 129, (*Figs*. 7.2–7.7) 130–6
  fixed-movable, (*Figs*. 7.8–7.10) 136–8
  span length, (*Fig*. 5.11) 73
Anterior region
  abutments, 130, 137
  arch curvature, (*Fig*. 6.5) 85, 129
  bite stop, (*Fig*. 17.5) 234–5
  crown
    full, faced, (*Fig*. 15.34) 208
    three-quarter, (*Fig*. 6.63) 116, 131, 137
      failure rate as retainer, (*Fig*. 6.13) 90
  dovetails, (*Fig*. 7.1) 129, (*Fig*. 7.9) 137, (*Figs*. 15.6–15.9) 191–3
  lower, bonded pontics in, 77
  occlusion, 114
  pontics, (*Fig*. 7.3) 131–2
  retainers, (*Fig*. 6.52) 110–11, 131, 136, (*Fig*. 7.10) 137
Antes' law, 40
Anticoagulant therapy, 38
Apicectomy, 83
Arch, (*Figs*. 20.1–20.2) 274
  curvature, (*Fig*. 6.5) 85, 129
Articulating strips, plastic, 241
Articulator, 230–1, 235
  early, 4
  face bow transfer, to, (*Fig*. 17.2*c*) 232, 233–4, (*Fig*. 17.6*b*) 236
  fully adjustable, (*Fig*. 17.1*b*) 231, 236, (*Fig*. 17.7) 237
  semi-adjustable, (*Fig*. 17.1*a*) 231, (*Fig*. 17.3*a*) 233
Assessment of patient, (*Figs*. 15.1–15.9) 191–5
Axial reduction, diamonds for, (*Fig*. 15.24) 203, (*Fig*. 15.29) 205

Ball and socket joint, 26, 145
Base metal alloys, 48, 51
  porcelain and, (*Fig*. 4.9) 50–1, 77
Bennett angle adjustment, (*Fig*. 17.3*b*) 233, (*Fig*. 17.7*a*) 237
Bevelling, (*Fig*. 6.58) 113, 116, 127
Biodent varnish, 108
Bite
  registration, paste and frame, (*Fig*. 17.4*b*) 233
  stop, anterior, (*Fig*. 17.5) 234–5
  transfers, 230, 234–5
Blade implant, (*Figs*. 2.12, 2.14, 2.15) 15–16
Bleeding, 194, 210–11, 216
Bone loss, (*Fig*. 2.14) 15, 16, 32, 39, (*Figs*. 15.1–15.2) 191
Box
  for dovetail, (*Fig*. 6.77*a*) 126–7, (*Fig*. 6.79) 127–8, 137, 141, 145, (*Figs*. 15.19–15.20) 200–1, 207–8, (*Fig*. 20.3*a*) 275
  finishing axial wall of, 207
  for joint, 251
Brass ligature wire, (*Fig*. 19.18) 257, 258
Bridge
  adjustment after trial, 238
  basic components, (*Fig*. 2.26) 24
  checking, 246–8
  construction materials, (*Figs*. 4.1–4.9) 43–51
  contraindications, 34–42
  failure
    age of patient and, (*Fig*. 3.4) 35–6, 38
    causes of, (*Figs*. 19.1–19.12) 294–54
    results of, 38
    treatment of, (*Figs*. 19.13–19.22) 255–61
  indications for, 30–4
  long-span, 61, (*Fig*. 5.11) 73, 77, 85, 137, 140–1, 269, 271
    abutments for, 39–41, 81, 140
  patient's care of, 245, (*Figs*. 18.7–18.8) 246
  placement, 238–40, (*Figs*. 18.1–18.6) 241–5
    See also Cementation
  records, 246–7
  removal, 255–6, (*Figs*. 19.14–19.19) 256–9
  replacement, (*Figs*. 19.20–19.21) 259
  stages in preparation of, 208–9
  types of, 24–5, (*Figs*. 2.27–2.31) 26–8
  uncemented 240
  unnecessary 139
  See also Acrylic; Anterior; Cantilever; Compound; Fixed; Fixed-fixed bridge, etc.
Brushes, (*Fig*. 14.5) 183, 245
Bruxism, 180
Buccal margins, supragingival, (*Fig*. 20.3*b*) 275–6
Bur
  half-round, 93, 98, 123
  multi-bladed, 207
  round, 98, 177
  tungsten-carbide, 258
  Whaledent, (*Fig*. 6.30) 98, (*Fig*. 6.34*a*) 99
Butyl methacrylate 223

Caledonian impressions, (*Fig*. 4.12) 60
Canine, 136
  replacement, (*Figs*. 9.3–9.4) 148–9, 264, 267, 269
  restoration, (*Fig*. 6.52) 110–11, 264
  as retainer, 86, 101–2, 141, (*Fig*. 8.1*a*) 142, 147, 267, 270–1
Cantilever bridge, (*Figs*. 2.30–2.31) 27–8, 146–50, (*Fig*. 19.13) 255

Cantilever bridge—*contd*
abutments, 40, 81, 137, 164
aesthetics, (*Fig.* 9.1) 147, 263
fixed-fixed bridge and, (*Fig.* 11.2) 163
incorporation with other designs, 150
indications and contraindications, 146
passing of dental floss beneath, (*Fig.* 5.6) 71, 150
porcelain, 25, 46, 78, 133, (*Fig.* 9.1) 147–9, 263, 266
uses of, (*Figs.* 9.1–9.4) 146–50, 263–7
Caries
in abutment tooth, 82, (*Fig.* 6.6) 85, 140–1, (*Fig.* 19.12) 254, 261
at margin of retainer, 30, (*Fig.* 19.9) 255, (*Fig.* 19.10) 254, 261
rate, 37–8
recurrent, prevention of, 104–5
subgingival, 186
under canine retainer, 154
See also Cementation failure
Case history, 272–3
Cementation, 230–1, 238–9, 243, (*Fig.* 18.6) 244–5
failure, 25, 37, 85, 110, 127, 171, 247, 253
caries following, (*Fig.* 19.9) 253, (*Fig.* 19.13) 255, 261
fixed-fixed bridge, (*Fig.* 6.9) 88, 249–50, (*Fig.* 19.10) 254
in long-span bridge, (*Fig.* 3.9) 41
pin fixation and, 92, (*Fig.* 19.2) 250
spring bridge, 160
testing, 243, 246–7
Cements, 63–6, 178, 220, 222–3
choice of, 243–4
mixing, 244
retention and strength (*Fig.* 4.13) 65, 89, 223, 243–4
See also Phosphates; Zinc
Centric relation, 230, 232
Cerebral thrombosis, dental treatment after, 35
Cervical caries, 38
Chamfer finish, (*Fig.* 6.50) 109–10, 112, (*Fig.* 6.57) 113, 207–8, 241
diamond for, (*Fig.* 15.24) 203, (*Fig.* 15.25) 204, (*Fig.* 15.32) 206
Charlton post/core unit, 119
Chem Bond cement, 178
Children
bridge contraindicated for, 12, 35–6
preservation of teeth, (*Fig.* 2.3) 8–10
space maintenance in, (*Fig.* 2.8) 11–12
Chisel, straight, 256, (*Fig.* 19.17) 257
Chloroplatinic acid, 60
Chrome-cobalt appliances, 12, 14, (*Fig.* 2.21) 20, 170, 271
Chromium alloys, 50
Citricon, 59
Clasps, 20, 22
Cleft palate, 19, (*Fig.* 3.3) 34
Coe-flex, 57, (*Fig.* 4.12) 60
Colour
matching, 4
recording, 219–20, (*Fig.* 16.8) 221
stability, pontic, 69
Compound bridge, (*Fig.* 2.31) 28, 162, (*Figs.* 11.1–11.4) 163–5, 268, 270
triple, (*Fig.* 11.4) 164–5
Condylar guidance adjustment, (*Fig.* 17.3*a*) 233–4, (*Fig.* 17.7) 237
Connectors
posterior, 142, (*Figs.* 8.2–8.5) 143–4
space for, 200, (*Fig.* 15.20) 201
Conservation, routine, 195
Contacts, (*Fig.* 15.26*b*) 204–6
checking, 239, 240
pontic, (*Figs.* 5.4–5.5) 70, 71, (*Fig.* 5.9*b*) 72, 74–5, 222, (*Fig.* 18.1) 241
Continuity of treatment, 272
precision retainers in, 168, (*Fig.* 12.4) 169
Convergence angle and retention, 36, (*Fig.* 3.6) 37, 87
Copings
acrylic, 53–4
transfer, 219
Copper
plating, 62–3
ring, 218
Copper-gold alloy, 46
Cores, (*Fig.* 5.15) 75–6
Countersink, mesial, (*Fig.* 6.79) 127, 136–7, 141
Crack propagation, (*Fig.* 6.54) 111, 142
Crismani rigid attachment, (*Fig.* 12.1) 166, 168, (*Figs.* 12.4–12.5) 169, (*Fig.* 12.8) 171, 265–6, 271–2
Crown
as abutment, (*Figs.* 6.1–6.2) 83–3, (*Fig.* 6.4*c*) 84
contraindications, 39, (*Figs.* 3.7–3.8) 40
anterior, (*Fig.* 6.13) 90, (*Fig.* 6.63) 116, (*Fig.* 15.34) 208
below prosthesis, 52
bonded alumina, 46
cementing, 64–5
constructed on model, (*Fig.* 16.14) 227
contour, 113, 127, 201
early, 5
length of, (*Figs.* 3.5–3.6) 36–7, 87
partial veneer, 173
pin-retained, 173
polyether impression of, 62
removal, acrylic in, 54
remover, 238, (*Figs.* 19.14–19.15) 256
restoration, (*Figs.* 15.12–15.15) 196–8
as retainer, (*Figs.* 6.12–6.15) 89–91, 126–7, 142, 148–9
See also Three-quarter crown
root surface insufficient for, 17
venting, (*Fig.* 18.6) 244–5, 250
weakening, (*Fig.* 19.19) 258
See also Full crown; Porcelain crown: Post crown; Three-quarter crown
Crowning
in cleft palate, (*Fig.* 3.3) 34
dichotomy treatment by, (*Fig.* 2.4) 9–10
instanding and imbricated teeth treated by (*Fig.* 2.6) 10–11
protrusive central treated by, (*Fig.* 2.5) 9–10
CSP precision retainer, (*Fig.* 12.2) 167

Dalbo, (*Fig.* 12.6) 169
Degudent gold alloy, 49, 107
Denar
articulator, (*Fig.* 17.1*b*) 231
pantograph, (*Fig.* 17.7*a*) 237
Dentatus
articulator, (*Fig.* 17.1*a*) 231, (*Fig.* 17.3*a*) 233, (*Fig.* 17.6*b*) 236

Dentatus—*contd*
  face bow, (*Fig.* 17.2*a*) 232, (*Fig.* 17.6*a*) 236
  screws, (*Fig.* 15.13) 197–8
Dentinogenesis imperfecta (*Fig.* 3.7) 40
Denudation, 187
Design, (*Figs.* 15.18–15.20) 198–202
  pontic, (*Figs.* 5.2–5.12) 69–73, (*Fig.* 14.3) 182, (*Fig.* 15.26*b*) 204–6, 260
  spring bridge, (*Figs.* 10.4–10.5) 153
Devitalization, 199
Diagnosis, 273
Diamonds, 202 (*Figs.* 15.21–15.22, 15.24) 203–4, (*Figs.* 15.25–15.26, 15.28–15.29, 15.31–15.32) 204–8
Dichotomy, crowning for, (*Fig.* 2.4) 9–10
Die materials, 52, 54, 56, 62–3
Discoloration, (*Fig.* 4.4) 44–5, 69, 259–60
Discs, 62–3, 180 (*Figs.* 15.26–15.27) 204, 205–6
Distal slices, (*Fig.* 15.30) 205, 206
Dolphin self-shearing threaded retention pin, 196, (*Fig.* 15.15) 197
Dovetail, 142 (*Fig.* 8.2) 143, (*Figs.* 15.6–15.9) 192–3
  anterior, (*Fig.* 7.1) 129, (*Fig.* 7.9) 137
  covered, 143, (*Fig.* 8.4) 144, 269
  double, (*Fig.* 7.9*a*) 138
  and slot, 25, (*Fig.* 2.28) 26, 138, 141, 200–1
  See also Box for dovetail
Drift of teeth, 7–8, 13, 139, 189
Drill bushings, (*Fig.* 6.72*b, e*) 124, (*Figs.* 6.73, 6.75) 125
Drills, 118 (*Fig.* 6.67) 119, (*Fig.* 6.74) 125, (*Fig.* 6.76) 126
  early, (*Fig.* 1.9) 5–6
  Whaledent, 100–1
Duralay resin 52–3, 219, 239

EBA cements, 63–4, 244
Eccentric precision retainer, (*Fig.* 12.10*a*) 172
Edentulous ridge, 186
Eggler post puller, 259
Elastic impression materials, early, 6
Elasticon, (*Fig.* 4.12) 60
Elderly people, 35–6
Electroplated dies, 62–3
Electroplating
  impression compound, 54
  polyether rubber, 61, 63
  polysulphides, 63
  silicones, 63
  tin, 178
Electropolishing, 240
Electrostripping, 240
Emoform, 246
Endodontic
  implants, (*Figs.* 2.16–2.17) 17–18
  therapy, 273, (*Figs.* 20.1–20.2) 275
Endosseous
  implants, (*Figs.* 2.12–2.15) 15–17
  pins, (*Fig.* 2.13) 15, 16
Endosteal implants, vitreous carbon, 16–17
Epithelium, junctional, 184 (*Fig.* 14.8) 185–6
Epithelization, 14
Etch-retained acrylic bridges, bonding failures, 180
Etruscan prosthesis, (*Fig.* 1.5) 2
Eugenol cement, 63, 244
Examination of patient, 273–4

Extraction of teeth, temporary bridge construction and, (*Fig.* 16.13) 226, (*Figs.* 16.14–16.17) 227–8
Ezz-Thru plastic loop, 245, (*Fig.* 18.8) 246

Face bow, (*Fig.* 17.2*a, c*) 232, (*Fig.* 17.6*a, f*) 236, 276
  recording, 231 (*Fig.* 17.2) 232
  transfer, (*Fig.* 17.2*c*) 232, 233–4, (*Fig.* 17.6*b*) 236
Facing
  failure, 242, (*Fig.* 18.4) 243, 260
    due to inadequate occlusal gold, (*Fig.* 5.1) 68, 250
  materials, 221
    acrylic, 68–9, 220, 251, 259
    porcelain, 220, 221, 261
  reverse pin, 75
Fenestration, periosteal, 187
Filling, root, 117. *See also* Restoration; Silicate fillings
Fit surface examination, 239
Fixed bridge
  contraindications, 34–42
  early, (*Figs.* 1.2, 1.4, 1.8) 1–4
  indications for, 30–4
Fixed-fixed bridge, (*Fig.* 2.27) 25, 28, 116, 239–40
  abutments for, 81, (*Fig.* 6.4*a*) 84, (*Figs.* 6.12–6.13) 90, 130, 200
  anterior, 129, (*Figs.* 7.2–7.7) 130–6
  cantilever bridge and, (*Fig.* 11.2) 163
  cementation failure, (*Fig.* 6.9) 88, 249–50, (*Fig.* 19.10) 254
  fixed-movable bridge and, (*Figs.* 11.3–11.4) 164–5
  lack of full occlusal coverage in, (*Figs.* 6.43–6.44) 104, 140
  porcelain, 46, 78
  porcelain/gold, (*Fig.* 5.15) 75–6
  posterior, 139, 140–1
  removal of second casting, (*Fig.* 19.16) 257
  retainers for, 131, 249
    inadequate, (*Fig.* 3.6) 37
  spring bridge and, 162, (*Fig.* 11.1) 163
  stress in, 140
  uses of, 262–72
Fixed-movable bridge, 25, (*Fig.* 2.28) 26, 28, 239
  abutments for, 81, (*Fig.* 6.4*b*) 84, 86, (*Fig.* 6.13) 90, (*Fig.* 20.3*a*) 275
  anterior region, (*Figs.* 7.8–7.10) 136–8
  connectors, 142, 200, (*Fig.* 15.20) 201
  early, 5
  fixed-fixed bridge and, (*Figs.* 11.3–11.4) 164–5
  occlusal view, (*Fig.* 20.5) 276
  posterior, 141, (*Fig.* 8.1) 142
  retainers for, 105, 115–16, 200
  uses of, 263–5, 267–9, 271
  with rotated or tilted abutments, (*Fig.* 6.4) 84, 200
Fixed prostheses, (*Figs.* 2.26–2.31) 24–8
  removal of, 255, (*Figs.* 19.14–19.19) 256–9
  replacement of, (*Figs.* 19.20–19.21) 259
Fixed-semimovable bridge, 26, 142, (*Fig.* 8.3) 143, 269
Flap procedures, 186–7, 189
Floss, dental, (*Fig.* 5.6) 71, 150, (*Fig.* 14.4) 183, 245
Fluorescence, 219
Foot engine, (*Fig.* 1.10) 5
Free-end saddle, 266
  and fixed bridge, incorporating Crismani patrix, (*Fig.* 12.5) 169, 272

Free-end saddle—*contd*
unilateral
support for, (*Fig.* 2.11) 14
treatment for, (*Fig.* 2.15*b–d*) 16
Frictional sleeves, 22, (*Fig.* 2.24) 23
Full crown
addition of rails to, 102, (*Figs.* 6.39–6.40) 102, 115–16
bonded, 202, (*Figs.* 15.33–15.34) 207–8, 275, (*Fig.* 20.4) 276
on central canine, 263
gold, (*Figs.* 6.46–6.47) 106–7, 275
faced, 107, (*Figs.* 6.48–6.60) 108–14, 208
acrylic and, 107
with precision retainer, 167

Gingiva
altering contour of, (*Fig.* 15.10) 194–5
attached, 187, 189
graft, 187
hyperplasia of, 38
inflammation of, (*Fig.* 14.1) 181, 182–3, (*Fig.* 14.7*a*) 185, 187, 189, 210
irritation of, 45–6, 50, 72, 78, 87, (*Fig.* 19.7) 252–3, 260
recession, 187, 253
retraction, 56–7, (*Fig.* 16.2) 210–11
cords, (*Figs.* 16.1–16.3) 210–12
sulcus, normal, 184, (*Fig.* 14.8) 185
trauma, diamond to reduce, (*Fig.* 15.31) 206
Gingivally-placed solder joints, (*Figs.* 5.16–5.17) 76
Gingivectomy, 87, (*Fig.* 15.10) 194–5, 260
Gingivitis, 38–9, (*Fig.* 19.7) 252
Gmür, (*Fig.* 12.9) 171
Gold
acrylic and, 49–50, 68, 107, 132, 227
aesthetics, (*Figs.* 6.41–6.42) 102–3, (*Fig.* 15.27) 204
alloys, 46, 48–51, 107, 109
bonding to, 65, (*Fig.* 5.9*a*) 72, 251–2
bridge, 32, 46–9, 89
cast, 118, (*Fig.* 19.3) 250
collar, 117–18
cutting, 258
degree of, to be displayed, 202, 242, (*Fig.* 18.5) 243
distortion, prevention of, 108, (*Fig.* 6.49) 109, 250–1
dovetail, 142, (*Fig.* 8.2) 143
heat treatment, (*Fig.* 4.7) 47–8, 89, 250
inlays, 5–6, 116–17
uncemented, (*Fig.* 6.44) 104, 140
margin, distortion of, (*Fig.* 6.56*c*) 112
occlusal, (*Fig.* 5.13) 74–5, 78, 103–4, 204
inadequate, (*Fig.* 5.1) 68, 250
perforation of, (*Fig.* 19.22) 261
tearing of, (*Fig.* 19.3) 250–1
pin fixation and, 94, 96, 98–100
polishing, 240–1
pontic, (*Figs.* 5.20–5.21) 78–9, 145, (*Fig.* 11.1) 163
porcelain and, 51, (*Fig.* 5.9*a*) 72, 74
bonded, 48, (*Fig.* 4.8) 49, 73, 77, 79, 89, 107–9, 112, (*Fig.* 6.59) 114, (*Fig.* 7.4) 132–3, 241
porous, (*Fig.* 19.3) 250
post/core units, 118–19
retainers, 46
subframe, (*Fig.* 5.19) 77, (*Fig.* 6.60) 114, (*Fig.* 7.4) 132–3
Gold—*contd*
with porcelain jacket crowns, (*Fig.* 5.15) 75, (*Fig.* 5.17) 76, 133, 263
teeth, 3–4, 20
thickness of, (*Fig.* 5.1) 68, (*Fig.* 6.56) 112, (*Fig.* 6.58) 113, (*Fig.* 6.68) 120, 250–1, 261
tissue contact, 71, 75
weak, interproximal, (*Fig.* 5.3) 70
wear, checking, 247
wire, 4
See also Full crown
Goldwork try-in, 239–40
Greek dentistry, 2, 3
Grinding of teeth, 86
Grooving of incisal edge, 116

Haemorrhagic diseases, 38
Heat treatment of gold, (*Fig.* 4.7) 47–8, 89, 250
Hebrew dentistry, 3–4
High spots, marking, (*Figs.* 18.2–18.3) 241–2
Hinge axis transfer bow, (*Fig.* 17.6*c*) 236
History
of fixed bridge appliances, (*Figs.* 1.1–1.10) 1–6
medical, 272–3
Horizontal pin fixation, (*Fig.* 6.26) 96, (*Figs.* 6.28–6.38) 97–101, 266–7, 270
positioning of pins, (*Fig.* 6.29) 97
uses of, 266–7, 270
using threaded pins and lingual plate, (*Fig.* 6.28) 97
Whaledent kit for, 96, (*Figs.* 6.27–6.28) 97, (*Figs.* 6.30–6.36) 98–101
Human teeth as pontics, 4
Hydrocolloids, 6, 62–3
irreversible, 57
reversible, 54, (*Fig.* 4.10) 55, 56
Hygiene, pontic, (*Fig.* 5.2) 69
See also Oral hygiene

Imbricated teeth, crowning for, (*Fig.* 2.6) 10–11
Implants, (*Figs.* 2.10–2.17) 13–18
endodontic, (*Figs.* 2.16–2.17) 17–18
endosseous, (*Figs.* 2.12–2.15) 15–17
endosteal, 16–17
subperiosteal, (*Figs.* 2.10–2.11) 14–15
Impregnum, (*Fig.* 4.12) 60, 61
Impression
checking, 219
compound, 54, 232
direct and indirect technique, 52
materials, 6, 51–4, (*Fig.* 4.10) 55, 56–7, (*Fig.* 4.11) 58, 59, (*Fig.* 4.12) 60, 61–2, 174, 223, 232
mixing, 21, (*Fig.* 16.4) 213–14, 215
special tray for, (*Fig.* 16.4*a*, *b*) 213–14, (*Fig.* 16.5) 215–16
plaster, 234, 235
properties required of, 51.2
quadrant and full arch, 276
for spring bridge bar, (*Figs.* 10.13–10.14, 10.17) 157–8
taking, 216 (*Figs.* 16.6–16.7) 217–18
early, 4
preparations for, 210, (*Figs.* 16.1–16.3) 211–13
reasons for, 51
for temporary bridge, 223, (*Fig.* 16.10*c*–i) 224–5

Incisal edge, 120, (*Fig.* 10.19) 159, (*Fig.* 13.4) 176
  grooving, 116
Incisor
  region, blade implants in, 16
  replacement
    central, 262–3, 266, 269–70
    lateral, 263–4, 266–7, 269–70
      with upper central, 269
    lower, 270–71
Inlay, 52
  Class II, 127, (*Fig.* 6.80) 128, 141–2, 265
  Class III, (*Fig.* 6.79) 127, (*Fig.* 7.8) 136–7, 141, (*Fig.* 8.1) 142
  gold, 5–6, (*Fig.* 6.44) 104, 116–17, 140
  incisal withdrawal type, 141
  uncemented, (*Fig.* 6.44) 104, 140
Instanding teeth, crowning for, (*Fig.* 2.6) 10–11
Instruments, dental, early, (*Figs.* 1.6–1.7, 1.9–1.10) 3–5
Intercuspation 230
Interdens 245
Inter-occlusal relationships, acrylic resin impression of, 33
Interproximal area
  preparation of, (*Figs.* 15.24, 15.26–15.32) 204–6
  wide embrasures, (*Figs.* 5.2–5.3) 69–70
Inverse bevel incision, 184, 186, 189
Iridioplatinum pins, 92–3, 100, (*Figs.* 6.71–6.72) 124, (*Fig.* 6.75) 125
Irrigator, oral, 245

Jaw relationship, 53

Keratinized tissue, 187
Kerr Bite Registration paste and frame, (*Fig.* 17.4*b*) 233
Kurer screw post system, 120

Labial
  aspect of full gold crown, (*Fig.* 6.55) 112
  gumwork, 154
  reduction, (*Figs.* 15.33–15.34) 207–8
Lactona hydrocolloids, (*Fig.* 4.10) 55
Lastic, 55, 59, 60, 61
Light-cured resins, 174
Loop, plastic, 245, (*Fig.* 18.8) 246
Loss of teeth
  methods of treating, (*Figs.* 2.10–2.31) 12–29
  prevention of, (*Figs.* 2.3–2.7) 8–11, 195
  reasons for treating, 12, (*Fig.* 2.9) 13
  in same arch, after bridge placed, 41
Lower
  arch, (*Fig.* 20.2) 274
  prosthesis, full, stabilizing, 171, (*Fig.* 12.10) 172
  teeth replacements
    multiple units, 271–2
    single units, 266–8

Maintenance of bridge, 41
Malocclusion, 132
Mandrel, paralleling, (*Fig.* 6.73) 125
Margins
  buccal, supragingival, (*Fig.* 20.3*b*) 275–6
  caries at, 30, (*Fig.* 19.9) 253, (*Fig.* 19.10) 254, 261

Margins—*contd*
  finishing, 111, (*Fig.* 6.55) 112, (*Figs.* 6.57–6.58) 113, 115, (*Fig.* 6.62) 116–17, 201–2, 221, 241
    diamond with curved tip for, (*Fig.* 15.32) 206
  gold, distortion of, (*Fig.* 6.56*c*) 112
  porcelain, finishing, (*Fig.* 20.3*c*) 275–6
  subgingival, 185–6, 187, 189, 272
  temporary bridge, 221, (*Fig.* 16.9) 222
Masticatory efficiency, 139, 140, 195
Materials
  bridge construction, (*Figs.* 4.1–4.9) 43–51
  dies, 53, 54, 56, 62–3
  pontics, 73, 105, 145, 147, 154
  retainers, 89, 105
  temporary bridge, 60, 78, 222, 225
  See also Cements; Impression materials
Mesial slices, (*Fig.* 15.30) 205, 206
Metal partial dentures, 20, 24
Methyl methacrylate resins, 225
Metric and English equivalents, 277–8
Mirror, for paralleling, 208, (*Fig.* 15.35) 209
Missing teeth
  effects of, (*Figs.* 2.1–2.2) 7–8, 178
  space maintenance, (*Fig.* 2.9) 11–13
  See also Replacement of teeth
Mobility, 247, 256, 261
  progressive, 189
MOD
  amalgam restorations, 109
  inlay
    flexion, (*Fig.* 6.9) 88, 89
    gold, uncemented, (*Fig.* 6.44) 104, 140
    removal of, 255
    as retainer, (*Figs.* 6.14–6.15) 91, (*Fig.* 6.17) 94, 103, 116–17, 128, 141–2
Model
  damage, 239
  localized, (*Fig.* 19.21) 259
  See also Crown constructed on model, Pottery; Stone
Molar
  as abutment, 265, 268–9, 271
  lower, missing, 146, 150
  replacement, 265–6, 268–9, 271
    with premolar, 269, 271–2
  restoration, 265
Monitoring of patient's tissue responses, 189
Moyco wax, 234, 235
Mucosal inserts, 14
Multirooted teeth as abutments, 186–7, 196
Muscle
  dysfunction syndrome, 273, 274
  spasm, 8

Needles for passing floss or tapes, 245, (*Figs.* 18.7–18.8) 246
Neo-plex, (*Fig.* 4.12) 60
Ney parallel-pin kit, 123, (*Figs.* 6.71–6.72) 124
Nickel-chromium alloy, 48, 77, 154, 160–1, 251
Nickel-cobalt-chromium post, 118
Nickel-silver pin technique, 96 (*Fig.* 6.27) 97, (*Fig.* 6.33) 99, 100

Occlusal
  adjustment, 261

Occlusal—*contd*
analysis, 188
coverage, full, for retainers, 103, (*Figs.* 6.43–6.44) 104, 140
gold, (*Fig.* 5.13) 74–5, 78, 103–4, 204
inadequate, (*Fig.* 5.1), 68, 250
perforation of, (*Fig.* 19.22) 261
tearing of, (*Fig.* 19.3) 250–1
groove, 115
indicator wax, (*Fig.* 18.3) 242
records, 229–37
articulators, 230–1 (*Figs.* 17.1–17.3) 231–5, (*Fig.* 17.6) 236–7
bite transfers, 230, 234–5
extensive bridge prostheses, 231–4
opposing quadrants, combined reconstruction of, 235
simple bridges, 229–31
wax additive technique, 235–6
reduction, 21, 23–4, 202–4, 230
diamond for, (*Figs.* 15.21–15.24) 203
stress, retainers and, 86, 87, (*Figs.* 6.8–6.9) 88–9
surface
pontic, (*Fig.* 5.7) 71, 247
porcelain, 14, 242
sandblasted, 230, 242
Occlusion
checking, (*Fig.* 18.2) 241, 247
correction of, 195, 230, 272, 274, (*Fig.* 20.4) 276
faulty, 251, (*Fig.* 19.6) 252
Opotow paste, 243
Opposing quadrants, combined reconstruction of, 235
Opposing teeth
over-eruption of, (*Fig.* 2.2) 8, (*Fig.* 6.7) 86
treatment of, 202
Optosil, 59, 61, 174
Oral examination, 273–4
Oral hygiene, 247, 252
poor, contraindicating bridgework, 30, (*Fig.* 3.1) 31, 37, 39, 193
Orthodontics, 136
reasons for fixed bridge, 31–2
in tooth replacement, (*Fig.* 2.9) 13
Ostectomy, 184–5
Osteoplasty, 184–5, 187
Overcrowding, (*Figs.* 2.4–2.5) 9, (*Fig.* 2.9) 13
Over-eruption
avoided by fixed bridge or splinting, 32
of opposing teeth, (*Fig.* 2.2) 8, (*Fig.* 6.7) 86
prevention of, 139, 261
Oxidation, 50–1

Pain-dysfunction syndrome, 12
Palatal collar in bonded full crown, (*Fig.* 6.51) 110
Palate
angulation, (*Fig.* 10.9) 156
resilience, (*Fig.* 10.12) 157
Pantograph, (*Fig.* 17.7*a*) 237
Paralleling
devices, 120, (*Figs.* 6.69–6.76) 121–6, 208
preparation, 208 (*Fig.* 15.35) 209
Parallelometer, (*Fig.* 12.2) 167
Partial denture
in gingival hyperplasia, 38
precision retained, 22, (*Fig.* 2.25) 23–4
sectional, (*Figs.* 2.22–2.24) 20–2, 271

Partial denture—*contd*
tooth-borne, (*Fig.* 2.21) 20
Patient
assessment of, (*Figs.* 15.1–15.9) 191–4
attitude of, 30, 35, 273
care of bridge by, 245, (*Figs.* 18.7–18.8) 246
habits of, 86
treatment of, 272–6
See also Age of patient
P.D. posts and pins (*Figs.* 6.66–6.67) 119, 218
Periodontal
breakdown, as cause of bridge failure, (*Fig.* 19.8) 253
cases, silicone impression in, 60
condition
abutments and, 37, 82, 86–7, 161, 186
assessment of, 194–5
factor affecting retention, 86–7, 105
contraindications to bridge, 37, 39
destruction, 182
disease
advanced, 39
chronic inflammatory, (*Figs.* 14.1–14.3) 181–2
implant with, (*Fig.* 2.17) 17–18
health, optimal, 182, (*Figs.* 14.4–14.6) 183–4
overloading, 260–1
pockets, (*Fig.* 14.2) 181, (*Fig.* 14.7) 185–6, 189
preparation of the mouth, (*Figs.* 14.1–14.7) 181–90
probing, 181, (*Fig.* 14.2) 182
reasons for fixed bridge, 32
splint, (*Fig.* 1.2) 1, 98
surgery, 189, 195
therapy, 188–90, 191, 210
splinting and bridgework after, (*Fig.* 6.18) 94, (*Fig.* 6.26) 96
Periodontics in therapy sequence, 188–90
Periodontitis, chronic marginal, 181, (*Fig.* 14.2) 182, 188
Periodontium, examination of, 188
Periosteal fenestration technique, 187
Permagum, 60
Permlastic, 57, (*Fig.* 4.12) 60
Phosphate cements, 63–4, 244
See also Zinc phosphate
Pin fixation
cementation failure and, 92, (*Fig.* 19.2) 250
gold and, 94, 96, 98–100
methods of, (*Figs.* 6.16–6.36) 92–101
See also Horizontal pin fixation; Vertical pin fixation
Pinholes
drilling, 93, 123, 198
multiple parallel, 120, (*Figs.* 6.69–6.76) 121–6
Pinlays 200, 270
cementing, 64–5
impression for, (*Fig.* 16.7) 218
multiple, alignment of, 120, (*Figs.* 6.69–6.76) 121–6
temporary bridge over, 225
three-quarter, (*Fig.* 6.68) 120, 131, (*Fig.* 19.2) 250
Pinledge, 131–2, 263
Pinning of restoration, (*Fig.* 6.49) 109, 196, (*Figs.* 15.12–15.17) 197–9
Pins
cast, 92, 93
endosseous, (*Fig.* 2.13) 15, 16
45° (*Fig.* 8.5) 144
impression for locating, 53

Pins—*contd*
multiple, indirect alignment of, 123, (*Figs.* 6.71–6.72) 124
nickel-silver, 96, (*Fig.* 6.27) 97, (*Fig.* 6.33) 99, 100
in pinlay impressions, 218
plastic, 93, (*Fig.* 6.19) 95–6, 98, 118, (*Fig.* 6.66) 119
pontic retention by, (*Fig.* 5.9*a*) 72, 75
retention of castings by, 91, (*Figs.* 6.16–6.17) 92–4, (*Figs.* 6.19–6.38) 95–101
self-shearing, (*Fig.* 6.38) 101, 196, (*Fig.* 15.15) 197
self-tapping, 198
threaded, 32 (*Fig.* 6.28) 97, (*Figs.* 15.13–15.15) 196–7, 226, (*Fig.* 19.20) 259
wrought, 92–3
Pipe-smoking, 86
Plaque, 181–2
control, (*Fig.* 5.6) 71, 150, (*Figs.* 14.4–14.6) 183, 187, 189–90, 245, (*Figs.* 18.7–18.8) 246
Point contact, (*Fig.* 15.26*b*) 204–6
pontic, (*Fig.* 5.5) 70
See also Contacts
Polycarboxylate cements, 64–6, 244
Polyether rubber impression, (*Fig.* 4.12) 60, 61–3)
allergy to, 61
Polygel, 61
Polymerization, 174, 226
gas production on, 60
Polymer tooth implants, 16
Polysiloxanes, 60
Polysulphide
impressions, 210, (*Figs.* 16.1–16.4) 211–15
special tray for, (*Fig.* 16.4*a*) 213, (*Fig.* 16.4*f*) 214, (*Fig.* 16.5) 215, 216
rubbers, 57, (*Fig.* 4.11) 58, 59, 61, 62–3, 213–15
dimensional stability of, (*Fig.* 4.12) 60, 61
heavy-bodied, (*Figs.* 16.4*g*, *h*) 214–15, 216, 218
light-bodied, 213, (*Fig.* 16.4*d*) 214, 216, (*Fig.* 16.6) 217
Pontic
acrylic, 77–9, 170, (*Figs.* 13.3–13.4) 175–6, 252–3
in adhesive bridges, 174, (*Figs.* 13.1–13.4) 175–6, (*Fig.* 13.6) 177, (*Figs.* 13.10, 13.15) 179
anterior region, (*Fig.* 7.3) 131–2
bonded, 49, 77, 145, 149
design, (*Figs.* 5.2–5.12), 69–73, (*Fig.* 14.3) 182, (*Fig.* 15.26*b*) 204–6
poor, (*Fig.* 14.3) 182, 260
failure, (*Fig.* 5.1) 68, 251, (*Fig.* 19.6) 252, 259–60
gold, (*Figs.* 5.20–5.21) 78–9, 145, (*Fig.* 11.1) 163
hygiene, (*Fig.* 5.2) 69
long-pin, (*Fig.* 5.9*a*) 72, 75, 132, 241
materials for, 73, 105, 145, 147, 154
See also Porcelain pontic
posterior bridge, 79, 145
properties required of, (*Fig.* 5.1) 68–9
removal of, 154, (*Fig.* 10.7) 155
retention by pins, (*Fig.* 5.9*a*) 72, 75
reverse pin, 132
sanitary, 34, (*Figs.* 5.20–5.21) 78–9
self-cleansing, 73
span (*Fig.* 5.11) 73
spring bridge, 154, (*Figs.* 10.6–10.8) 155
porcelain jacket type, (*Fig.* 5.18) 77, 79, 154
too deep, (*Fig.* 5.10) 72
types of, 73, (*Figs.* 5.13) 5.21) 74–9
choice of, 79, 147

Pontic—*contd*
width, lack of, 136
Pontostructor, 120–1
Porcelain
aluminous, 46, 133, 135, 263
baked on, (*Fig.* 13.6) 177, 178
base metal alloys and, (*Fig.* 4.9) 50–1, 77
bonded
faced full crown, 107, (*Fig.* 6.48) 108–9, (*Fig.* 6.56*a*, *b*) 112, (*Fig.* 6.59) 114
failure of, 252
to gold, 48, (*Fig.* 4.8) 49, 73, 77, 79, 89, 107–9, 112, (*Fig.* 6.59) 114, (*Fig.* 7.4) 132–3, 241
bonding to, poor, 65
bridge, 45–6, 78, 133, (*Figs.* 7.5–7.7) 134–5, (*Fig.* 9.1) 147–9, 263, 266
aluminous, (*Fig.* 4.6) 46, 133
cantilever, 25, 46, 78, 133, (*Fig.* 9.1) 147–9, 263, 266
reinforcement of, 133, (*Fig.* 7.5–7.7) 134–5, 148
crown, 46, 50
jacket (*Fig.* 5.18) 77, 154, (*Fig.* 14.1) 181, 263
over gold subframe, (*Fig.* 5.15) 75, (*Fig.* 5.17) 76, 133, 263
rigidity of, 87
facing, 220, 221
detaching, 261
finishing margins, (*Fig.* 20.3*c*) 275–6
gold and, 51, (*Fig.* 5.9*a*) 72, 74, (*Fig.* 5.15) 75–6
occlusal surfaces, 114, 242
pontics, (*Fig.* 5.14) 74–5, 78, 147, 220, 245–6, 251
jacket-type (*Fig.* 5.16) 76, (*Fig.* 5.18) 77, 79, 148, (*Fig.* 9.4) 149, 245–6
occlusal, 251
tissue contact, 71, (*Fig.* 5.9*b*) 72, 74
thickness of, (*Fig.* 5.19*b*) 77, 141, 145, 220, 252
Post/core units, 118–20
Post crown, 198
impression for, 218
retainers, 91, (*Figs.* 6.64–6.65) 117, 118, (*Figs.* 6.66–6.67) 119–20, 131, 136–7
removal of, 258–9
root filling for, 117
temporary bridge, 225
Posterior bridge, 139–45
after root canal therapy, 83
cantilever, 27, 40, 146
connectors, 142, (*Figs.* 8.21–8.25) 143–4
fixed-fixed, 139, 140–1
fixed-movable, 141, (*Fig.* 8.1) 142
fixed-semimovable, 142, (*Fig.* 8.3) 143
pontics, 79, 145
reasons for, 139
short-span, 26
Posterior region
chamfer finish in, 208
crowns
bonded full, finishing margins (*Fig.* 6.55) 112, (*Fig.* 6.57) 113
three-quarter, (*Figs.* 6.61–6.62) 115–16, 141
failure rate as retainers, (*Fig.* 6.12) 90
teeth replacements, 149–50
Posts
cast, reinforcing abutment, (*Fig.* 19.11) 254
screw, 120
Potash alum, 211
Pottery model, (*Fig.* 1.3) 1

P.P. paralleling instrument, (*Fig*. 6.69) 121
Prec-in-Dent paralleling instrument, 121, (*Fig*. 6.70) 122
Premolars
as abutments, 153, 265, 267–8, 270–1
replacement of, 264–5, 267–8, 271
with molars, 269, 271
President polysiloxane, 60
Protrusive centrals, crowning, (*Fig*. 2.5) 9–10
Psychological
contraindications for bridge, 35
indications for bridge, 31
Pulp
chamber, lowering of pH in, by cement, 64
size and position of, 199
tests, electric, 247–8
Pulpal necrosis, 254
Pulpitis, 238
Pulpotomy, bridge made after, (*Fig*. 3.2) 33

Rails, 207
addition of, to crown, 102, (*Figs*. 6.39–6.40) 102, 115–16
retention of pontic by, 73, (*Figs*. 5.13–5.14) 74–5
Records. *See* Bridge; Colour; Occlusal; Shade
Refractory model, 134, (*Fig*. 7.7) 135
Reimplantation of teeth, (*Fig*. 2.7) 10–11
Reinforcement
abutments, (*Fig*. 19.11) 254
cantilever bridge, 133, (*Figs*. 7.5–7.7) 134–5, 148
rods and sheets, (*Fig*. 4.6) 46, (*Fig*. 7.5–7.7) 134–5
Reliability of pontics, 68
Removable prostheses, (*Figs*. 2.18–2.25) 18–24, 33–4, 41, (*Fig*. 12.7) 170, 252
precision retainers in, (*Fig*. 12.6) 169, (*Figs*. 12.7–12.8) 170
Removal
of fixed prosthesis, 255, (*Figs*. 19.14–19.19) 256–9
of pontic, 154, (*Fig*. 10.7) 155
of temporary bridge, 238
Replacement
of bridge, (*Figs*. 19.20–19.21) 259
of teeth, (*Figs*. 2.1–2.31) 7–29, 32, 86, 147, 262–76
multiple units, 268–72
single units, 262–8
space for, lacking (*Fig*. 3.3) 34
Resin, 174
acrylic, 52–3, 173, 180, 226
self-curing, 174, 222, 234
tooth
pontic, (*Figs*. 13.3–13.4) 175–6
replacement, (*Fig*. 13.1) 175
Restoration
abutments, 34, 82, (*Figs*. 15.11–15.15) 196–8
bonded porcelain, 148
canine, (*Fig*. 6.52) 110–11, 261
crown, (*Figs*. 15.12–15.15) 196–8
molar, 265
pinning of, (*Fig*. 6.49) 109, 196, (*Figs*. 15.12–15.17) 197–9
post crown, 198–9
as retainer, gold chamfer beyond, (*Fig*. 6.50) 109–10
Retainer(s) 20, 26–7, 38, 85–128
aesthetics of, 102, (*Figs*. 6.41–6.42) 103, (*Fig*. 6.45) 105, 111, 115

Retainer(s)—*contd*
anterior, (*Fig*. 6.52) 110–11, 131, 136, (*Fig*. 7.10) 137
caries in, untreated at margin, 30
checking alignment of, 239–40
choice of, (*Fig*. 6.45) 105, 147
definition of, 85
fixed-fixed bridge, 131, 249
fixed-movable bridge, 105, 115–16, 200
in fixed-prosthesis removal, (*Figs*. 19.14–19.19) 256–9
gold, 46
impressions for locating, 53
major, 106, (*Figs*. 6.46–6.47) 106, 107, (*Figs*. 6.48–6.76) 108–26, 137, 141
relative failure rates, (*Figs*. 6.11–6.13, 6.15) 89–91
margins, faulty, (*Fig*. 19.7) 252
materials for, 89, 105
minor, (*Fig*. 6.15) 91, 106, (*Figs*. 6.77–6.80) 126–8, 137, 141
multiple, 85
occlusal stress, 86–7, (*Figs*. 6.8–6.9) 88–9
precision, (*Fig*. 2.20) 19–20, 22, (*Figs*. 2.24–2.25) 23–4, 25, (*Fig*. 7.10) 137, 144–5, 150, 154, (*Fig*. 10.6) 155, 165–8, (*Figs*. 12.4–12.6) 169, 201
in fixed-bridge prostheses, (*Figs*. 12.1–12.10) 166–72, 271
in removable prostheses, (*Fig*. 12.6) 169, (*Figs*. 12.7–12.8) 170, 269–71
relative retention of, 89, (*Fig*. 6.45) 90–105
rigidity of, 89, (*Figs*. 6.8–6.10) 88–9
spring bridge, (*Fig*. 10.5) 153–4
strength required, according to type of bridge, 85–6
uncemented, 140–1, (*Fig*. 19.9) 253, (*Fig*. 19.13) 255
upper incisor, faced gold crown for, (*Fig*. 6.53) 111
See also Canine; Crown; Full crown; Post crown; Three-quarter crown
Retention
cements and, 64, (*Fig*. 4.13) 65, 89, 223, 243–4
convergence angle and, 36, (*Fig*. 3.6) 37, 87
crown shape and surface as factors, (*Fig*. 6.1–6.2) 82–3
factors affecting, 85–9
mechanical, 77–8
methods of increasing, 91, (*Figs*. 6.16–6.40) 92–102
pontic
by pins, (*Fig*. 5.9*a*) 72, 75
by rails, 73, (*Figs*. 5.13–5.14) 74–5
sandblasting to aid, (*Fig*. 13.8) 177
tooth eruption and, 82
Reverse pin facing, 75
Ridge forms, pontic design and, (*Fig*. 5.12) 73
Rigidity, 249, 251
lack of, 87, (*Fig*. 6.10) 88–9
retainers, 87, (*Fig*. 6.8–6.10) 88–9
Rochette bridge, (*Fig*. 13.4*a*) 176, (*Figs* 13.5–13.15) 177–9
Rod-span technique, 134 (*Fig*. 7.7) 135
Roman dentistry, (*Figs*. 1.6–1.7) 3
Root
canal
caries in, (*Fig*. 6.3) 84
early, 4

Root canal—*contd*
post crown and, 54, 117, 198
post through, for endodontic implant, 16
therapy, 33, 83, 254, 259
condition of abutments, 39, 83, (*Fig*. 6.3) 84
resorption, (*Fig*. 16.11) 226
surface area, 17, 81–2
access to, 184
Rotated teeth, 34, (*Fig*. 20.2) 274, (*Fig*. 20.3*a*) 275
abutments, 41, (*Fig*. 6.4) 84–5, 136, (*Fig*. 15.18) 200
Rotherman precision retainer, (*Fig*. 12.10*a*) 172
eccentric, (*Fig*. 2.20) 19–20

Saddle area, recession in, due to blade implant, 16
See also Free-end saddle
Saliva control, 216, 218
Sandblasting. *See* Occlusal surface; Retention
Sanitary pontic, 34, (*Figs*. 5.20–5.21) 78–9
Screw(s), (*Figs*. 15.13–15.14) 197–8
acrylic-headed, (*Fig*. 6.27) 97, 100
self-threading, 96
threaded, 258
posts, 120
Scutan, 61
Sectional partial denture, (*Figs*. 2.22–2.24) 20–2, 271
Sensodyne, 246
Shade
alteration at fit stage, 221, 242
guides, 220–1
recording, 220, (*Fig*. 16.8) 221
Shimstock, plastic, 242
Sign, dental, early, (*Fig*. 1.1) 1
Silicate fillings, (*Fig*. 19.9) 253, 261
Silicone
impression materials, 59–60, 62–3, 174, 223, (*Fig*. 16.10*c*) 224
paste, 243
technique, 60–1, 225
Silver
plating, 63
polysulphides, 59
wire, 4
Slots
in all-porcelain bridge, 134
double, in three-quarter crown, 101, (*Figs*. 6.39–6.41) 102, 115
and dovetails, 25, (*Fig*. 2.28) 26, 138, 141, 200–1
mesial and distal, cutting of, 207
Soft tissue
contact, (*Fig*. 5.6) 70
irritation, 69, (*Fig*. 5.8) 71, 145, 225
ridge, 186
See also Tissue
Solder joint, 114, 133
failure of, (*Fig*. 19.5) 251, 260
gingivally-placed, (*Figs*. 5.16–5.17) 76
Space
for connectors, 200, (*Fig*. 15.20) 201
lack of, (*Fig*. 3.3) 34, (*Fig*. 16.12) 226
maintainers, (*Fig*. 2.8) 11–12, 32, 38
Span, length of, 39–40, (*Fig*. 3.9) 41, 61, (*Fig*. 5.11) 73, 77, 85, 137, 140, 206, 251
Spastics, 35
Spatula, wooden, impression material on, (*Fig*. 19.21) 259–60

Speech
defects, correction of, 129
problems
due to tooth loss, 12–13
with removable prosthesis, 33
Spirco drills, 93, 123
Splint fixation, (*Fig*. 6.27) 97, (*Fig*. 6.34*b*) 99, (*Fig*. 6.35) 100, (*Fig*. 6.37) 101
Splinting, over-eruption avoided by, 32
Splints, periodontal, (*Fig*. 1.2) 1, 98
Split post technique, 22, (*Fig*. 2.24) 23, 105, (*Fig*. 15.16) 198
Spoon denture, (*Fig*. 2.18) 18
Spring bridge, 26–7, (*Fig*. 2.29) 27, 33, (*Fig*. 3.8) 40, 151
abutments, 81, 90, 151, 153, 161
aesthetics, 151, (*Fig*. 10.1) 152
bar, 154–5, (*Figs*. 10.9–10.10) 156, (*Figs*. 10.13–10.16) 157–8, (*Figs*. 10.20–10.21) 159–60, 246, 262
bent, 152, ((*Fig*. 10.3) 153, 161, 247, (*Fig*. 19.4) 251
cleaning, 160, 161
construction stages, (*Figs*. 10.4–10.5) 153, (*Figs*. 10.12–10.19) 157–9
contraindications, (*Fig*. 10.2) 152, 262
design, 153, (*Figs*. 10.4–10.5) 153
fitting, (*Fig*. 10.19) 160
fixed-fixed bridge and, 162, (*Fig*. 11.1) 163
indications for use, 151 (*Fig*. 10.1) 152
lower, 161
pontic, 154, (*Figs*. 10.6–10.8) 155
porcelain jacket type, (*Fig*. 5.18) 77, 79, 154
retainers, 153, (*Fig*. 10.5) 154
two together, 156, (*Fig*. 10.11) 157
uses of, 262–4, 270
yearly checks, 160–1
Stainless steel
pins, 93
wire, 176, 218
Steeles all-porcelain occlusal pontic, (*Fig*. 5.14) 74–5
Stone
dies, 62, 93
model, (*Fig*. 6.20) 95
Storra, 61
Straight bevel finish, (*Fig*. 6.58) 113
Subperiosteal implants, (*Figs*. 2.10–2.11) 14–15
Sulphonates, aromatic, 61
Surgery, periodontal, 189, 195
Surgident hydrocolloids, (*Fig*. 4.10) 55
Syncron pins, (*Fig*. 6.38) 101
Syringe for injecting impression material, (*Fig*. 16.4*b*, *c*) 213, (*Fig*. 16.4*e*) 214, 223, (*Fig*. 16.10*b*) 224
uses of, 216, (*Fig*. 16.6) 217
Systemic disease, fixed prosthesis indicated in, 31

Telescopic full-crown technique, (*Fig*. 6.4*c*) 84
Tempbond, 223, 276
Temporary bridge, (*Figs*. 15.4–15.5) 192, 221, 259
abutments for, 222, 223
gold/acrylic, 227
long-term, 225, (*Figs*. 16.11–16.17) 226–8
margins, 221, (*Fig*. 16.9) 222
materials for, 60, 78, 222, 225
methods of construction, 222–3, (*Fig*. 16.10) 224–5

Temporary bridge—*contd*
removal of, 238
short-term, 222–3, (*Fig.* 16.10) 224–5
Temporary denture, (*Fig.* 16.12) 226–7
Temporomandibular joint dysfunction, 8, 12
Tempspan, 223
Therapy
periodontal, (*Fig.* 6.18) 94, (*Fig.* 6.26) 96, 191, 210
sequence, periodontics in, 188–90
Thermal coefficients, (*Fig.* 4.1) 44
Three-quarter crown
anterior, (*Fig.* 6.63) 116, 131, 137
double slots in, 101, (*Figs.* 6.39–6.41) 102, 115
lack of rigidity, 87, (*Fig.* 6.10) 88–9
posterior, (*Figs.* 6.61–6.62) 115–16, 141
preferred to full crown, 272
as retainer, 101–2, (*Fig.* 6.42) 103, 105, (*Fig.* 6.77) 126–7, 147–8, 154, (*Fig.* 19.10) 254, 263–4
failure rate, 86, (*Figs.* 6.12–6.13) 89–90, (*Fig.* 6.15) 91, 140
Selberg modification, (*Fig.* 6.78) 127, 137, 141, 202, 264
stages in preparation of, (*Fig.* 15.30) 205
Tilted teeth, 34
as abutments, 41, (*Fig.* 6.4) 84–5, 136
Tin, 178
Tissue
contact
pontic, (*Fig.* 5.4) 70, 71–2, (*Fig.* 5.9*b*) 72, 74–5, 222, (*Fig.* 18.1) 241
porcelain, 71, (*Fig.* 5.9*b*) 72, 74
loss, 227
in missing tooth region, 41
preservation, 109, 114, 127
reduction, (*Fig.* 6.14) 91, 104, (*Fig.* 5.57*c*) 113, 131, 153, 202–4, 206
supporting, re-evaluation of status of, 189
See also Soft tissue
Tissue-borne prostheses, (*Figs.* 2.18–2.20) 18–20, 33
TMS pins, 94, 196–7
kit for, self-tapping, (*Fig.* 15.17) 199
Toothache, (*Fig.* 19.1) 249
Tooth-borne removable prostheses, (*Figs.* 2.21–2.25) 20–4
Toothpaste, desensitizing, 246
Transfer
bow, (*Fig.* 17.6*b, c*) 236
copings, 219
Trim, 223
Trupontic, (*Fig.* 5.13) 74, 77
Try-in of goldwork, 239–40

Ultraviolet radiation, 219
Under-eruption, 8, (*Fig.* 2.3) 9
Upper
arch, (*Fig.* 20.1) 274
central, missing, 148–9, (*Figs.* 10.4–10.5), 153
incisors, as retainers, faced gold crown for, (*Fig.* 6.53) 111
teeth replacements
lateral, 147
multiple unit, 269–70
single unit, 262–6

Vale sliding bar, (*Fig.* 8.3) 143
Varnish, 108, 240, 244
Venting, (*Fig.* 18.6) 244–5, 250
Verone, 61
Vertical pin fixation, 92–6
Vitreous carbon implants, 16–17
VSMS self-threading screws, 96

Water-repellant impressions, 62
Wax, 240
additive techniques, 235, 236
bite transfers, 234
impression, 52, 232
occlusal indicator, (*Fig.* 18.3) 242
patterns, strengthening, 53
simulation of pontic, 223
wafers, (*Fig.* 17.4*a*) 233, (*Fig.* 17.5*b, c*) 234–5
Wax-up, 134, (*Figs.* 10.15–10.16) 158, (*Fig.* 16.10*a, b*) 224–5
pins in, 93, 94, 96, (*Figs.* 6.32–6.33) 99–100, 126
Whaledent kit for horizontal pin fixation, 96, (*Figs.* 6.27–6.28) 97, (*Figs.* 6.30–6.36) 98–101
Wheelstone, (*Fig.* 15.23) 203
Whip-Mix articulator, 232
Wiptam technique, 17, 218

Xantopren, 59, 61
X-rays, 194, 197–200
bite-wing, 247

Young people, bridge contraindicated for, (*Fig.* 3.4) 35–7

Zinc acetate accelerator, 63
Zinc chloride, 211
Zinc oxide
cements, 63, 222–3, 243–4
impression paste, 234, 235
Zinc phosphate cements, 64–4, 101, 243–4
ZON plastic needle, 245, (*Fig.* 18.7) 246